IMAGING the Central Nervous System of the Fetus and Neonate

IMAGING the Central Nervous System of the Fetus and Neonate

Edited by

Paul D. Griffiths
University of Sheffield
Sheffield, U.K.

Martyn N. J. Paley
University of Sheffield
Sheffield, U.K.

Elspeth H. Whitby
University of Sheffield
Sheffield, U.K.

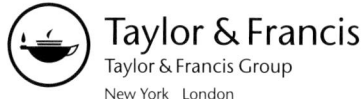

Taylor & Francis
Taylor & Francis Group
New York   London

Taylor & Francis an imprint of the
Taylor & Francis Group, an informa business

Published in 2006 by
Taylor & Francis Group
270 Madison Avenue
New York, NY 10016

International Standard Book Number-10: 0-8247-2856-4 (Hardcover)
International Standard Book Number-13: 978-0-8247-2856-4 (Hardcover)
Library of Congress Card Number 2005046685

Library of Congress Cataloging-in-Publication Data

Imaging the central nervous system of the fetus and neonate / edited by Paul Griffiths, Martyn Paley, Elspeth Whitby
    p. ; cm.
Includes bibliographical references and index.
ISBN-13: 978-0-8247-2856-4 (alk. paper)
ISBN-10: 0-8247-2856-4 (alk. paper)
    1. Ultrasonics in obstetrics. 2. Central nervous system--Diseases--Diagnosis. 3. Fetus--Abnormalities--Ultrasonic imaging. I. Griffiths, Paul, 1960 Feb. 27- II. Paley, Martyn. III. Whitby, Elspeth
    [DNLM: 1. Central Nervous System Diseases--diagnosis. 2. Central Nervous System--abnormalities. 3. Fetus. 4. Infant, Newborn. 5. Magnetic resonance Imaging--methods. 6. Ultrasonography, Prenatal--methods. WS 340 I31 2006]

RG628.3.U38I43 2006
618.2'07543--dc22   2005046685

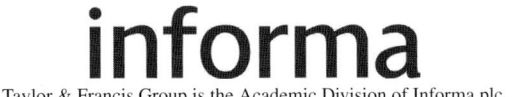

Taylor & Francis Group is the Academic Division of Informa plc.

**Visit the Taylor & Francis Web site at
http://www.taylorandfrancis.com**

Preface

One of the most significant areas of advance in clinical medicine over the last 20 years has been in the imaging technologies. It is difficult to point to the single method or application that has benefited most from those advances because nearly all specialities in medicine have been involved. Perhaps the most significant trend, however, has been the development and introduction of imaging methods that do not use ionizing radiation, such as ultrasonography (US) and magnetic resonance imaging (MRI). Imaging methods using x-rays or nuclear medicine products are the largest single man-made source of radiation burden to the population. Research and development into other methods that can replace techniques that use ionizing radiation is a justifiable goal in itself, for the benefit of both patients and hospital staff involved in imaging. It is difficult/impossible to provide accurate estimates of risk of imaging with ionizing radiation on an individual basis, but suffice it to say, the risks are small but present and must be taken into account when devising imaging policies.

The effects of ionizing radiation used in medical imaging in adults are divided into two types depending on the mechanism of risk accumulation with increasing dose. Non-stochastic effects occur in body areas such as the cornea where radiation will definitely have a deleterious effect that is dose-dependent. This is not usually a concern for patients but it is for staff involved in high-exposure procedures such as interventional angiography. Most of the concern for patient risk is the induction of malignant processes, which are described as being stochastic events, i.e., they are chance occurrences with the risk increasing with exposure. The risk of tumor development is not equal all over the body, some parts being quite resistant to radiation and others being very sensitive (ova, bone marrow, breast, thyroid, etc.). Irradiation of the ovaries and testicles presents concerns other than tumor generation in the individual, as there is risk of DNA damage that will be passed to a future offspring and could manifest as malformation or tumor.

When experts in radiation biology produce dose-related risks for radiation exposure in a medical environment they take account of the relative exposures of different parts of the body with different imaging methods because of the variation of radiation sensitivity, as described above. They take account of the patient's age as well, as it is highly likely that cells that are dividing rapidly are more susceptible to the damaging effects of radiation. Because an induced malignancy may take many years to develop, a lower age is an increased risk because there is more time for a problem to develop. Hence clinical imagers are very keen to limit radiation exposure in children wherever possible. It is imperative that the developing fetus should not be exposed to unnecessary radiation because of the known risks of teratogenicity and tumor formation. Although x-ray based methods of accessing the fetus have been used in the past, this is not the case now and even irradiating the mother during pregnancy should be performed only for well-considered reasons. Fetal assessment by imaging, therefore, is the realm of methods that do not use ionizing radiation.

The introduction of obstetric US into clinical practice in the late 1970s and early 1980s and its subsequent expansion has had a major effect on clinical practice. The majority of women are offered fetal screening in the second trimester, which may be supplemented by detailed anomaly scanning if problems are found. The widespread use of ultrasonography in neonatal imaging has cemented that method as the primary method of assessing the fetus and neonate. It is easy to predict that MRI should have a role in fetal and neonatal evaluation, if it is reasonable to extrapolate from the pediatric and adult population where US and MRI are used in a complementary fashion. The problems with using MRI have been many-fold including price, limited access, and practical issues that frequently require anesthesia/sedation in neonates and, until recently, have made imaging of the fetus a non-option. Many things have changed and the introduction of ultrafast MR imaging in the late 1990s made MRI of the fetus a realistic option. MRI generally is exceptionally good for neuroimaging and it is not surprising that most of the early work in fetal MRI has concentrated on the brain and spine.

This book describes the status of ultrasonography and MRI of the central nervous system of the fetus and neonate in the early part of the new millennium and attempts to explore the relative roles of each method. We have tried to be as current as possible and have included a section where we describe our view of future developments, but this is a rapidly expanding field and still driven by technological refinements in a major way.

We do have one request for workers who are active in this field or who are contemplating becoming involved, and that is the continuing need for vigilance about safety issues. All imaging methods work by perturbation of human tissues by the input of energy—be it x-rays in CT, sound waves in US, or radiofrequency (RF) pulses in MRI—and none of these can be considered totally safe. US, is thought to be totally safe for the majority of pregnant mothers and very few doctors using US are concerned about damaging effects of any description and they are probably right. Most of the new developments in US technology use greater power deposition when compared to the studies confirming the safety of US in earlier studies and continuing safety studies are required. MRI presents a range of potential safety issues, the two most important being temperature increases due to RF deposition and acoustic noise damage from the very noisy sequences used. Both of these are unresolved at present and are surprisingly difficult to study in the current environment. The acoustic effects on subsequent hearing acuity should be very easy to study; however, it must be appreciated that, as far as we know, "normal" pregnancies are not referred for fetal MRI. Any study, therefore, must rely on the small number of cases where a brain problem has been described on US but no abnormality was shown on in utero MRI or post-natal imaging and the child is shown to be otherwise developmentally and neurologically normal. Unless there are obvious and gross effects on hearing (which seems unlikely), that study will require a long-term multicenter study.

Paul D. Griffiths
Martyn N. J. Paley
Elspeth H. Whitby

Contents

Contributors

Susan I. Blaser   The Hospital for Sick Children, Toronto, Ontario, Canada

T. M. Bohnen   LMT Lammers Medical Technology GmbH, Luebeck, Germany

Dan Connolly   Sheffield Children's Hospital, Royal Hallamshire Hospital, Sheffield, U.K.

Paul D. Griffiths   Academic Unit of Radiology, University of Sheffield, Sheffield, U.K.

Stephen L. Kinsman   Department of Pediatrics and Neurology, University of Maryland School of Medicine, Baltimore, Maryland, U.S.A.

Pam Loughna   Academic Division of Obstetrics and Gynaecology, Nottingham City Hospital, Nottingham, U.K.

Pamela Ohadike   Department of Neonatology, Neonatal Intensive Care Unit, Sheffield Teaching Hospitals, Sheffield, U.K.

Martyn N. J. Paley   Academic Unit of Radiology, University of Sheffield, Sheffield, U.K.

Marysia Placzek   Department of Biomedical Science, School of Medicine and Biomedical Sciences, University of Sheffield, Sheffield, U.K.

Ashley J. Robinson   The Hospital for Sick Children, Toronto, Ontario, Canada

Michael Smith   Department of Neonatology, Neonatal Intensive Care Unit, Sheffield Teaching Hospitals, Sheffield, U.K.

Alan Sprigg   Sheffield NHS Trust, Sheffield, U.K.

Tobias Tsai   C/O Department of Pediatrics and Neurology, University of Maryland School of Medicine, Baltimore, Maryland, U.S.A.

Elspeth H. Whitby   Academic Unit of Radiology, University of Sheffield, Sheffield, U.K.

Elysa Widjaja   Academic Unit of Radiology, University of Sheffield, Sheffield, U.K.

SECTION 1

An Overview of Normal and Abnormal Brain Development

1.1

Early Development of the Neural Tube

Marysia Placzek

Department of Biomedical Science, School of Medicine and Biomedical Sciences,
University of Sheffield, Sheffield, U.K.

INTRODUCTION

The adult human body can be defined in terms of its three axes: anterior-posterior (future rostral-caudal), dorso-ventral, and, within the context of these, left-right. These axes are readily apparent in the external body appearance of the head, neck, trunk, back, and front. In addition, many of the internal body systems display similar axial form, and of these, the nervous system stands out as a pivotal example of a structure with defined anterior-posterior (A-P) and dorso-ventral (D-V) polarity. Indeed, an understanding of the development of the nervous system, and of the differentiation of the many discrete cell types within it, depends critically on an understanding of how a neural tube develops with A-P and D-V polarity.

NEURAL PLATE FORMATION AND NEURULATION

The central nervous system (CNS) (the presumptive brain and spinal cord) and peripheral nervous system both derive from an embryonic structure termed the neural tube. In humans, a neural tube with recognizable A-P and D-V axes is already apparent in the four-week-old embryo, neural tube development being initiated in Weeks 2 to 3 of embryogenesis. The neural primordium forms when a small cluster of specialized cells termed node cells, situated in the midline of the embryo beneath the embryonic epiblast (ectoderm), secrete antagonists of bone morphogenetic proteins (BMPs). BMP signaling causes epiblast cells to adopt an epidermal ectoderm fate, while antagonism of BMP signaling results in epiblast cells adopting a neural fate (1). Thus, under the influence of BMP antagonists, a cohort of cells within the epiblast ectodermal sheet, close to the midline node, are instructed to adopt a neural fate, becoming neuroectodermal cells of the neural plate (Fig. 1). Immediately after its induction, the neural plate elongates and, concomitant with this elongation, the node itself differentiates. Node-derived cells undergo convergent extension and ingression, and differentiate into a rod of axial mesoderm that underlies the midline of the induced neural plate (Fig. 1) (2). In posterior regions of the body axis, this rod of axial mesoderm is composed of notochord cells.

The powerful convergent extension movements of the embryo are a primary driving force behind the process of neurulation— the folding of the neural plate and fusion of its lateral edges to form the neural tube (Fig. 2). Neurulation transforms the medio-lateral axis of the neural plate into the ventro-dorsal axis of the neural tube. During neurulation, notochord cells continue to lie immediately beneath midline regions of the induced neural plate, and so come to underlie ventral-most regions of the neural tube while, as a result of delamination of the neural tube, surface epidermal ectoderm comes to overlie dorsal-most regions of the neural tube (Fig. 2).

Neural plate formation

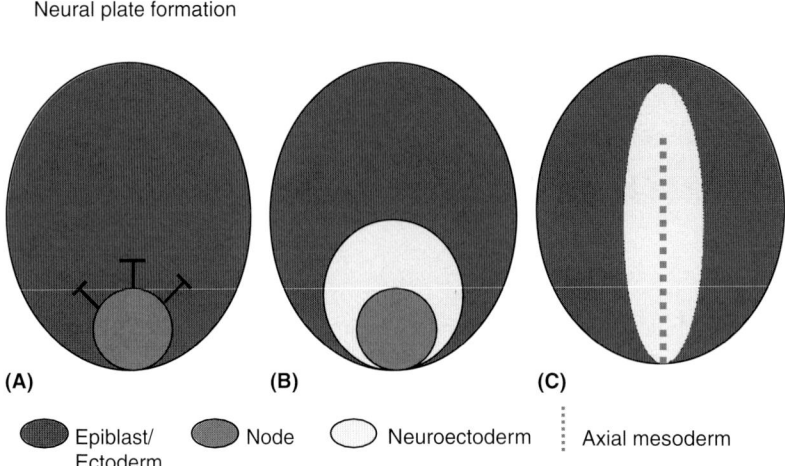

Figure 1. Neural plate formation. (**A**) Node cells secrete BMP antagonists. (**B**) Epiblast ectodermal cells adjacent to the node differentiate into a plate of neuroectoderm, termed the neural plate. (**C**) The neural plate elongates; concomitantly, node-derived cells undergo convergent extension, self-differentiating into axial mesoderm, and ingressing to underlie the midline of the induced neural plate.

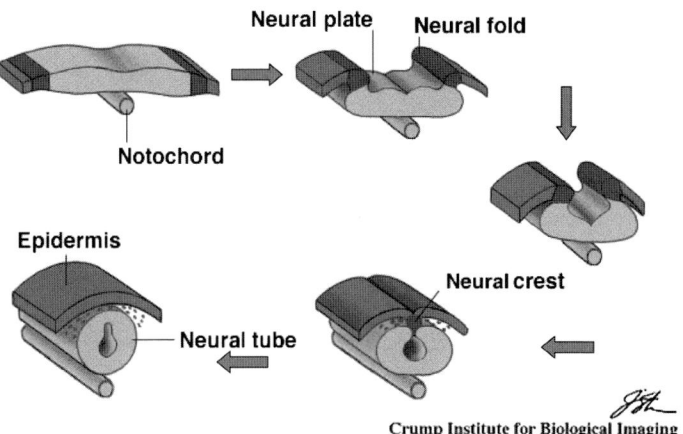

Figure 2. Neurulation transforms the medio-lateral aspect of the neural plate into the ventro-dorsal aspect of the neural tube. Notochord cells that lie beneath the medial aspect of the neural plate lie beneath the ventral aspect of the neural tube. *Source*: Modified from Ref. 4.

In the human, neural tube closure—the coming together of the lateral edges of the neural plate and formation of the dorsal-most aspect of the neural tube— initiates in more than one place. A primary site of closure occurs in hindbrain (rhombencephalic) regions, between somites 4–6, and proceeds both anteriorly and posteriorly (Fig. 3). A second site of closure, forming slightly later, initiates anterior to the optic chiasm and proceeds posteriorly. Final closure of the cranial anterior neuropore occurs at around 25 days, while closure of the caudal neuropore occurs approximately 2 days later (3). Neurulation is followed by formation of the cephalic flexures, converting the A-P axis into the rostro-caudal (R-C) axis that remains throughout fetal and post-natal life.

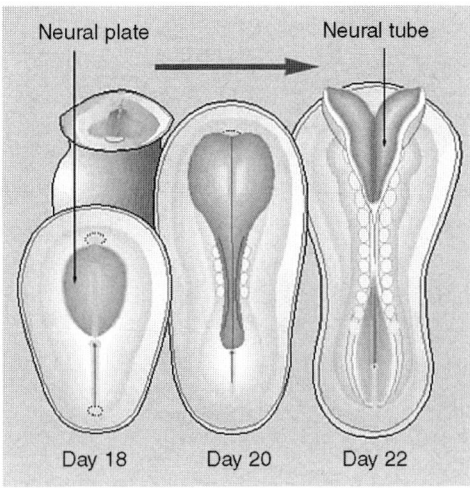

Figure 3. In the human, neural tube closure is initiated around Day 20, final closure occurs around Day 25. *Source*: From www.sciencemuseum.org.uk.

NEURAL PATTERNING

Immediately after neural plate induction and neurulation, signals act to pattern the induced neural tissue. The key function of these signals is to polarize the neural tissue, converting a plate/tube of overtly identical cells into a neural tube with recognizable A-P and D-V polarity. This, ultimately, will result in the correct formation of the many different neuronal and glial subtypes within the brain and spinal cord. The polarization of neural tissue is recognizable, first, in the early regionalization of neural tissue into distinct domains, and subsequently in the differentiation of the distinct neuronal and glial cells—all of which differentiate in a spatially and temporally predictable manner. This exquisitely regulated differentiation underlies the later co ordinated function of cells within the nervous system.

NEURAL PATTERNING: VENTRALIZATION IN THE POSTERIOR NEURAL TUBE

Among the processes that lead to polarization of the neural plate into a structure with A-P and D-V character, the best understood are the events responsible for ventralization of the neural tube. The appreciation of these events derives largely through experimental analyses of animal model systems, in particular, chick and mouse. However, the concepts and principles derived through these studies apply equally to human neural tube patterning.

Experimental embryological approaches in chick embryo have shown that the newly-diferentiated notochord acts as an "organizer" of adjacent tissues, including the overlying developing nervous system (5). The notochord secretes a signaling molecule called Sonic hedgehog (Shh) that appears to emanate away from the notochord in the form of a concentration (morphogen) gradient, such that very high levels of Shh protein are present close to the notochord, with low levels of Shh further away (6,7). A triangular wedge of cells in ventral-most regions of the neural tube therefore encounter the highest concentrations of Shh and, by a process of homeogenetic induction, these are induced to form a specialized group of cells, termed floor plate cells, that themselves secrete Shh (5). Subsequently, Shh synthesized by both the notochord and floor plate diffuses away from these two ventral sources, and establishes a concentration gradient within the neural tube, with highest concentrations ventrally, and diminishing concentrations more dorsally (Fig. 4A). Shh acts as a morphogen—a secreted signal capable of eliciting distinct and predictable changes in cell fate in responding cells at distinct threshold concentrations (8,9). The fate changes are first instigated in neural cells by alterations in their transcription factor profile. Class 1 transcription factors which, prior to the action of Shh are expressed broadly in the neural plate and neural tube, are particularly sensitive to Shh signaling, and are repressed in response to low threshold concentrations of Shh. Class II transcription factors are induced, or de-repressed, in response to high threshold concentrations of Shh, and so come to be expressed in cells that occupy ventral regions of the neural tube (Fig. 4B).

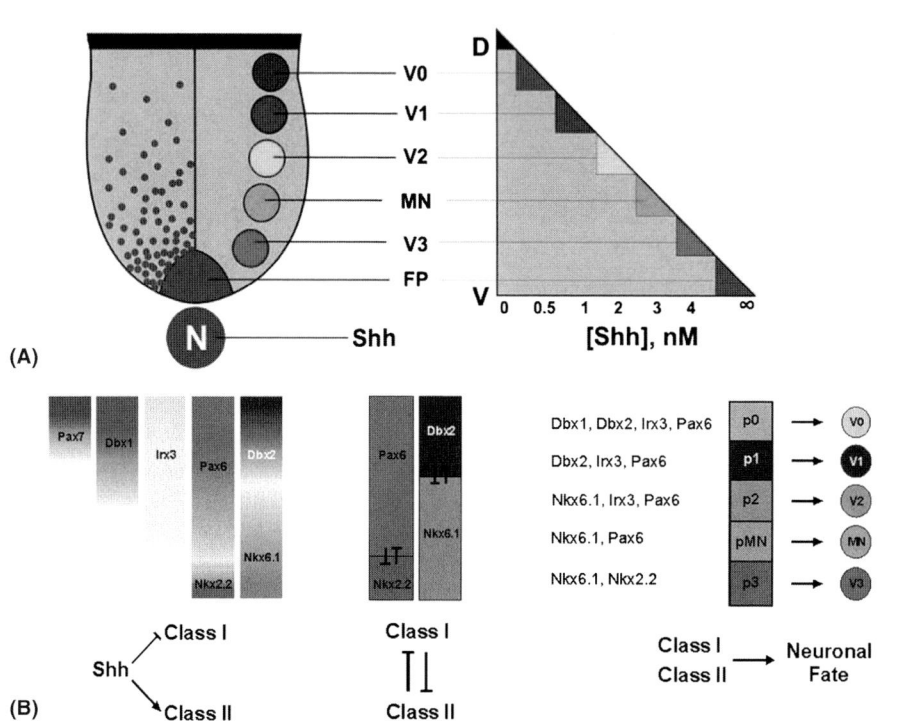

Figure 4. Sonic hedgehog (Shh) regulated transcription factors define ventral neural progenitor domains of the spinal cord. (**A**) A concentration gradient of Shh protein is established in the neural tube, in response to which five distinct progenitor domains are established. These predict the five distinct ventral neuronal subtypes that arise in the ventral spinal cord. (**B**) Shh regulates a series of transcription factors, repressing class I genes and de-repressing, or inducing, class II genes at distinct threshold concentrations (*left*). Negative cross-regulatory interactions refine and maintain progenitor domains (*center*). The combinatorial expression of homeodomain transcription factors in distinct progenitor domains determines the neuronal subtype that arises from each domain (*right*). *Abbreviations*: D, dorsal; Dbx, developing brain homeobox transcription factor; FP, floor plate; Irx, Iroquois homeodomain transcription factor; MN, motor neuron; N, notochord; Nkx, Nkx homeodomain protein; Pax, paired homeodomain protein; V, ventral; V0–V3, ventral interneurons 0–3. *Source*: From Ref. 10.

Distinct class I and class II transcription factors display differing sensitivities to the Shh morphogen, as a result of which Shh is able to elicit a complex transcription code in cells along the D-V axis, which in turn define distinct regional territories along the D-V axis. Importantly, this transcription factor code is instructive in neuronal and glial fate determination, and pre-figures and predicts the genesis of defined classes of differentiated neurons and glia. In this manner, the bilaterally symmetric organization of the ventral CNS comes to form, with V3 interneurons differentiating closest to the floor plate, followed by (ventral to dorsal) motor neurons, V2, V1, and V0 interneurons (Fig. 4).

An outstanding question remains that of whether Shh acts alone to govern neuronal identity. Recent studies, in fact, indicate that additional signals may provide positional information, acting either in sequence or in parallel to Shh. Zinc finger proteins of the GLI family, which act as transcriptional mediators of Shh signaling, may play a crucial role in integrating the distinct signaling inputs, to effect a coherent program of neurogenesis (10,11).

NEURAL PATTERNING: DORSALIZATION OF THE CAUDAL NEURAL TUBE AND FORMATION OF THE PERIPHERAL NERVOUS SYSTEM

The principles involved in dorsalization of the neural tube are largely similar to those involved in its ventralization; however the signaling molecules required to pattern the dorsal neural tube are different from Shh (12). Members of the transforming growth factor β (TGFβ) family of signaling molecules, including BMPs, are expressed within the surface ectoderm (epidermis) that overlies the neural tube (Fig. 2). These appear to act, via a homeogenetic process, to induce their own expression within dorsal parts of the neural tube. TGFβs expressed in the surface ectoderm and dorsal neural tube signal to cells within the neural tube, changing their fate and inducing distinct classes of dorsal interneurons, including D1A, D1B, D2, D3, and D4 interneurons. The ability of TGFβs to induce distinct dorsal neurons appears to reflect, at least in part, their ability to elicit fate changes in response to distinct concentration thresholds. A widely accepted model thus suggests that a graded distribution of TGFβ signals is present in the dorsal neural tube, and induces a dorsal transcription factor code in a concentration-dependent manner. Numerous lines of evidence have suggested an antagonism between the ventralizing gradient of Shh and the dorsalizing gradient of TGFβs. Thus, the integration of Shh and TGFβ signaling patterns the dorso-ventral axis of the neural tube (10,11).

One facet of dorsalization that is very distinct to ventralization of the neural tube is the induction of neural crest cells. Neural crest cells are induced in dorsal-most regions of the neural tube, but do not remain confined to it. Instead, they migrate out of the dorsal aspect of the neural tube, follow a number of discrete migratory pathways, before settling in final target areas where they undergo terminal differentiation into the discrete components of the peripheral nervous system (13).

NEURAL PATTERNING: VENTRALIZATION OF THE ROSTRAL NEURAL TUBE

A wealth of evidence shows that Shh is required, not just for the differentiation of motor neurons and ventral interneurons in the spinal cord, but for the differentiation of classes of ventro-lateral neurons along the whole R-C axis. However, Shh elicits different outcomes in cell fate in the brain versus the spinal cord. Thus, for instance, in the hindbrain, serotonergic neurons form ventro-laterally, adjacent to Shh-expressing floor plate cells, and in the midbrain, dopaminergic neurons differentiate ventro-lateral to the floor plate. This occurs because a large degree of anterio-posterior (rostro-caudal) identity is already imposed on neural tissue, prior to its exposure to Shh. Final neuronal identity reflects the position of a cell within a Cartesian-grid of information, supplied by the patterning morphogen, Shh, and signals that convey distinct A-P identities on neural plate cells (6,14).

The signaling sources and signals that polarize the neural tissue along its A-P axis, and interact with Shh to impart distinct neuronal identities are beginning to be defined (15,16). Evidence suggests that members of the Wnt and FGF families of signaling molecules, together with retinoids, posteriorize the neural plate and neural tube, the antagonism of these signals required to produce anterior identities. It is likely that anterior endoderm that borders the anterior edge of the induced neural plate, and a variety of posterior tissues, act as the source of such antagonistic signals, their integrated action producing an A-P regionalized neural plate, within which forebrain (telencephalon and diencephalon), midbrain (mesencephalon), hindbrain (rhombencephalon), and spinal cord domains exhibit distinct identities, manifest in their expression of distinct transcription factor codes (Fig. 5).

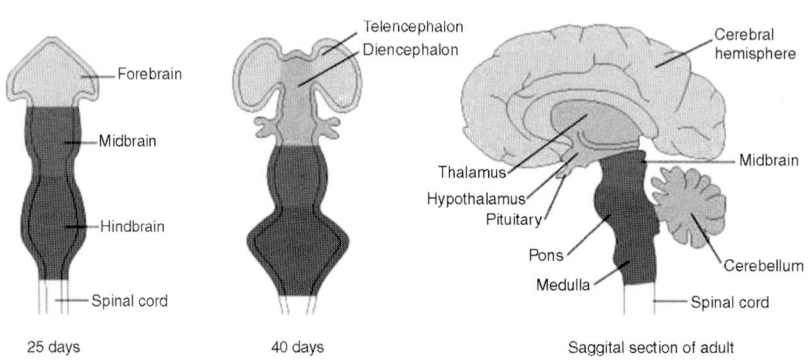

Figure 5. Antagonistic signals act along the A-P axis to produce a neural tube that is regionalized along the R-C axis. *Source*: From somna.npa.uiuc.edu.

PRECHORDAL MESODERM AND DEVELOPMENT OF THE HYPOTHALAMO-PITUITARY AXIS

In addition to imparting forebrain identity to neural tissue through its antagonism of posteriorizing signals, the anterior endoderm affects the character of extending axial mesoderm. Thus, although most of the node-derived axial mesoderm will form notochord, a small portion of anterior-most axial mesoderm encounters anterior endoderm and consequently differentiates into a structure termed the prechordal mesoderm (Fig. 6).

The prechordal mesoderm lies beneath the forebrain, and plays a pivotal role in patterning the forebrain, notably the hypothalamus (16,17). The concepts of hypothalamic patterning by prechordal mesoderm are broadly similar to those of neural patterning by the notochord. Signals from the prechordal mesoderm induce a floor plate-like structure in ventral-most regions of the hypothalamus that will form the infundibulum (median eminence), and initiate a transcription factor code within ventral hypothalamic territory that is translated into the differentiation of discrete classes of hypothalamic neurons. However, the signaling molecules that derive from prechordal mesoderm are distinct from those of the notochord. In particular, prechordal mesoderm expresses signaling factors of the TGFβ superfamily, including nodal and BMPs, that are not expressed by notochord. These co-operate with Shh to mediate the ability of prechordal mesoderm to induce and pattern both the hypothalamic infundibulum and neurogenic regions of the hypothalamus (16). The induction of the hypothalamus converts cells in the early eye field into hypothalamic cells, and hence splits the eye field into its predictable bilaterally symmetric arrangement. Subsequent to inducing the infundibulum and hypothalamus, the prechordal mesoderm retreats caudally. Consequently, the infundibulum comes to appose the underlying oral ectoderm, and induces immediately adjacent oral ectoderm to differentiate into Rathke's pouch, the precursor of the anterior pituitary (18). Thus, both the normal bilateral organization of the eyes, and the normal development

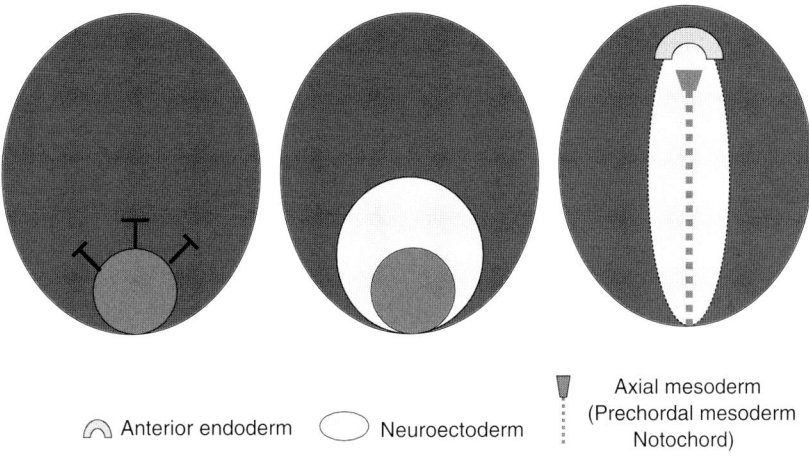

⌒ Anterior endoderm   ⬭ Neuroectoderm   ▼ Axial mesoderm (Prechordal mesoderm Notochord)

Figure 6. Anterior endoderm patterns the forebrain and prechordal mesoderm. Signals from the anterior endoderm appear to act on axial mesoderm after it has undergone convergent extension, specifying axial mesoderm to a prechordal mesoderm identity.

of the hypothalamo-pituitary axis are established through a series of inductive interactions that are initiated by the prechordal mesoderm.

SHH AND HOLOPROSENCEPHALY

The multiple effects of signals that derive from prechordal mesoderm and that act within the forming brain were first appreciated through analyses of the Shh-null mouse. This mutant mouse shows multiple dysmorphologies, including a lack of ventral cell types, holoprosencephaly, a nasal-like proboscis, cyclopia, and lack of a pituitary gland (19). The importance of Shh signaling in the human brain was recognized almost immediately afterwards, when studies revealed that holoprosencephaly in humans can be caused by Shh haploinsufficiency (20). This defect is characterized by an incomplete separation of the ventral forebrain, so that distinct cerebral hemispheres fail to form, and associated craniofacial abnormalities, including a proboscis-like nasal structure, cyclopia, cleft lip, and palate (Box 1 and Fig. 7). The severe lethality associated with these defects means that, although holoprosencephaly has an incidence as high as 1 in 250 conceptuses, only 1 in 16,000 live births are seen.

BOX 1. HOLOPROSENCEPHALY: Holoprosencephaly covers a wide spectrum of phenotypes, characterized by the incomplete cleavage of the forebrain (prosencephalon) into the right and left hemispheres, and the malformation of the diencephalon, telencephalon, olfactory, and optic bulbs. In the most severe case of holoprosencephaly, termed cyclopia, a single forebrain vesicle is formed without any evidence of division into left or right hemispheres. Here, a nose-like proboscis extends over a single, medial eye. In the next grade of holoprosencephaly, ethmocephaly, the eyes show a partial bilateralization, again separated by a proboscis-like structure. In cebocephaly, closely spaced eyes lie above a nose with a single nostril. In none of these cases does the prosencephalon divide to form the left and right hemispheres. In milder forms of holoprosencephaly, the prosencephalon splits to a varying, but not normal, degree. In such cases, the eyes are still close together, the nose is flat, and there is a cleft lip. The lesser grades of holoprosencephaly include various "midline" abnormalities including abnormally spaced eyes and dental anomalies such as a single central incisor. As detailed in the text, a variety of genetic and environmental factors can contribute to holoprosencephaly. Depending upon the genetic background and on the environmental factors to which an individual is exposed at a critical sensitive time-point, the same loss-of-function allele can give a wide variety of phenotypes.

Mutations in the Shh gene have been shown to cause both familial and sporadic cases of holoprosencephaly, but do not account for all cases. However, other genes that have been implicated in holoprosencephaly (21,22) have been shown to be crucial for normal forebrain development, and appear to govern the expression of Shh in the ventral forebrain. Several families with holoprosencephaly have a defect in the SMAD2 (TGIF) gene that is downstream of nodal signaling (23). Intriguingly, a number of studies suggest that nodal governs expression of Shh in the ventral forebrain (16). In a second group of families with familial holoprosencephaly, a chromosomal break-point interrupts the SIX3 gene (24). SIX3 appears to antagonize WNT signaling, and so allow the formation of early forebrain-like tissue. In mice with a targeted ablation of SIX3 (a SIX3 "knock-out" mouse), the ventral forebrain, including ventral-most Shh-expressing regions, fails to form properly (16).

Holoprosencephaly has also been seen as part of the Smith-Lemli-Opitz (SLO) syndrome (25). This syndrome is caused by loss-of-function alleles of the sterol delta-7-reductase gene (DHCR7) gene, a gene whose product acts in the final step of cholesterol biosynthesis. Cholesterol plays a critical role in the the production and reception of the Shh signal, and a prosaic interpretation of the holoprosencephaly seen in SLO syndrome patients is that the defects in cholesterol metabolism impact on Shh signaling, and so produce the same types of phenotypes as the lack of Shh. Indeed, using drugs to deprive pregnant mice of cholesterol will produce such syndromes in their offspring.

In addition to the genetic component to holoprosencephaly, environmental factors are also critical (26). Several teratogens can cause holoprosencephaly, one of them being the alkaloids of the plant *Veratum californicum*, another being ethanol. Veratrum alkaloids, such as cyclopamine block cholesterol synthesis and function, and prevent the reception of Shh, while ethanol is believed to impair the development of the prechordal mesoderm and neural plate.

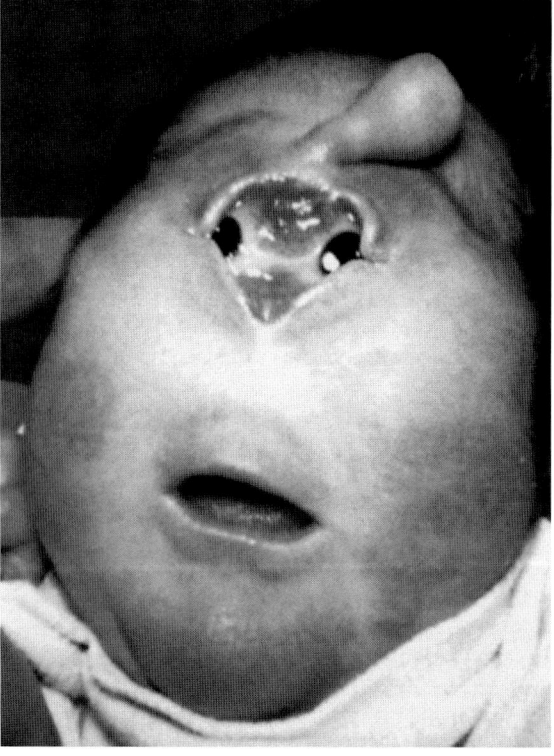

Figure 7. Cyclopia in a newborn. A proboscis-like structure is seen above the partially fused eye. *Source*: From M. Barr, Ann Arbor, Michigan.

In summary, holoprosencephaly shows phenotypic heterogeneity (one gene causing different phenotypes depending on the other genes in the organism), genetic heterogeneity (different genetic loci being able to create the same abnormal phenotype), and environmental causation (wherein teratogens are able to disrupt the genetic pathways required to form the normal phenotype). However, aberrancies in ventral midline Shh-expressing cells, or in the Shh pathway, both of which are critical to the normal development of the forebrain, appear to play a pivotal role in this disorder.

SUMMARY

Cell signaling plays a key role in the development of the nervous system, governing the differentiation of the numerous different neuronal and glial cells that are formed in embryogenesis. Critical groups of cells act as organizers of the developing neuro-epithelium, providing sources of secreted signaling molecules that polarize the developing neural plate and neural tube, setting up a Cartesian-like grid of positional information. Key amongst these secreted signals are Shh, TGFβs, WNT, and retinoids. According to their position on the grid, cells acquire a distinctive signature of transcription factors, which ultimately directs their differentiation into distinct neuronal and glial subtypes. Our understanding of the embryonic development of cells within the neural tube has profound implications for our understanding of human congenital abnormalities and disease states that are manifest as dysmorphology and dysfunctions of the brain and spinal cord.

REFERENCES

1. Harland R. Neural induction. Curr Opin Genet Dev 2000; 10:357–362.
2. Keller R. Shaping the vertebrate body plan by polarized embryonic cell movements. Science 2002; 298:1950–1954.
3. Copp AJ, Greene ND, Murdoch JN. The genetic basis of mammalian neurulation. Nat Rev Genet 2003; 4:784–793.
4. Pelps P. http://biology.kenyon.edu/courses/biol114/Chap14/Chapter_14.html.
5. Placzek M. The role of the notochord and floor plate in inductive interactions. Curr Opin Genet Dev 1995; 5:499–506.
6. Patten I, Placzek M. The role of Sonic hedgehog in neural tube patterning. Cell Mol Life Sci 2000; 57:1695–1708.
7. Ho KS, Scott MP. Sonic hedgehog in the nervous system: functions, modifications and mechanisms. Curr Opin Neurobiol 2002; 12:57–63.
8. Jessell T. Neuronal specification in the spinal cord: inductive signals and transcriptional codes. Nat Rev Genet 2000; 1:20–29.
9. Ingham P, McMahon AP. Hedgehog signaling in animal development: paradigms and principles. Genes Dev 2001; 15:3059–3087.
10. Jacob J, Briscoe J. Gli proteins and the control of spinal-cord patterning. EMBO Rep 2003; 4:761–765.
11. Ruiz I, Altaba A, Nguyen V, Palma V. The emergent design of the neural tube: prepattern, Shh morphogen and Gli code. Curr Opin Genet Dev 2003; 13:513–521.
12. Lee KJ, Jessell TM. The specification of dorsal cell fates in the vertebrate central nervous system. Annu Rev Neurosci 1999; 22:261–294.
13. Lien RJ, Naidich TP, Delman BN. Embryogenesis of the peripheral nervous system. Neuroimaging Clin N Am 2004; 14:1–42.
14. Marti E, Bovolenta P. Sonic hedgehog in CNS development: one signal, multiple outputs. Trends Neurosci 2002; 25:89–96.
15. Lumsden A, Krumlauf R. Patterning the vertebrate neuraxis. Science 1996; 274:1109–1115.
16. Wilson SW, Houart C. Early steps in the development of the forebrain. Dev Cell 2004; 6:167–181.
17. Kiecker C, Niehrs C. The role of prechordal mesendoderm in neural patterning. Curr Opin Neurobiol 2001; 11:27–33.

18. Burgess R, Lunyak V, Rosenfeld M. Signalling and transcriptional control of pituitary development. Curr Opin Genet Dev 2002; 12:534–539.

19. Chiang C, Litingtung Y, Lee E, et al. Cyclopia and defective axial patterning in mice lacking Sonic hedgehog gene function. Nature 1996; 3:407–413.

20. Roessler E, Belloni E, Gaudenz K, et al. Mutations in the human Sonic hedgehog gene cause holoprosencephaly. Nat Genet 1996; 14:357–360.

21. Muenke M, Beachey PA. Genetics of ventral forebrain development and holoprosencephaly. Curr Opin Genet Dev 2000; 10:262–269.

22. Wallis D, Muenke M. Mutations in holoprosencephaly. Hum Mutat 2000; 16:99–108.

23. Gripp KW, Wotton D, Edwards MC, et al. Mutations in TGIF cause holoprosencephaly and link NODAL signaling to human neural axis determination. Nat Genet 2000; 25:205–208.

24. Wallis DE, Roessler E, Hehr U, et al. Mutations in the homeodomain of the human SIX3 gene cause holoprosencephaly. Nat Genet 1999; 22:196–198.

25. Kelley RL, Roessler E, Hennekam RC, et al. Holoprosencephaly in RSH/Smith-Lemli-Opitz syndrome: does abnormal cholesterol metabolism affect the function of Sonic hedgehog? Am J Med Genet 1996; 66:478–484.

26. Edison R, Muenke M. The interplay of genetic and environmental factors in craniofacial morphogenesis: holoprosencephaly and the role of cholesterol. Congenit Anom (Kyoto) 2003; 43:1–21.

1.2

The Supratentorial Brain

Paul D. Griffiths
Academic Unit of Radiology, University of Sheffield, Sheffield, U.K.

THE SUPRATENTORIAL BRAIN

The classification of development of the human brain put forward in most clinical texts describes a series of sequential mechanisms occurring in utero. As well as helping to understand normal development this scheme allows many of the brain abnormalities seen in clinical practice to be explained (at least in part). The approach is useful but a number of points should be remembered:

■ The described events do not occur sequentially but overlap to a considerable degree. This explains the coexistence of different types of malformation and why they are associated. It is virtually impossible to give the exact gestational age at which the abnormality was formed.
■ Some of the more common brain malformations are difficult to explain using the simplistic classification.
■ Considerable alteration in microscopic structure occurs after the brain has formed on a macroscopic scale. Myelination and synaptic organization are examples that commence before birth but continue post-delivery that can produce a wide range of clinical problems.

In spite of those problems the traditional approach outlined below is helpful in the clinical environment.

PRIMARY NEURULATION

Around 15–17 days post-conception, the embryo has the form of a trilaminar disc consisting of endodermal, mesodermal, and ectodermal elements. The central portion of ectoderm undergoes structural changes, influenced by the mesodermal element called the notochord. The specialist ectoderm is called the neural plate and this undergoes considerable thickening when compared to the adjacent non-neural ectoderm. The neuroectoderm begins to fold and after 20 days post-conception the edges meet in the midline, fuse, and separate from the non-neural ectoderm. This process is called dysjunction and occurs at different times at different levels of the central nervous system but the cephalic end of the neural tube should be closed by 26 days post-conception. The whole process of forming the neuroectoderm and closing the neural tube is called primary neurulation.

Failure of primary neurulation at the cranial end of the neural tube produces abnormalities such as anencephaly and cephalocoeles. Anencephaly occurs when the majority of the neural tube at the cranial end fails to form. This is a severe malformation that often results in spontaneous abortion or therapeutic abortion after detection or

13

screening. It is very unusual for these children to have post-natal imaging, as extra-uterine life is usually very short.

A cephalocoele is defined as protrusion of intra-cranial contents through a bony defect in the skull. They are classified by which contents pass through the bone (meninges, brain, ventricles) and named after the bones through which it protrudes (e.g., a parietal meningoencephalocoele refers to protrusion of meninges and brain through the parietal bone). Not all cephalocoeles are due to abnormalities of primary neurulation although many of the severe cases are (Fig. 1).

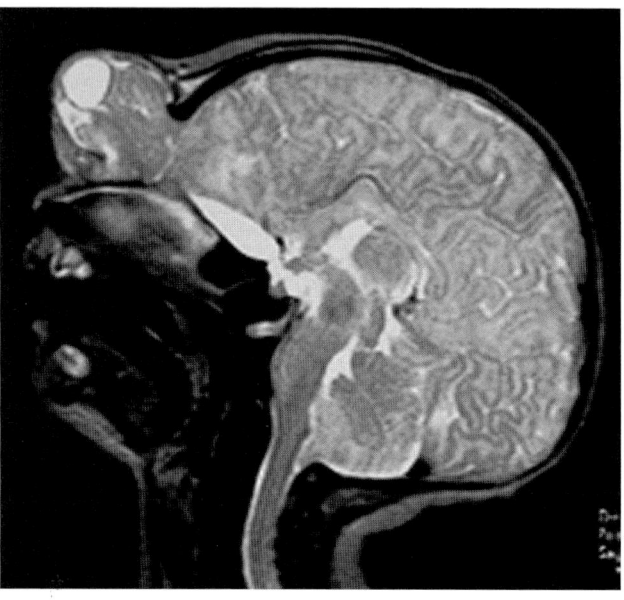

Figure 1. Sagittal T2 weighted image of a child with a fronto-nasal meningoencephalocoele.

VENTRAL INDUCTION

By the time the cranial end of the neural tube has closed (26 days) a series of constrictions and angulations begin to form in the cephalic end of the tube, which indicate the regions that will become structures within the posterior fossa (rhombencephalon), the mid brain (mesencephalon), and forebrain structures (prosencephalon). Two features characterize this stage of development: (1) massive expansion of the prosencephalon, particularly the portion that will become the cerebral hemispheres, and (2) cleavage in the sagittal plane. Cleavage is virtually complete in the forebrain (cerebral hemispheres and thalamus) but only partial in the brain stem and cerebellar structures. This process is underway by 35 days post-conception and continues at the same time that new connections between the cerebral hemispheres are being formed by the lamina reuniens (which will form the corpus callosum and the other commissural pathways).

The prosencephalon (forebrain) undergoes the most significant changes during ventral induction and therefore the structures derived from the prosencephalon are affected most severely. Maturation of the prosencephalon divides it into two clearly defined structures, the diencephalon (future thalamus and globus pallidus), and the telencephalon (future cerebral hemispheres, putamen, and caudate). The group of disorders that are produced by incomplete expansion and cleavage of the forebrain derivatives are called the holoprosencephalies. There is a wider spectrum of abnormalities that fall into this category as described by DeMyer (1). In the severest form, alobar holoprosencephaly, there is virtually no sagittal cleavage of the forebrain.

The thalami consist of a fused mass, the lateral ventricles form a monoventricle, and there is no interhemispheric fissure or falx (Fig. 2). Many of these fetuses are aborted; those that go to delivery are frequently stillborn and long-term survival is not possible. At the less severe end of the DeMyer classification is lobar holoprosencephaly. The typical features of this disorder are poorly formed frontal lobes, frontal horns of lateral ventricles, and anterior falx. These can produce comparatively subtle radiological findings but the septum pellucidum is always absent. Disorders that fall between the ends of the spectrum are called semilobar holoprosencephaly (Fig. 3).

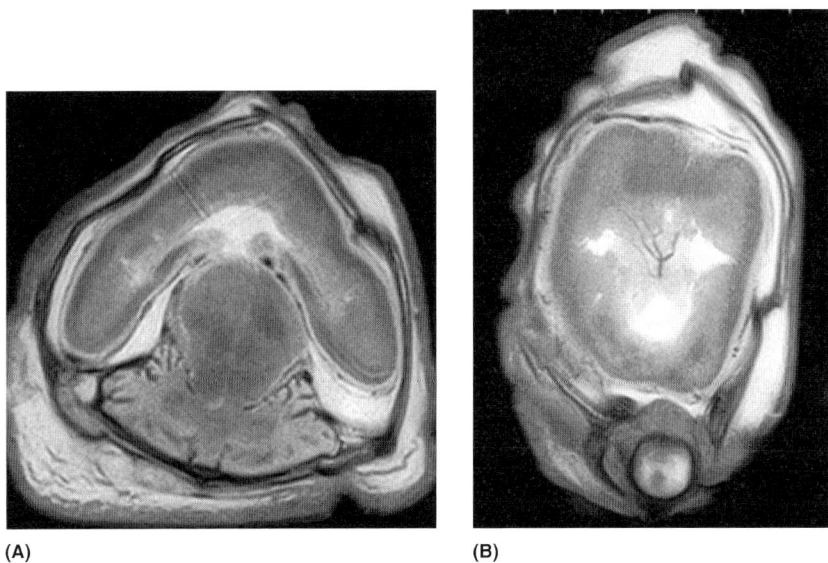

(A) (B)

Figure 2. Post-mortem T2-weighted MR images of a 16-week gestational age fetus with alobar holoprosencephaly in the axial (**A**) and coronal (**B**) planes. Note that there is no attempt at sagittal cleavage with the thalami consisting of a single mass centrally (**A**) and no inter-hemispheric fissure. A single globe is present in the midline and a single anterior cerebral artery is present (**B**).

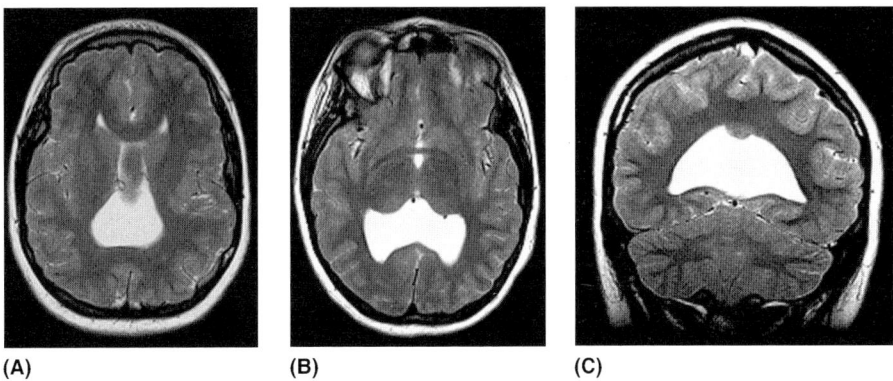

(A) (B) (C)

Figure 3. T2-weighted images from a child of 8 years with semilobar holoprosencephaly in the axial (**A**,**B**) and coronal (**C**) planes. In this case there is some attempt at sagittal cleavage; note the interhemispheric fissure and the falx is present posteriorly. The lateral ventricles, however, are incompletely separated and white matter is continuous over the midline (**C**) with a subependymal heterotopion present superiorly.

Many authors describe overlap between mild holoprosencephaly and septo-optic dysplasia (de Morsieur syndrome) and some describe it as a mild form of holo-prosencephaly (2). The features of septo-optic dysplasia include absent septum pellucidum and hypoplasia of the optic nerves and chiasm. It is usually the optic nerve hypoplasia that alerts the clinician to the presence of the abnormality. Septo-optic dysplasia illustrates some of the problems in trying to classify brain abnormalities. Clinicians with wide experience with children with septo-optic dysplasia recognize different subgroups to the disorder. For example, previous reports describe a high association with schizencephaly and hypothalamic dysfunction but only hypogenesis of the septum pellucidum, whereas some cases have agenesis of the septum pellucidum and other features of lobar holoprosencephaly but without cortical migration anomalies. It is likely that the origins of the two subgroups are different, possibly a vascular cause in the former and a "true" development variant of holoprosencephaly in the latter. Advances in the understanding of genetic mechanisms controlling brain development may help unravel these issues.

FAILURE OF COMMISSURATION (AGENESIS/HYPOGENESIS OF THE CORPUS CALLOSUM)

Commissural fibers are those that connect the two cerebral hemispheres. In humans there are four main structures: the anterior commissure, posterior commissure and the larger corpus callosum (Fig. 4), and a hippocampal commissure is also present that unites the two fornices.

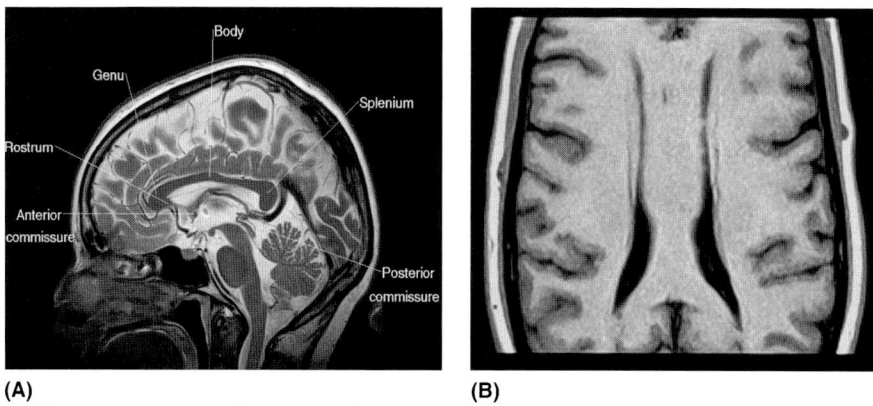

(A)   **(B)**

Figure 4. The appearance of a normal corpus callosum on a sagittal T2-weighted image (**A**) defining the portions of the callosum and the other commissural tracts. (**B**) is a non-orthogonal reformation of T1-weighted volume data reconstructed along the long axis of the normal corpus callosum. This method demonstrates the overall morphology exceptionally well, including the forceps major and minor.

Abnormalities in the formation of the commissures usually affect the corpus callosum, presumably because this is last to form embryologically (3). Indeed abnormalities of the anterior and posterior commissures appear to be comparatively rare. The separation of the developing cerebral hemispheres by ventral induction has already been described but the medial portions do not separate completely, remaining connected by the structures at the cranial end of the neural tube (lamina terminalis and lamina reuniens). The lamina reuniens contains exceptionally metabolically active cells and produces a number of important structures such as the septal region, anterior, and posterior commissures, and the commissural plate. By 7 weeks post-conception axons from the developing hemispheres have started to cross the commissural plate usually attempting to get from one cerebral hemisphere to an equivalent point on the opposite side. The cranio-caudal extent of the mature corpus callosum is best appreciated in the mid sagittal plane (Fig. 4A) and is described as having four regions, a thick anterior region (genu), a thicker posterior region (splenium) joined by a relatively thin body. The smallest region, the rostrum, extends backwards from the genu to the lamina terminalis.

The anatomical relationship between the normal corpus callosum and the hemispheric white matter is best shown on non-orthogonal reformations of 3D-volume data (Fig. 4B).

During Weeks 8–20 there is a significant increase in the length of the corpus callosum as it forms in a cranio-caudal direction, therefore the genu, body, and splenium form in that order. There has been some debate about the timing of the development of the rostrum. In spite of those arguments clinical observation appears to agree that the corpus callosum forms in the order genu, body, splenium, and rostrum. Patterns of failed commissuration reflect this, i.e., mildest forms are absence of the rostrum, followed by absent rostrum and splenium, rostrum splenium and body and so on through complete absence of crossing fibers (Fig. 5). Rakic and Yakovlev (3) have argued against the term agenesis of the corpus callosum because the fibers have formed, they simply have not crossed the midline and persist as a thick band of white matter on the mesial aspect of the hemisphere as the bundles of Probst. It should be noted that absence of the septum pellucidum is an inevitable consequence of failure of commissuration.

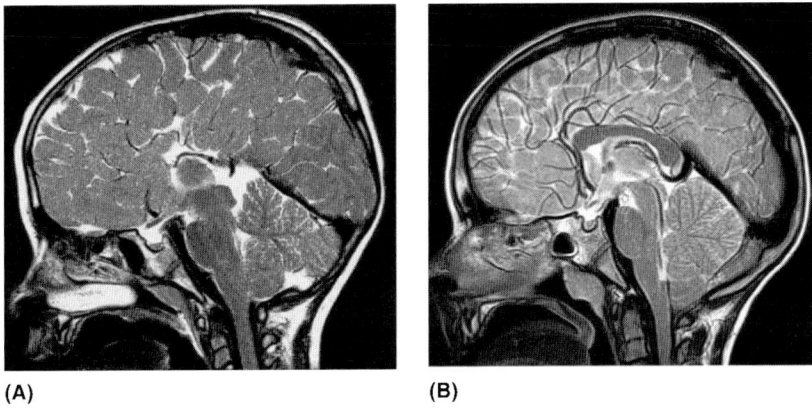

(A)   **(B)**

Figure 5. Two sagittal T2-weighted images from different people showing the range of failed commissuration. (**A**) shows agenesis of the corpus callosum with no crossing fibers above the ventricles, while (**B**) shows absence of the rostrum only (see Fig. 4**A**), which is the mildest variety of hypogenesis of the corpus callosum.

One important radiological observation is a consequence of the ordered sequence of formation of the corpus callosum. A focal defect in the body of the corpus callosum must be an acquired pathology resulting from destruction of part of the hemisphere and is often seen in stroke or multiple sclerosis. There are two notes of caution, one anatomical and one developmental. There is normally a noticeable decrease in thickness at the junction of the middle and posterior thirds of the corpus callosum that should not be interpreted as abnormal. There is one known developmental anomaly that appears to contradict the developmental sequence of the corpus callosum: middle interhemispheric fusion variant of holoprosencephaly in which the genu and splenium form but the body of the corpus callosum does not. This is an extremely rare anomaly (the author has only seen two new cases in 10 years) but one case is shown in Figure 6.

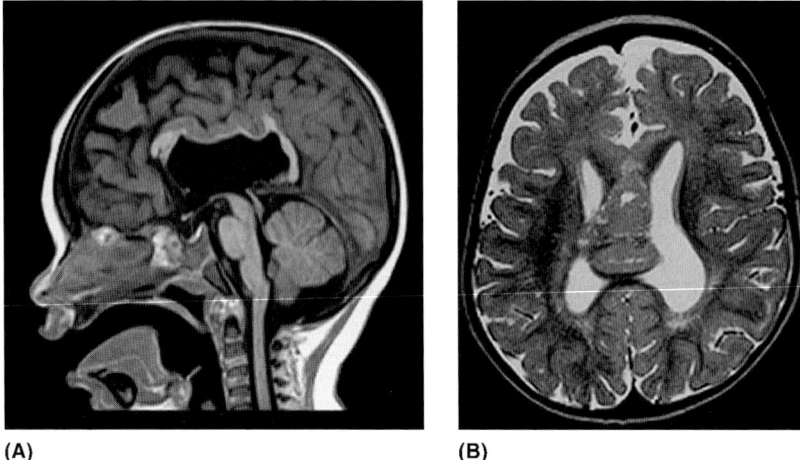

(A)   (B)

Figure 6. An exceptionally unusual pattern of callosal hypogenesis is shown on sagittal T1-weighted (**A**) and axial T2-weighted (**B**) MRIs from a child with marked developmental delay and seizures. The genu and splenium are present but the body is absent. This is the middle inter-hemispheric fusion variety of holoprosencephaly.

The demonstration of failed commissuration usually presents no problems on diagnostic imaging when severe, and can be shown on CT or MRI. However, good quality, thin sagittal sections are required for milder forms. Other structural abnormalities that occur with high frequency can be classified as anatomical deformities that result from a direct consequence of lack of commissuration, or associated malformations.

ANATOMICAL DEFORMITIES

Deformities of the ventricular system occur for several reasons. The bundles of Probst run lateral to the cingulate gyrus and deform the frontal horns particularly, which accounts for the "steer-horn" appearance of the frontal horns described on ultrasound and also seen on coronal MRI (Fig. 7). The absence of the corpus callosum causes the third ventricle to be abnormally high and deficiencies in the posterior portion of the corpus callosum allow the trigone and occipital horns to dilate causing a deformity known as colpocephaly. The temporal horns are also often dilated due to associated poor development of the mesial temporal structures, and the head of the hippocampus is usually malrotated. The cingulate gyrus is not inverted, as is normal, when there is failure of commissuration. Sometimes increased thickness of the anterior and/or posterior commissures is found.

MALFORMATIONS ASSOCIATED WITH FAILED COMMISSURATION

Other malformations are commonly associated with failure of commissuration and are in some ways more important as they usually indicate more severe neurological problems (4,5). These include:

1. Midline anomalies. Failure of commissuration is found in conjunction with many of the other midline anomalies including Dandy-Walker malformation, cephalocoeles, and facial anomalies.
2. Disorders of cortical formation. Failed commissuration is often found in conjunction with the developmental cortical abnormalities outlined below, most commonly poly-microgyria and heterotopia.

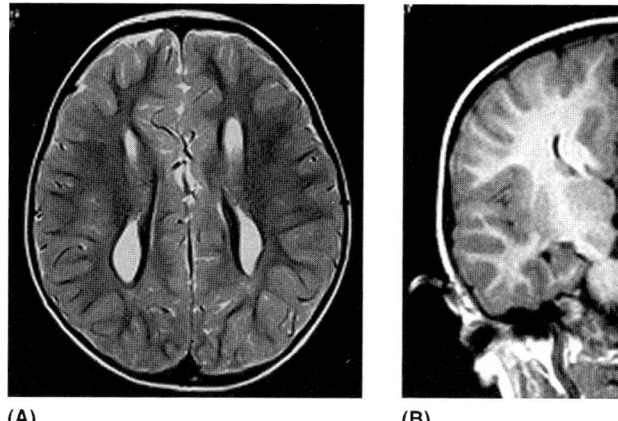

(A)　　　　　　　　　　　　(B)

Figure 7. Axial T2-weighted (**A**) and coronal T1-weighted images (**B**) from an MR examination of a child with agenesis of the corpus callosum showing the bundles of Probst. These appear as low signal tracts on (**A**) and high signal tracts on (**B**) running medial to the frontal horns, body and trigone of the lateral ventricles. Note the "steer horn" appearance of the frontal horns on the coronal image.

3. Extra-axial "cysts." Fluid-containing structures are commonly associated with failure of commissuration, particularly posteriorly. Barkovich and colleagues (6) have recently proposed a classification for this type of abnormality. The majority of the cysts communicate with the ventricular system (third ventricle, lateral ventricles or both) and these are termed type 1 cysts. Further subdivisions are made based on the presence or absence of abnormalities of cortical migration (Fig. 8).
4. Lipomas. 40–50% of intracranial lipomas (Fig. 9) occur in the interhemispheric fissure and are most frequently associated with failure of commissuration of some severity (7). These frequently show peripheral curvilinear calcification.

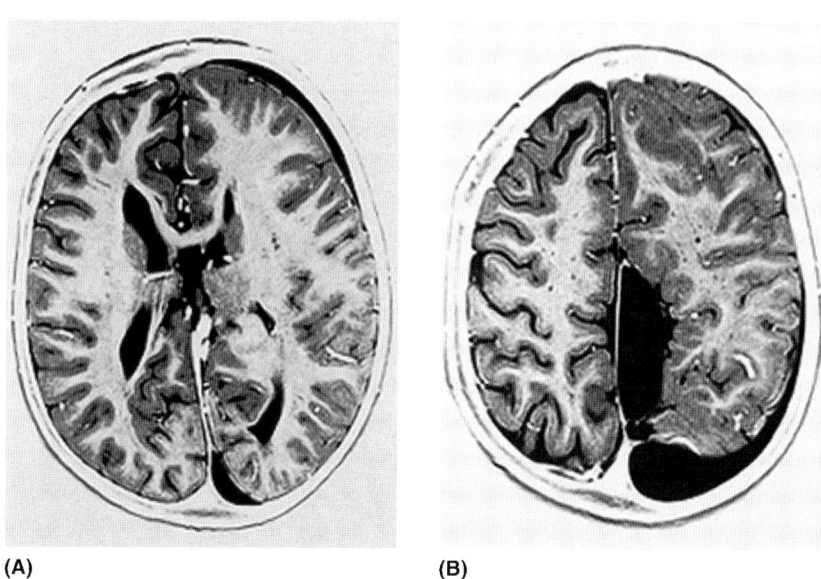

(A)　　　　　　　　　　　　(B)

Figure 8. T2-weighted (video reversed) axial images of a child with hypogenesis of the corpus callosum (**A**) and an associated interhemispheric cyst posteriorly (**B**). The left hemisphere also shows extensive abnormalities of cortical formation.

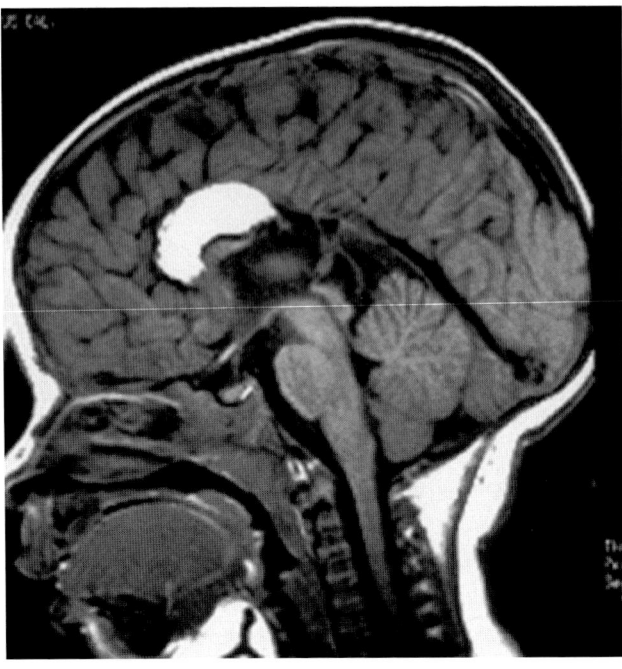

Figure 9. A case of marked hypogenesis of the corpus callosum with an associated lipoma on a sagittal T1-weighted image.

ABNORMALITIES OF CORTICAL FORMATION

When the brain has undergone ventral induction successfully the next major process is the formation of the future gray matter structures from mature neurons and glia. This starts at around 7 weeks by a rapid formation of neurons at the ventricular surface. Most of the gray matter in the brain is formed from rapidly-dividing progenitor cells located in the subependymal regions of the ventricles. These areas are often referred to as the "germinal matrix" in the clinical literature and are present around all areas of the ventricular system. Those cells around the lateral ventricles produce the future cerebral cortex and putamen/caudate. The globus pallidus, thalamus, and hypothalamus are formed from germinal matrix around the third ventricle, while the germinal matrix around the fourth ventricle forms the deep cerebellar nuclei and a component of the cerebellar cortex.

Once future neurons and glial elements have been 'born' in the germinal matrix they migrate to the future cortex (7). Most cells migrate in a radial fashion along glial fibres to a predetermined site on the cortex (Fig. 10). This can be studied in experimental animals by "fate-mapping"; i.e., labeling an immature neuron and finding its ultimate site. This type of work has shown that the destination of the neuron is predetermined before the neuron is born. This means that if the germinal matrix from the tectum, whose developing neurons are destined for the occipital cortex, are transplanted to another point in the brain the neurons will still find their way to the original destination. This is in marked distinction to the developing neurons of the neural crest, for example, which will alter their morphology and connections depending on local surroundings.

Barkovich and colleagues (8) have presented work that attempts to classify the group of abnormalities that are manifest by failure to form a normal future cerebral cortex. Three processes are specified: failure of cellular proliferation, failure of migration, and failure of cortical organization. The principle of the classification is that a malformation should be grouped with the earliest failed mechanism demonstrable. This is appropriate as, e.g., failure of proliferation is likely to have major effects on migration and cortical organizations.

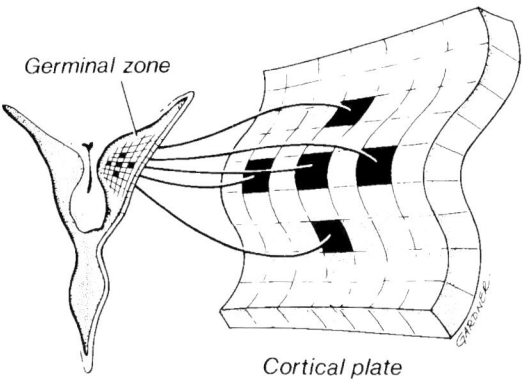

Figure 10. Line diagram showing the migration pathway of neurons and glia from the germinal matrix adjacent to the ventricles along radial glial fibres to a predetermined site on the cortex.

Failure of Cellular Proliferation

This is the earliest type of abnormality that results in malformation of the cerebral cortex. The process starts in the seventh gestational week and abnormalities can be generalized or focal. Subclassifications include the number of neurons and glia formed, for example, global reduction of cellular proliferation produces microcephaly vera while unilateral overproduction of neurons/glia produces hemimegalencephaly. It is likely that congenital brain tumors and the intracranial manifestations of tuberous sclerosis originate at this stage.

Failure of Migration

Migration commences at 8 weeks and continues until approximately Week 22. Like cellular proliferation failure, this process can be generalized or focal. The most extreme forms produce lissencephaly and agyria/pachygyria (Fig. 11).

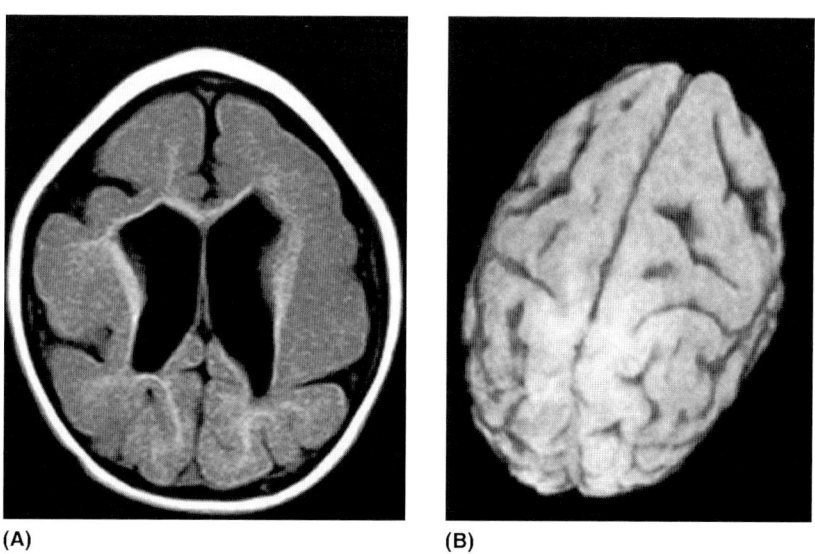

(A)   **(B)**

Figure 11. A single axial T1-weighted image from a gradient echo volume (**A**) acquisition shows lissencephaly. The segmented surface reconstruction (**B**) shows the extent of the cortical abnormality and the anterior to posterior gradient in the severity of the malformation.

One of the most interesting groups of disorders to result from failed migration are heterotopia. These are characterized by abnormal collections of gray matter at anatomically inappropriate sites. These are discussed in detail below.

Failure of Cortical Organization

Once the neurons and glia arrive at the surface of the brain they must organize into the normal six-layer form of the normal neocortex. Recent work has shown that more neurons and glia migrate to the cortex than are found in the mature cortex, therefore another important process is programmed cell death (apoptosis) of the neurons that are surplus to requirement. Failure of appropriate cortical lamination and insufficient apoptosis may produce the irregular thickened cortex found in polymicrogyria. Even at this stage extensive cellular organization and synaptogenesis is required to form the normal future cortex.

It is reasonable to assume that extensive derangement of an early process (cellular proliferation) will produce more macroscopic involvement of the brain than a focal derangement of a later process (e.g., failure of cortical organization). This has major implications for the chances of being able to detect a malformation in utero at the time of antenatal screening (19–20 weeks after the last menstrual period). For example, there are two reasons why a small area of polymicrogyria might not be detected in utero:

1. The imaging method used does not have sufficient anatomical and contrast resolution. Note that polymicrogyria can be exceptionally difficult to detect post-natally even with extremely high-resolution volume imaging (see below).
2. It is possible that the defect causing the polymicrogyria has not manifested as early as 18–20 weeks and the abnormality is not detectable by an imaging method.

A detailed description of all of the abnormalities of cortical formation is beyond the scope of this book, but one disorder from each of the three processes involved in cortical formation has been selected for detailed discussion.

Hemimegalencephaly—A Disorder of Cellular Proliferation

Hemimegalencephaly is a rare congenital brain anomaly characterised by enlargement of one cerebral hemisphere, its ventricular system and hemicranium (9). The disorder may be an isolated finding (dysplastic HME) and is usually due to a non-transmissible somatic mutation. It may be associated with a heterogenous group of hemihypertrophy syndromes than can occur in conjunction with Wilms tumor, adrenal or hepatic tumors of infancy. The abnormality may also be found in conjunction with some of the phakomatoses, including neurofibromatosis Sturge-Weber, Klippel Treneuny syndrome, tuberous sclerosis complex, hypomelanosis of Ito, epidermal nevus syndrome and Proteus syndrome (10). Macroscopic changes include unilateral hemispheric enlargement with anomalous cortical formation including agyria/pachygyria, polymicrogyria, and gray matter heterotopias. Microscopically the main features are of disordered neocortical architecture, which may contain only four layers, and clusters of abnormal large neurons. The white matter contains swollen, multinucleated astrocytes with fibrillary gliosis. Many cells are present that can not be classified as being neurons or glia but are thought to be embryologically primitive.

Hemispherectomy has been suggested as a valid treatment in cases of HME with intractable seizures. Two of our cases received this surgery, both of which had catastrophic intraoperative bleeding which was fatal in one case. Both of these children had disorders of neuronal migration and/or cortical organization with associated areas of abnormal venous drainage shown on the surgical specimens. Barkovich and Chuang (9) demonstrated abnormal arteriovenous shunting in two out of three patients with HME who received angiography, both of which had cardiac failure. The high incidence of cortical dysplasia and migrational disorders in HME should lead to careful assessment by MRI prior to any surgical intervention (Fig. 12).

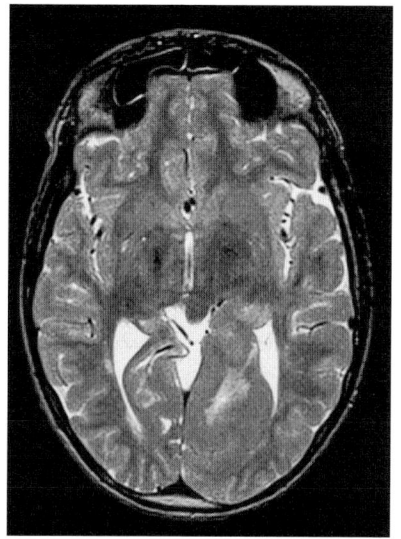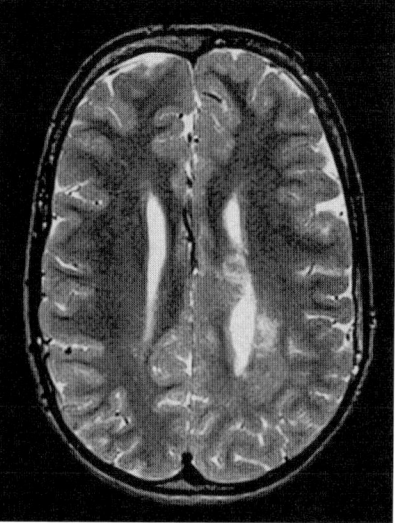

Figure 12. Axial T2-weighted images in a case of left hemimegalencephaly. Note the increased size of the left hemicranium, hemisphere, and trigone. There is an extensive cortical malformation in the left occipital and parietal lobe.

Heterotopia—Disorders of Cellular Migration

In this context heterotopia refers to the presence of neurons located outside the normal cortical or deep gray matter structures, usually in the white matter of the cerebral hemispheres. In the scheme described previously this implies incomplete migration of neurons and glia (or embryologically primitive cells in tuberous sclerosis) at some point along the radial glial fibres. On anatomical grounds heterotopia are classified into subependymal, focal subcortical ("nodular") or band heterotopia (Fig. 13). Irrespective of the anatomical site, heterotopia have characteristic MR imaging features, having an MR signal identical to normal gray matter on all sequences, no enhancement and no mass effect or edema. Subependymal heterotopia often involve a high proportion of the periventricular region of the lateral ventricles and appear as smooth ovoid areas. Clinically, these varieties of heterotopia often have mild manifestations or are sometimes found incidentally (11).

Occasionally, subependymal heterotopia will have a familial association but only affect females. It has been suggested that in these families affected males are usually under spontaneous abortion in utero because of more severe developmental brain abnormalities such as lissencephaly. Patients with focal subcortical heterotopia usually have seizures and frequently are developmentally delayed.

Band heterotopia produces one of the most striking of any characteristic MRI findings of any condition. Recent work in animals has shown that neuronal migration is

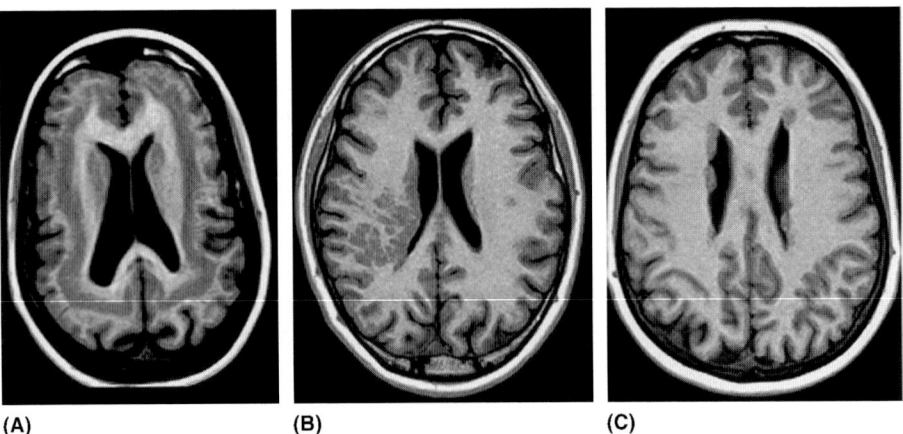

(A)   (B)   (C)

Figure 13. Three patients with different varieties of heterotopia shown on axial T1-weighted images. (**A**) is a case of band heterotopia with a complete band of abnormally sited gray matter in the hemispheric white matter. (**B**) shows nodular heterotopia in the right frontal white matter and (**C**) shows multifocal subependymal heterotopia.

an extensive process over a long period of time but has two discrete peaks. It is likely that band heterotopia is brought about by arrested migration of the second wave of neurons and glia. This produces the following layers (from deep to superficial):

1. Ventricular surface
2. Periventricular and deep white matter
3. Band of arrested neurons/glia
4. Superficial white matter

The cortical ribbon may be thinner than normal with shallow sulci and patients with this variety of heterotopia are often severely clinically affected. Genetic abnormalities have been demonstrated in patients with band heterotopia and some authorities view this as a variety of lissencephaly (12).

Polymicrogyria—Abnormal Cortical Organization

This developmental abnormality results from aberrant organization of the cortical ribbon and is named for the propensity to form multiple small, shallow gyri. The amount of brain tissue that is involved is exceptionally variable and the imaging detection of small areas of polymicrogyria are among the most difficult diagnoses to make. The usual appearance, on MR imaging, is an area of thickened cortex with an irregular gray/white border. The cortex itself has signal characteristics identical to normal gray matter on all sequences, but the subjacent white matter often has T2 prolongation and 5% can show macroscopic calcification. Some areas of polymicrogyria produce an inward buckling of the cortex leaving a prominent V-shaped cerebro spinal fluid space that often contains an enlarged, abnormal venous channel. Although standard spin echo/fast spin echo imaging should always be performed in cases being investigated for localization-related epilepsy, gradient echo T1-weighted volume acquisitions should always be performed. This allows multiplanar reconstructions in non-orthogonal planes and evaluation of the cortical surface by surface-rendering software. These methods tend to increase the detection rate and detection certainly of areas of polymicrogyria (Figs. 14 and 15).

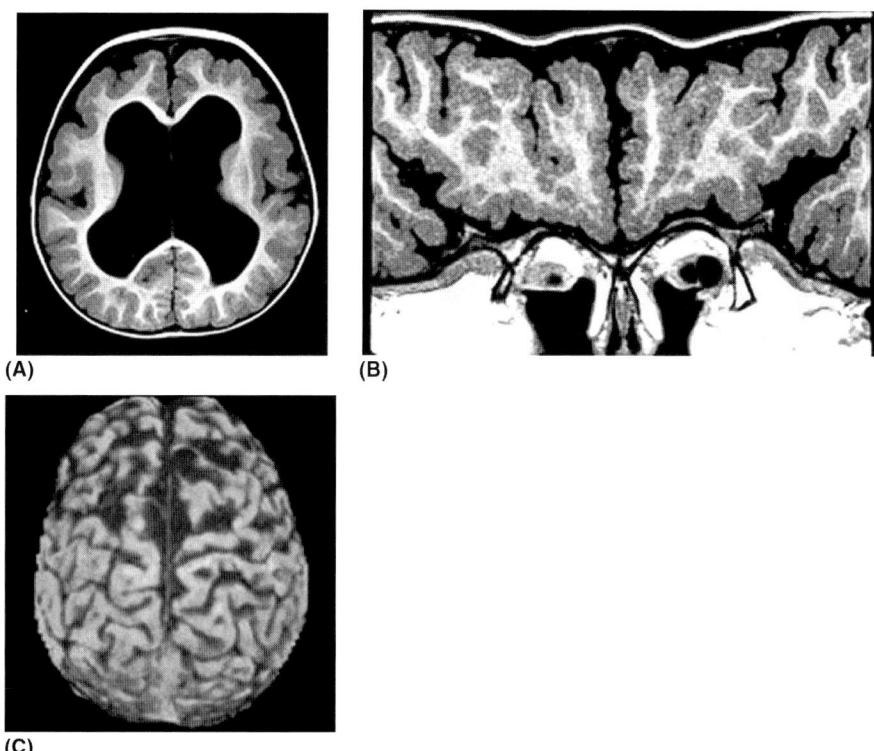

Figure 14. A 12-month-old child with Dandy–Walker malformation (not shown), ventriculomegaly and bilateral frontal polymicrogyria. The axial T1-weighted image (**A**) shows a difference in the pattern of the cortical ribbon between the frontal lobes and the parietal lobes. The non-orthogonal reformation (**B**) and surface reformation (**C**) confirms polymicrogyria and the full extent of the process.

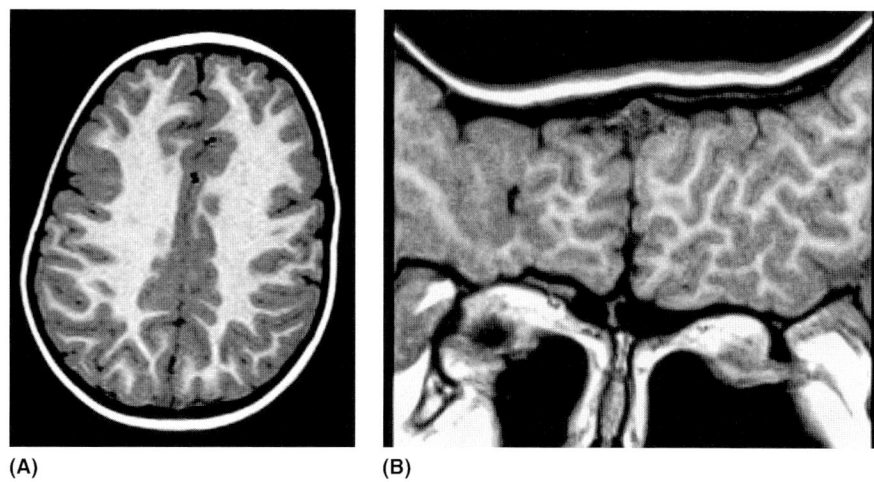

Figure 15. A more subtle, focal area of polymicrogyria in the right frontal cortex. An axial T1-weighted image (**A**) shows a suspicious appearance to the cortex on the right inferior frontal gyrus that is easily confirmed on the non-othogonal reformation of the volume data (**B**).

In summary, knowledge of the normal developmental processes of brain formation greatly assist the recognition and classification of brain malformations. Many of the clinically relevant abnormalities are subtle and require MR imaging of the highest quality in order to make an accurate diagnosis.

REFERENCES

1. DeMyer W. Holoprosencephaly (cyclopia–arhinencephaly). In: Myrianthopoulos N, ed. Malformations. New York: Elsevier, 1987:225–244.
2. Barkovich AJ, Fram EK, Norman D. Septo-optic dysplasia: MR imaging. Radiology 1989; 171:189–192.
3. Rakic P, Yakovlev PI. Development of the corpus callosum and cavum septae in man. J Comp Neurol 1968; 132:45–72.
4. Byrd S, Radkowski M, Flannery A, McLone D. The clinical and radiological evaluation of absence of the corpus callosum. Eur J Radiol 1990; 10:65–73.
5. Ettlinger G. Agenesis of the corpus callosum. In: Viniken PJ, ed. In: Handbook of Clinical Neurology, Vol. 30, Amsterdam: North Holland, 1977:285–297.
6. Barkovich AJ, Simon E, Walsh CA. Callosal agenesis with cyst: a better understanding and new classification. Neurology 2001; 56:220–227.
7. Barkovich AJ. Congenital malformations of the brain and skull. In: Barkovich AJ, ed. Pediatric Neuroimaging. New York: Raven Press, 1995:177–275.
8. Barkovich AJ, Kurniecky RI, Dobyns WB, et al. A classification scheme for malformations of cortical development. Neuropediatrics 1996; 27:59–63.
9. Barkovich AJ, Chuang SH. Unilateral megalencephaly. AJNR 1990; 11:523–531.
10. Griffiths PD, Welch RJ, Gardner-Medwin D, et al. The radiological features of hemimegalencephaly. Neuropediatrics 1994; 25:140–144.
11. Barkovich AJ, Kjos BO. Gray matter heterotopia. Radiology 1992; 182:493–499.
12. Dobyns WB, Truwit CL. Lissencephaly and other malformations of cortical development: 1995 update. Neuropediatrics 1995; 26:132–147.

1.3

The Infratentorial Brain

Paul D. Griffiths
Academic Unit of Radiology, University of Sheffield, Sheffield, U.K.

THE INFRATENTORIAL BRAIN

The rhombencephalon (or hindbrain) is the caudal-most portion of the developing brain and is marked cranially by the mid-brain flexure and caudally by the cervical flexure where it is continuous with the spinal cord. The rhombencephalon will eventually form the pons, medulla, and cerebellum. Six transverse grooves appear in the ventral surface of the hindbrain by four weeks post-conception, which produce segments called rhombomeres that are closely related to the development of cranial nerve nuclei 5–10. A transverse crease (plica choroidea) forms in the roof of the developing fourth ventricle, which has intense neuroblastic activity laterally (alar plates). These form the rhombic lips at around Week 6 post-conception and contain the primordia of the cerebellar hemispheres. For detailed descriptions of cerebellar development see references (1,2). The cerebellar hemispheres contact in the midline and start to fuse during Week 9 (post-conception) to form the cerebellar vermis, therefore the vermis cannot form if the cerebellar hemispheres have not developed. The vermis is fully formed by the end of Week 15 post-conception (corresponding to approximately 17 weeks after the last menstrual period, which is the timing schedule used in clinical practice). The anatomy of the adult vermis is shown in Figure 1C. The nodulus forms first but after the vermis develops from superior to inferior, in a way analogous to the corpus callosum, vermian hypoplasia involves the lobules in a predictable fashion, the lobules of the posterior lobe being involved before those of the anterior lobe.

Classification of malformations/deformations of the brain stem and cerebellum is difficult because there are many factors that affect their development and that of the bony posterior fossa, and there is marked confusion of terminology in the published literature. Three of the four mechanisms described in the previous chapter do occur in the posterior fossa (neurulation, ventral induction and gray matter production, and migration), however these are less relevant in producing a clinically useful classification of hindbrain abnormalities for a number of reasons:

- Failure to close the neural tube does occur in the region of the rhombencephalon but this is exceptionally rare. This is probably because the neural tube in the vicinity of the hindbrain and cervical region is the first to close.
- The process of ventral induction does occur in the posterior fossa structures, i.e., expansion of the cerebellum and partial sagittal cleavage of the cerebellar hemispheres and brain stem. However these do not produce a large number of malformations seen in clinical practice.
- Abnormalities of formation of the cerebellar cortex do occur but are uncommon (discussed later in this chapter). The process is complicated in the cerebellum because the periventricular germinal matrix producing radial migration is not the only neurogenetic mechanism and new neuron production continues after birth.

27

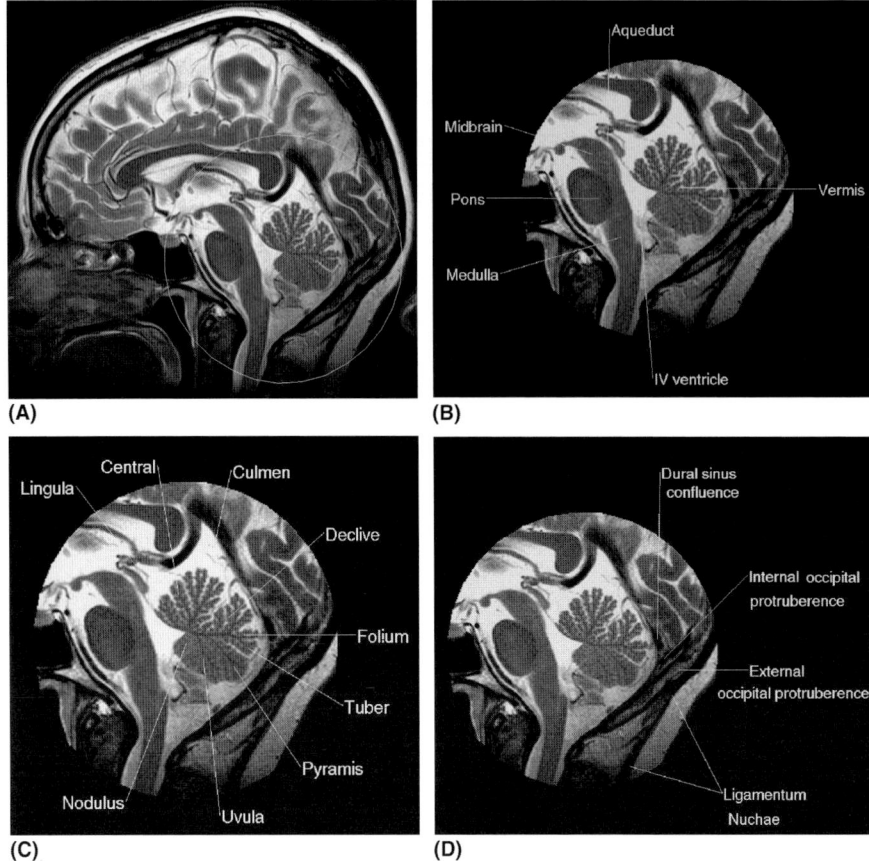

Figure 1. High resolution sagittal T2-weighted images of the whole brain (**A**) and focused on the posterior fossa (**B–D**) showing the anatomical features of the infratentorial brain (**B**), subdivisions of the cerebellar vermis (**C**) and the anatomical relationships around the confluence of the dural sinuses (**D**).

■ The commonest malformations/deformities of the brain stem and cerebellum of clinical relevance (Dandy–Walker malformations, Chiari 1 and Chiari 2) cannot be easily explained by those mechanisms.

This has led some authorities, notably Raybaud et al. (unpublished), to develop a more pragmatic approach to the classification based on the size of the posterior fossa and this is the method will use in this chapter.

Why Is the Size of the Posterior Fossa Important?

The development of the skull and its appropriate growth and modeling relies on several mechanisms and in the supratentorial compartment the effect of cerebral hemispheric growth appears to be a major factor. Our recent work using post mortem MR imaging in fetuses has shown a close correlation between the growth of the cerebral hemispheres and the growth of the supratentorial skull (3). There are several differences between the development of the cerebellar and cerebral cortices that may explain the different mechanisms of posterior fossa development. The majority of cerebral cortex forms by radial migration of neurons and glia from the periventricular germinal matrices to a predetermined site on the future cerebral cortex. In contrast, cerebellar neurons and glia form via two sources: radial migration, similar to that of the cerebral cortex, which forms the deep cerebellar nuclei and the Purkinjie cell layer. Other generative cells situated laterally form a second germinal zone during Weeks 11–13 post-conception and become the granular layer and, in contrast to the cerebral cortex, birth of neurons continues in the cerebellum after birth. Therefore, the growth of the cerebellum tends to lag behind that of the cerebral hemispheres. Our work showed that significant growth of the vermis does not commence until 16–17 weeks after the last menstrual period and at a slower rate than the cerebral cortex (significant growth starting at 13 weeks). In addition, there does not appear to be correlation between the rate of growth of the vermis and the rate of growth of the bony elements of the posterior fossa, as the absolute area and rate of growth of the bony structures are far ahead of the cerebellar vermis. This argues against a causal link between cerebellar growth and development of the bony posterior fossa (Fig. 2).

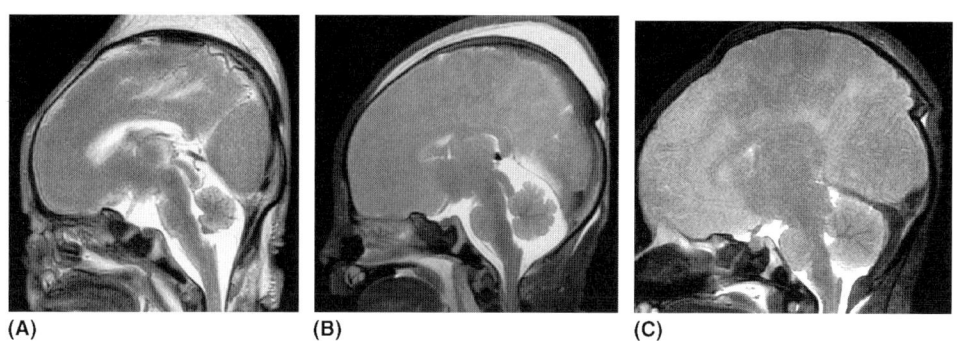

(A)   (B)   (C)

Figure 2. Differential growth of the cerebellar vermis compared to the bony posterior fossa shown on post mortem MR imaging. Sagittal T2-weighted images in fetuses of 20 (**A**), 26 (**B**) and 32 weeks (**C**) gestational age. Note the relative small size of the vermis at earlier gestational ages.

An explanation for the relatively advanced development of the bones of the posterior fossa over the neural structures has been advanced in the hydrostatic theory of McLone (4). By this mechanism the posterior fossa develops in response to cerebro spinal fluid (CSF) pressure instead of growth of the cerebellum itself. The CSF pressure in the fetal posterior fossa is increased by a physiological restriction of CSF flow within the developing spinal cord in the second trimester. This is supported by observation of what is sometimes called a "physiological hydrocephalus" at 16–17 weeks in the ultrasound literature. Therefore the extra pressure exerted on the developing bones of the posterior fossa causes extra growth at that period. This is important because when the cerebellum does start to grow significantly, the ability of the bones to grow and remodel is limited later in pregnancy and the cerebellum will attempt to grow into a space that is too small. This has major relevance for developmental abnormalities of the hindbrain and the surrounding bone, in particular for Chiari 2 deformities. The vast majority of Chiari 2 cases are found in conjunction with open spinal dysraphic processes, mainly myelomeningocoele. The association is explained by proposing that CSF pressure cannot be increased in the posterior fossa during the second trimester because the spine malformation allows CSF to disperse elsewhere and pressure in the cisterna magna cannot be raised. As a result the mesenchyme overlying the cerebellum does not form adequately and a small bony fossa results. The Chiari 2 deformity and its associations described below are the result of the cerebellum attempting to grow into a restricted space.

Our current post-mortem MRI work supports McLone's hypothesis on a mechanistic level in normals, and early results studying fetuses with myelomeningocoeles, in utero and post-mortem, is also consistent. It is also interesting to speculate on how the increased size of the posterior fossa is produced in the Dandy–Walker malformation, a condition associated with marked hypoplasia of the neural structures of the posterior fossa. It is possible that the cystic dilatation of the IV ventricle occurs early in pregnancy due to, at least in part, failed formation of the exit foramina that allows normal CSF circulation and the early raised pressure in the posterior fossa produces significant overgrowth of the surrounding bones. The anatomy of the dural sinus confluence and bony prominences on the occipital bone support this view (Fig. 1D).

Assessment of Bony Posterior Fossa Size

Volume measurements of the bony confines of the posterior fossa are possible using cross-sectional imaging and MR volume acquisitions are ideally suited to this. However, these are time-intensive and not routinely carried out in clinical practice. Some groups, including our own, have used area measurements in the mid-sagittal plane as a surrogate marker of posterior fossa volume (3), however robust large numbers of age-related control data are not available. Neuroradiologists have a large internal database of normality but this subjective assessment is difficult to use in scientific studies. One useful method is to assess the size of the posterior fossa by looking at the anatomical relationship between the external occipital protuberance, the internal occipital protuberance and the dural confluence (sagittal sinus, straight sinus and transverse sinuses).

The external occipital protuberance is a midline bony prominence on the posterior portion of the occipital bone and the fibers of the ligamentum nuchae insert into the inferior portion of that protuberance. There is usually close congruence between the external occipital protuberance and the bony prominence on the internal aspect of the occipital bone (internal occipital protuberance). This indicates the site of dural sinus confluence which usually lies at the level of the internal occipital protuberance but to one side (usually right). The dural sinuses develop early in early fetal life and it would be expected that malformations/deformities that have their effects after that time would not displace the position of the dural confluence. In contrast, malformations forming before or at the time of the condensation of the dural sinuses would be expected to produce an abnormal site of the dural confluence. This can be assessed indirectly by looking for lack of congruence between the external occipital protuberance and the dural sinus confluence. This approach can be useful but is not the complete picture in assessing the size of the posterior fossa. The dural sinus external occipital protuberance congruence is important for the upper portion of the bony posterior fossa. The development of the skull base, however, is the most important factor that influences growth of the bony posterior fossa around the foramen magnum and a different range of developmental abnormalities can affect that process. Examples of this are found in patients with some varieties of Chiari 1 malformation who have normal internal/external occipital protuberance congruity and small posterior fossae. This situation is brought about by failure of formation of the mesoderm that forms the basal portion of the occipital bone.

Developmental Abnormalities Associated with a Large Posterior Fossa

The signature malformation that produces a large posterior fossa is the Dandy–Walker malformation. The Dandy–Walker malformation consists of vermian aplasia or hypoplasia, patulous exit foramina of the fourth ventricle, cystic abnormality behind the cerebellum that is continuous with the fourth ventricle, and hydrocephalus. It should be noted, however, that hydrocephalus does not usually develop until after birth and ventriculomegaly may be mild or absent in utero. There is a high association with other brain abnormalities (failed commissuration, cortical formation malformations, and encephalocoeles). The cerebellar hemispheres may be hypoplastic as well as the vermis. The developmental abnormalities that give rise to Dandy–Walker malformation are likely to arise early in pregnancy, before the venous confluence has formed. This is supported by the observation that the internal occipital protuberance and dural confluence are displaced away superiorly from the foramen magnum producing a large posterior fossa volume (Fig. 3). This feature can often be recognized on plain radiographs when the internal occipital protuberance can be seen superior to the junction of the lambdoid sutures (torcula-lamboid inversion).

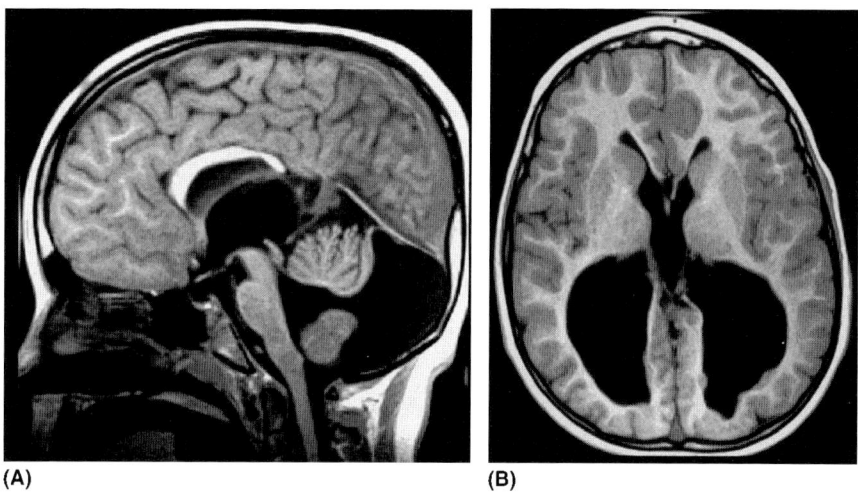

(A)   **(B)**

Figure 3. A child with Dandy–Walker malformation and subependymal heterotopia. The sagittal T1-weighted image (**A**) shows marked vermian hypoplasia (compare with Fig. 1C), a patulous egress from the fourth ventricle and an enlarged posterior fossa as shown by superior displacement of the venous confluence (compare with Fig. 1D). The corpus callosum is also hypoplastic. The axial T1-weighted image (**B**) shows enlarged ventricles and gray matter protrusions into the left trigone and occipital horn consistent with heterotopia.

The diagnosis of Dandy–Walker malformation is usually straightforward on cross-sectional imaging, particularly on MRI with its capacity to image in the sagittal plane. A significant number of cases seen in clinical practice do not have all of the features described above and this often causes semantic confusion. Less-pronounced malformations are often termed Dandy-Walker varianta and Barkovich describes "typical" Dandy–Walker variants to consist of minor vermian hypoplasia, a retro-cerebellar cystic structure continuous with the fourth ventricle that does not necessarily enlarge the posterior fossa, and no hydrocephalus (5).

There are other developmental cystic abnormalities in the posterior fossa that may give rise to further confusion in nomenclature and significance. These include:

■ Mega cisterna magna
■ Arachnoid cysts in the posterior fossa
■ Retrocerebellar cysts of Baker

The cisterna magna is the basal cistern behind and below the cerebellum and Mega cisterna magna is formed by abnormal enlargement of that CSF-containing space behind the cerebellum and medulla. The vermis is fully formed and the exit foramina from the fourth ventricle are normal. The posterior fossa may be enlarged and the mass effect can cause hydrocephalus.

Arachnoid cysts are thought to be true developmental abnormalities in most cases, however, they usually present later in life because they show interval growth of CSF collections within the pia-arachnoid. Approximately 25% of arachnoid cysts occur in the posterior fossa but only 9% are related to the vermis (the others being in the cerebello-pontine angle, quadrigeminal cistern or prepontine cistern) (6). They often present early because of their large size and prominent effects on cerebellar function because of the restricted space for expansion in the posterior fossa. Hemorrhage may occur into arachnoid cysts but invariably the cyst has signal characteristics identical to CSF on all standard MR sequences and CT examinations. This can give rise to further diagnostic confusion with a mass lesion—the epidermoid tumor. The abnormality often has signal characteristics identical to CSF on spine echo, fast spin echo and gradient echo imaging sequences but can usually be distinguished from arachnoid cysts by diffusion-weighted imaging. An arachnoid cyst does not show any restriction to diffusion of water and will appear low signal on diffusion-weighted images and high signal on maps of apparent diffusion coefficients. In contrast, epidermoids show diffusion restriction with lower apparent diffusion coefficients than intraventricular CSF.

There can be few examples of a more confused literature than that surrounding Blake's cysts that should feature in the differential diagnosis of retro-cerebellar cystic structures. Altman et al. describes a Blake's pouch to be a persistent diverticulum of the fourth ventricle, which may enlarge the posterior fossa and produce hydrocephalus (7). Strand et al. put forward the theory that Blake's pouch cyst and retrocerebellar arachnoid cysts are the same entity because at some stage the communication with the fourth ventricle is lost and contact with the developing arachnoid matter is made (8). Calabro et al. clearly distinguish between Blake's pouch cysts and retrocerebellar arachnoid cysts although they recognize differentiation of the two on imaging is difficult and can only be resolved on histological analysis (9).

Developmental Abnormalities Associated with Normal Sized Posterior Fossa

Chiari 1

The Chiari 1 malformation refers to ectopia of the cerebellar tonsils, which is displacement of the tonsils below the foramen magnum. It is generally reserved for developmental abnormalities and distinguished from:

1. Tonsillar herniation which implies an acquired compartmental shift due to the presence of a mass lesion, most often with the posterior fossa.
2. Acquired abnormalities that produce basilar invagination often resulting from a disorder that causes "bone-softening."

Some degree of tonsillar descent is seen in adults and children without clinical implications and the standard texts state that 6 mm of tonsillar descent can be considered within normal variation. However careful assessment is always required of the degree of "crowding" of the medulla/upper cervical cord. This is best done by looking for the amount of residual CSF around the cord on axial images (Fig. 4).

In many patients the Chiari 1 malformation is associated with other abnormalities detectable on imaging. Most frequently these are bony abnormalities of the craniocervical junction. These include skull base malformations such as platybasia, assimilation of the C1 vertebrae onto the occipital bone, and other segmentation anomalies of the cervical spine. Some authorities have suggested that these patients have defects produced exceptionally early in fetal life at the time of transverse segmentation.

In patients with Chiari 1 but no evidence of craniocervical bony abnormalities it has been suggested that the tonsillar ectopia is due to intrauterine hydrocephalus. The raised intracranial pressure at that time produces tonsillar herniation. The hydrocephalus does not persist after delivery, but the tonsils do not return to their normal intracranial position. In these cases the cerebellar tonsils often have a pointed "peg-like" configuration. Irrespective of the cause of the tonsillar descent, the detection of Chiari 1 malformations should prompt investigation of the whole spine using MRI because of high association (up to one-quarter of cases) with syringohydromyelia.

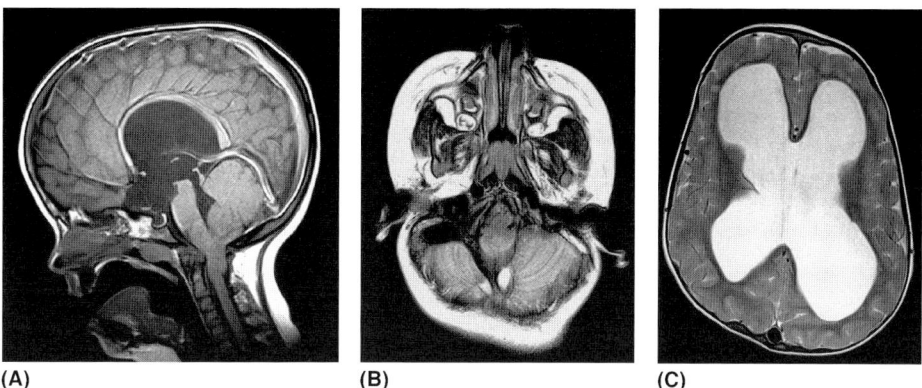

(A)   **(B)**   **(C)**

Figure 4. Imaging from a child with a severe Chiari 1 malformation. A sagittal T1-weighted image (**A**) shows the cerebellar tonsils to be at the level of mid C2 with marked impaction around the foramen magnum shown on an axial T2-weighted image (**B**). There is marked hydrocephalus (**C**). Note that the skull base is abnormally flat (platybasia) but the size of the posterior fossa is normal.

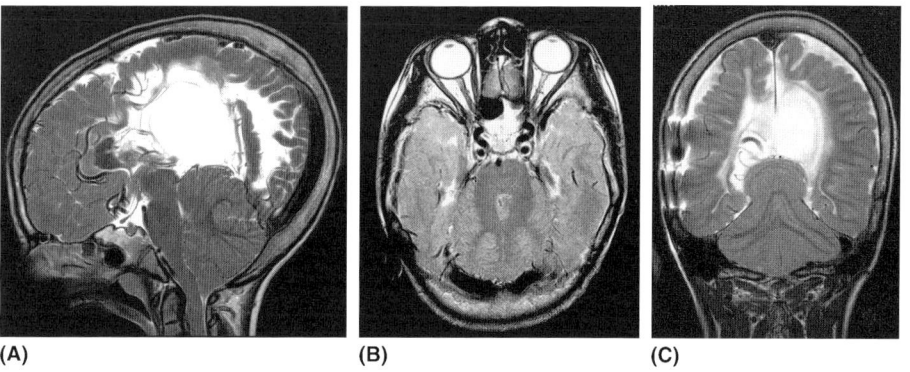

(A)   **(B)**   **(C)**

Figure 5. A child with severe developmental brain problems including rhombencephalosynapsis. T2-weighted images in the sagittal (**A**), axial (**B**) and coronal (**C**) planes shown no vermian structure at all, the two cerebellar hemispheres are fused directly. There is mild tonsillar descent. Supratentorially there is severe hypogenesis of the corpus callosum and a large posterior inter-hemispheric cyst.

When size of the posterior fossa is used to classify malformations, as used here, most Chiari 1 patients have normal sized posterior fossae. However, there are several situations when the Chiari 1 malformation will be associated with small bony posterior fossae (5). Craniosynostosis syndromes and occipital encephalocoele may produce the association of Chiari 1 and small fossae. In some cases of fetal hydrocephalus a small posterior fossa forms and the later growth of the cerebellum results in tonsillar ectopia.

Rhombencephalosynapsis

This is a rare disorder of the cerebellum that, in our experience usually has a normal-sized posterior fossa although Altman et al. describe their cases as having small posterior fossa (8). The vermis does not form but the cerebellar hemispheres are fused across the midline. As well as the cerebellar hemispheres being fused, the dentate nuclei and superior cerebellar peduncles are also fused. The diagnosis of this malformation is best seen on sagittal imaging where the complete absence of the normal vermian anatomy is recognized on the mid-sagittal section (Fig. 5). Supratentorial abnormalities

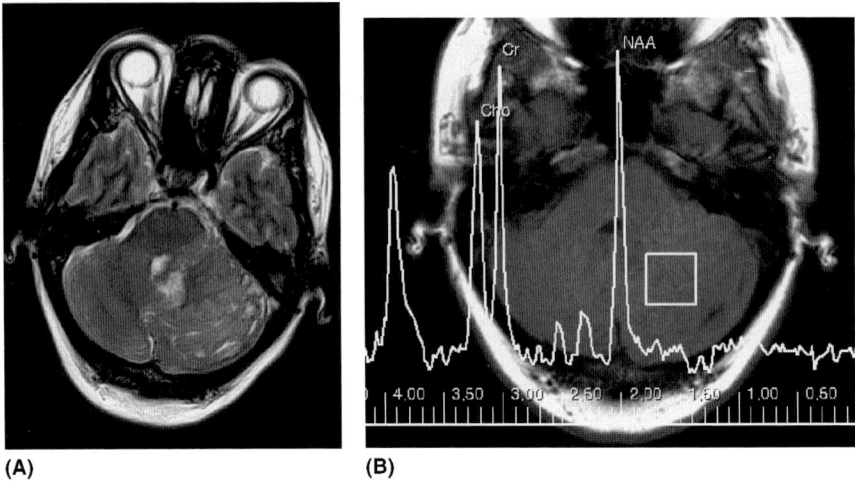

(A)   **(B)**

Figure 6. An adult patient with Lhermitte–Duclos syndrome. An axial T2-weighted image through the cerebellum (**A**) shows the typical, layered heterogenous signal characteristics in the left cerebellar hemisphere and vermis. Proton spectroscopy in that region (**B**) shows reduced NAA groups and a small lactate doublet.

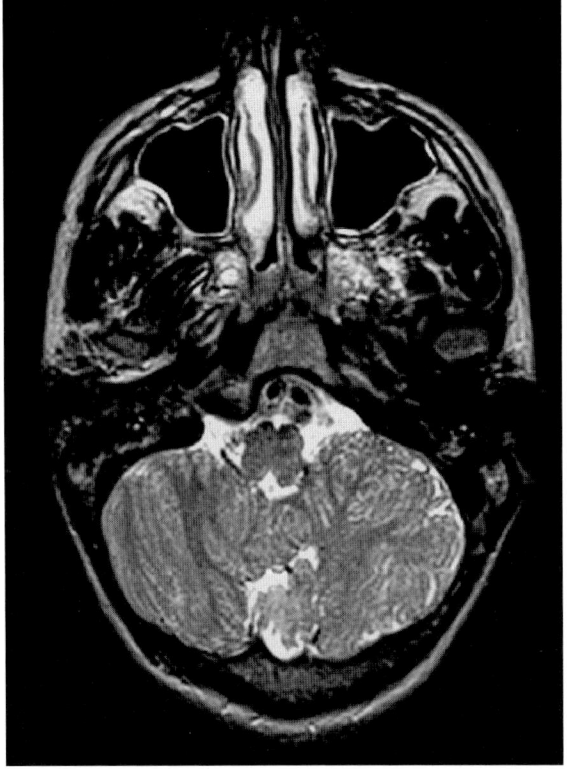

Figure 7. A patient with a disordered left cerebellar hemisphere due to a severe disorder of formation of the cerebellar cortex.

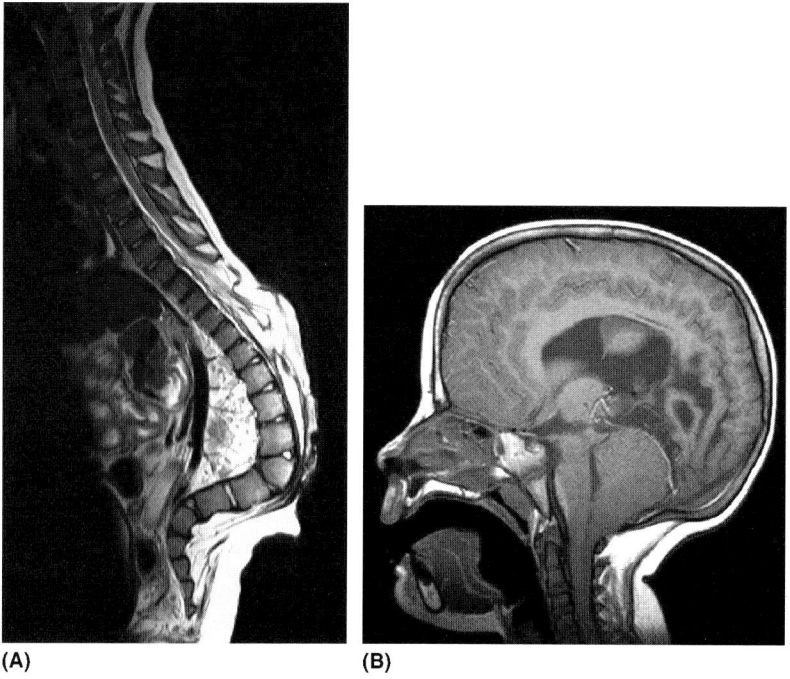

(A) **(B)**

Figure 8. A child with a low thoracic/high lumbar myelomeningocole shown on sagittal T2-weighted images of the spine (**A**) has a moderately severe Chiari 2 deformity shown on a sagittal T1-weighted image of the brain (**B**). Note the low-placed cerebellar tonsils and the vertical fourth ventricle. The posterior fossa is small as indicated by the displacement of the venous confluence toward the foramen magnum.

are commonly found in conjunction with rhombencephalosynapsis including thalamic fusion and absence of the septum pellucidum.

Lhermitte–Duclos Syndrome

Lhermitte–Duclos syndrome is a rare condition of the cerebellum that often becomes clinically apparent in the third and fourth decade, but the age of manifestation varies from birth to the sixth decade with no sex predilection. Forty percent of patients with Lhermitte–Duclos syndrome also have Cowden's disease and this association of two rare diseases has prompted the hypothesis that Lhermitte–Duclos syndrome and Cowden's disease are a single phakomatosis. This is supported by genetic analysis that showed a single abnormal locus within chromosome 10q23 in both disorders There has been much debate in the literature as to the nature of this cerebellar anomaly but it is thought to have both developmental and proliferative elements, hence the earlier terminology "dysplastic cerebellar gangliocytoma."

There are several reports in the literature concerning magnetic resonance imaging (MRI) appearances of Lhermitte–Duclos syndrome and these appear to be highly characteristic for the disorder.

We have recently performed proton spectroscopy in two confirmed cases of Lhermitte–Duclos syndrome (Fig. 6), which showed differences in the cerebella from controls of a similar age group (10). The NA/Cho ratio was 1.2 in both patients when compared to 1.7 ± 0.3 (mean $\pm$ standard deviation) in the controls. The NA/Cr ratio showed a similar difference measured at 1.0 and 1.1 respectively compared to 1.4 ± 0.3 in the controls. Inverted doublets centred at 1.43 ppm representing lactate were present in one patient's spectra.

Joubert's Syndrome

The original description of this syndrome was a familial association of patients with neonatal hyperpnea/apnea, abnormal eye movements and developmental delay (11). Agenesis or hypogenesis of the cerebellar vermis was found on post mortem examination and these have been supplemented by detailed radiological studies (12). Kendall et al. described 16 children with Joubert syndrome, all of which had varying degrees of hypogenesis of the cerebellar vermis. Other features recognizable on MRI included, dilated fourth ventricle, the inferior and superior cerebellar peduncles were small, and the superior peduncles were close to right angles to the brainstem.

Disorders of Formation of the Cerebellar Cortex

Many of the neurons that form the cerebellar cortex are formed in a similar fashion to those in the supratentorial compartment, i.e., born in the germinal matrix (around the fourth ventricle), undergo radial migration to the future cortex and then must organize to form a highly organized structure. It is not surprising, therefore that MRI examinations show cases in which there is abnormal formation of the cortex (Fig. 7) in comparable way to the supratentorial compartment. Many of these are associated with supratentorial cortical abnormalities in our experience. Understanding of the clinical effects of these abnormalities is in its early stages.

Rostral Vermian Cortical Dysplasia

This is a relatively recently described condition (13) in which there is defective foliation of the rostral vermis (and to a lesser extent onto the hemispheres) best seen on coronal images. Demaerel and colleagues described 15 patients who showed varying degrees of this abnormality on MR imaging, three of which also had supratentorial abnormalities of cortical formation as well. The clinical effects of this abnormality in isolation are uncertain at present.

Developmental Abnormalities Associated with a Small Posterior Fossa

A small bony posterior fossa is the characteristic finding of the Chiari 2 deformity, which is found invariably associated with open spine malformations such as myelomeningocele (Fig. 8). This association has caused much discussion in the embryology literature and the leading theory that accounts for the two is the hydrostatic theory of McLone (4). This theory is centred upon how the bones of the future skull are directed to develop and grow, which is important for the Chiari 2 deformity because the fundamental abnormality in the cranial compartment is a small bony posterior fossa. One important factor that influences bone growth is the growth of the underlying brain, possibly by a combination of growth factors produced by the brain and direct pressure. These are probably the main factors that influence the growth of the supratentorial skull and this view is supported by observation of fetuses imaged post mortem (3). The growth of the bone of the posterior fossa appears to be less dependent on growth of the cerebellum, mainly because the growth of the cerebellum is delayed in relation to the rest of the brain. The growth of the bony fossa appears to be promoted by the pressure exerted through the pressure of the CSF, mainly in the cisterna magna. McLone's theory suggests that a physiological obstruction to CSF flow in the spine occurs in the second trimester and the resulting increased pressure of the intracranial CSF expands the cisterna magna and promotes bony growth of the occipital bones. The theory is extended to explain the high frequency of association between Chiari 2 deformity and myelomeningoceles or other developmental spinal processes which does not allow the build up of CSF pressure. Therefore in later pregnancy/early infancy the cerebellum attempts to grow into a space that is not large enough. This results in the herniation of the cerebellum through the tentorium (towering cerebellum) and tonsillar descent into the upper cervical region.

This theory is supported by a number of indirect pieces of information from fetal and neonatal imaging:

■ Chiari 2 malformations do not occur with closed spinal dysraphic processes e.g., lipomyelomeningocele, presumably because CSF pressure can be maintained.
■ In utero MRI demonstrates significantly reduced extra-axial CSF in both the infra- and supratentorial compartments. (NB: The supratentorial CSF reduction can be difficult to appreciate on ultrasound).
■ There is loss of the normal congruence between the external/internal occipital protuberance and sinus confluence in cases of Chiari 2 with the sinus confluence being displaced towards the foramen magnum.

In summary, the developmental abnormalities involving the posterior fossa structures result from a wide range of different etiologies and it is impossible to come to a unifying theory at present. Classification systems are imperfect at best and confusing at worst, but we have described one approach that uses the size of the bony compartment of the posterior fossa.

REFERENCES

1. Rakic P, Sidman RL. Histogenesis of cortical layers in human cerebellum. J Comp Neurol 1970; 139:473–500.
2. Larroche J-C. Malformations of the nervous system. In: Adams J, Corsellis J, Duchen L, eds. Greenfield's Neuropathology. 4th ed. New York: Wiley, 1984:385–450.
3. Griffiths PD, Wilkinson ID, Variend S, Jones A, Paley MNJ, Whitby E. Differential growth rates of the cerebellum and posterior fossa assessed by postmortem MR imaging of the fetus: implications for the pathogenesis of the Chiari 2 deformity. Acta Radiol 2004; 45:1–6.
4. McLone DG, Naidich TP. Developmental morphology of the subarachnoid space, brain vasculature, and contiguous structures and the cause of the Chiari II malformation. AJNR 1992; 13:463–482.
5. Barkovich AJ. Congenital malformations of the brain and skull. In: Barkovich AJ, ed. Pediatric Neuroimaging. New York: Raven Press, 1995:177–275.
6. Naidich TP, Radkowski MA, Bernstein RA, Tan WS. Congenital malformations of the posterior fossa. In: Taveras JM, Ferrucci JT, eds. Radiology. Philadelphia: Lippincott, 1986:1–17.
7. Altman N, Naidich TP, Braffman BH. Posterior fossa malformations. AJNR 1992; 13:691–724.
8. Strand RD, Barnes PD, Young Pouissaint T, Estroff JA, Burrows PE. Cystic retrocerebellar malformations: unification of the Dandy–Walker complex and the Blake's pouch cyst. Pediatr Radiol 1993; 23:258–260.
9. Calabro F, Arcuri T, Jinkins JR. Blake's pouch cyst: an entity within Dandy–Walker continuum. Neuroradiology 2000; 42:290–295.
10. Nagaraja S, Wilkinson ID, Powell T, Griffiths PD. MR imaging and spectroscopy in Lhermitte-Duclos disease. Neuroradiology 2004; 46:355–358.
11. Joubert M, Eisenring N, Robb JP, Andermann F. Familial agenesis of the cerebellar vermis. Neurology 1969; 19:813–825.
12. Kendal B, Kingsley D, Lambert SR, et al. Joubert syndrome: a clinico-radiological study. Neuroradiology 1990; 31:502–506.
13. Demaerel P, Wilms G, Marchal G. Rostral vermian cortical dysplasia: MRI. Neuroradiology 1999; 41:190–194.

1.4

Studies of Malformations of the Posterior Fossa

Stephen L. Kinsman and Tobias Tsai
Department of Pediatrics and Neurology, University of Maryland School of Medicine, Baltimore, Maryland, U.S.A.

STUDIES OF MALFORMATIONS OF THE POSTERIOR FOSSA

As with the study of other central nervous system (CNS) malformations, determining the timing of when posterior fossa structural development veered from its normal course and embarked on the events that led to the resultant abnormal architecture of the malformation in question is central to understanding the malformation and its consequences (1). When studying malformations of the posterior fossa, one must not only consider neural development, but also the development of the surrounding structures. In the posterior fossa, neural tissue— the cerebellum and brainstem— exist within the posterior fossa, a tight cranial vault space bounded by bone and tentorium (2). Cross-sectional studies of the growth of the posterior fossa vault and the neural contents of the vault, i.e., cerebellum and brainstem, indicate different growth trajectories for each component with that the posterior fossa growing first by expansion of cerebrospinal fluid under pressure and only later does the cerebellum grow into the expanded posterior fossa vault (3). The relationship between the two growth trajectories remains incompletely studied. Magnetic resonance imaging (MRI) has opened the door to this type of detailed study of the development of the posterior fossa and its contents, even during the fetal period (4–9). Quantitative approaches to MRIs allow detailed analysis of cerebellum, brainstem, and surrounding structures (10). Our group has begun to use newer methods of size and shape analysis using this detailed MRI-acquired anatomic data to test hypotheses about (1) the degree of and cause(s) of anatomic variability seen in this group of malformations particularly the Chiari 2 malformation (11), and (2) the relationship between the observed and quantified anatomic variability and the degree of clinical symptoms/signs manifested in these conditions.

Despite decades of knowledge of the existence of posterior fossa malformations and efforts to understand their pathogenesis, there is little consensus about how these malformations occur and how they cause clinical symptoms/signs (12–19). There remains debate about whether the observed anatomic features are indeed the result of malformation or whether deformation also plays a role, perhaps even a dominant one (19,20). Studies have been limited due to the imaging techniques available. Autopsy studies are another approach that has been used but are limited due to population biases and are by nature retrospective with regard to clinical information. Also, autopsy studies are limited in their ability to collect quantitative anatomic data, particularly in three-dimensions, and are prone to fixation artifact. Earlier radiographic techniques were limited to examination of bony anatomy and landmarks, with no or limited ability to characterize neural structures. Computed tomographic (CT) studies increased anatomic detail, but are limited in their ability to define neural structures within the posterior fossa due to artifacts introduced by bone. Improvements in magnetic resonance neuroimaging allow the study of these malformations/deformations in larger populations, in greater detail, and with the potential for longitudinal analysis. This allows us to test hypotheses we could not in the past. Also, these studies may even shed light on causation, of the conditions themselves as well as the symptoms and signs they cause. They may also allow a testing of the efficacy of neurosurgical and other interventions in a more direct manner.

Our group has begun to explore the use of MRI to test hypotheses about Chiari 2 malformation in groups of patients with myelomeningocele (MMC) (11). Chiari 2 malformation remains an important source of morbidity and mortality in MMC (19). The malformation is characterized by cerebellar vermian herniation with or without herniation (also described as elongation/caudal descent) of the brainstem below the foramen magnum. Surgical decompression of the posterior fossa continues to be performed on many individuals with this condition, but debate continues on its role (20). Indications for decompression are mostly based on the presence of clinical symptoms and signs particularly if progression is apparent. Neuroimaging is used as much to rule out other causes of neurological impairment, e.g., hydrocephalus and/or syrinx, as to measure the severity of the Chiari malformation and to determine the need for surgery. However, debate continues as to the important components of the Chiari 2 malformation, as well as whether the mechanism of symptoms/signs is compression or traction of neural structures. Also, there remains controversy as to whether brainstem and/or cerebellar function can worsen over time in Chiari malformation from causes that are non-mechanical in nature (21). These might include premature cell death, abnormalities in the structure and/or function of white matter, and alterations in nuclear and synaptic development (22). In this author's experience, there appears to be an increased willingness to attribute neurological symptoms and/or signs in people with MMC to the Chiari 2 malformation (including as an explanation for at least part of the increased mortality in MMC). This results in various neurosurgical posterior fossa decompression approaches to treating these problems, despite very little work proving a cause and effect relationship for many of them. This is not, however, a denial of the importance of neurosurgical decompression in the management of Chiari 2 malformation in cases where clear clinical progression, particularly of signs, has been documented and other causes of dysfunction adequately ruled out.

In addition to this, recent advances in fetal closure of MMC have shown that the anatomy of the Chiari 2 malformation in MMC is significantly changed after fetal surgery (23–25). It appears that closure of the cele during the fetal period leads to a more normal CSF accumulation within the fetal posterior fossa. Some authors have suggested that this "normalization" of the posterior fossa leads to a "reversal" of the Chiari 2 condition, including ameliorization of symptoms and signs (24). However, only a few small series have been published to date and there remains uncertainty about whether the decrease in vermian herniation and larger posterior fossa protect against development of brainstem dysfunction in those who had fetal closure in MMC. Hopefully some of this uncertainty will be cleared up with the completion of the MOMS trial in the United States (26).

There is a more direct relationship between anatomy and clinical features in Chiari 1 malformation, where MRI-based studies have shed light on the pathogenesis of the condition (27,28). These studies show a small posterior fossa in Chiari 1, suggesting a compressive mechanism as a cause of symptoms/signs in the condition.

To better understand Chiari 2 malformation, our group undertook an analysis of the anatomic variability in Chiari 2 malformation as a first step towards designing better studies of both the pathogenesis of the malformation/deformation and of the relationship between symptoms/signs and definable anatomic abnormalities of the posterior fossa. We assessed traditional biometric measures of the posterior fossa using digitized images of MRI scans to assess size variability within a randomly selected population of individuals with Chiari 2 malformation and MMC. This study population was obtained from individuals followed in our large outpatient program at the Kennedy Krieger Institute in Baltimore, Maryland, U.S.A., after institutional approval of our study (n=25 for subjects and controls). We also used these digitized images to study shape variability within a subset of the group using an approach called thin-plate spline analysis (n=14 for subjects and controls) (11).

Analysis of the relationship between cross-sectional areas and lengths of various structures in the posterior fossa in Chiari 2 malformation is rational as this approach has been used successfully in Chiari 1 malformation as discussed above. The "unified" hypothesis put forth by McLone suggests that an inverse relationship should be seen between posterior fossa size and the degree of vermian herniation in Chiari 2 malformation (16). Another feature of the Chiari 2 malformation, brainstem herniation, was studied by Emery in an autopsy series where he found no relationship between the degree of brainstem herniation and the degree of vermian herniation (13). Therefore, the relationship between these different features of the condition remains incompletely understood and warrants further study. Also, an understated finding of these studies is the large amount of variability seen in the anatomic abnormalities of Chiari 2 malformation. The nature of this variability and its significance is likely to hold clues for both better approaches to classify and hopefully to manage this perplexing malformation.

MRI analysis is easily accomplished with either digitalized files obtained from radiographs or direct import of the digital files of the MRI scanner into a suitable image analysis program. Given the preliminary nature of our studies to date, we used digitalized files, allowing us to sample our extensive film archive of MRI images on patients with Chiari 2 malformation. Future studies will likely use the digital files directly from the scanner and be designed to collect volumetric and three-dimensional data for greater accuracy, much like the technique used to obtain our control data [for details of techniques used see Tsai and Kinsman (11)].

Another feature of the studies of the Chiari 1 malformation and the posterior fossa in other conditions is that they have helped define both landmarks and structures important for analysis of posterior fossa malformations. For details the reader is pointed to the publications of Christophe (28) and DiMario (29). For the purpose of our Chiari 2 studies we defined the mid-sagittal posterior fossa area as the area enclosed by a polygon whose vertices included the basion, opisthion, torcula, top of the tentorium, midpoint of the midbrain, and the top the dorsum sellae (Fig. 1). Our studies of posterior fossa area and length variables confirms the hypothesis that the posterior fossa is smaller than normal in Chiari 2 malformation and that this smallness correlates with the degree of vermian herniation in the condition (Tables 1 and 2). Our analysis also confirms the findings of Emery that the degree of brainstem herniation does not correlate with the size of the posterior fossa, suggesting a different pathogenesis for this important component of the condition (13).

Although there is a strong possibility that the causes of brainstem herniation lie outside the posterior fossa and may relate to such variables as dentate ligament length and/or degree of spinal cord tension (13,15,30), we hypothesized that shape alterations between the neural and bony components of the posterior fossa might also play a role. Qualitative analysis of a large series of Chiari 2 cases suggested to us a large amount of variability in the shape of the major components of the posterior fossa in individuals with the condition compared to controls. This included the shape of the midline vermis, the shape and positioning of the tentorium cerebellum, and the shape of the brainstem. Also, the relationships between all these structures and their relative positions appeared to be highly variable as well.

To investigate this qualitative finding further, we applied a method of analysis designed to study shape variability (31,32). This approach had the added advantage of being statistically powerful enough to be applied to small sample sizes and to study whether changes in landmark position vary independently or dependently (33). This

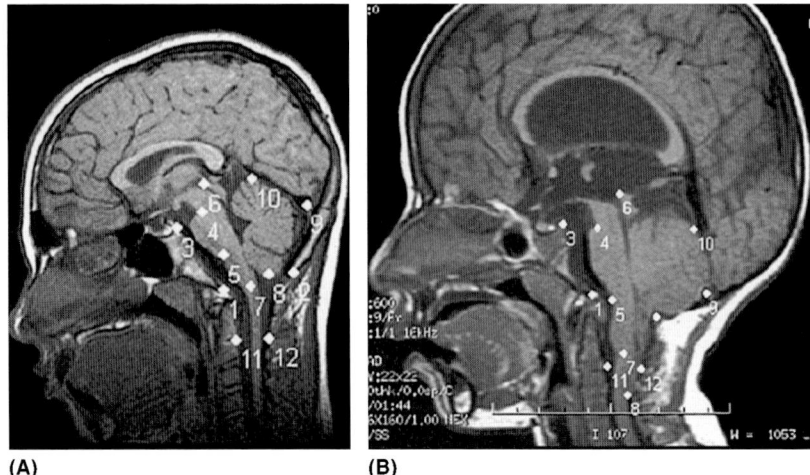

(A)   **(B)**

Figure 1. (**A**) shows the 12 landmarks on the midsagittal SPGR MRI of a control subject. (**B**) shows those same 12 landmarks on the midsagittal T1-weighted MRI of a Chiari 2 patient. The landmarks are, in order: (1) Basion; (2) Opisthion; (3) Top of dorsum sellae; (4) Superior pontine notch (SPN); (5) Inferior pontine notch (IPN); (6) Iter (rostral portion of sylvian aqueduct); (7) Cervicomedullary junction (CMJ); (8) Caudalmost extent of midline cerebellar tissue (vermis ± tonsils); (9) Torcula; (10) Top of tentorium cerebelli; (11) Anterior border of cervicospinal canal at the level of the C2 vertebrae; (12): Posterior border of cervicospinal canal at the level of the C2 vertebrae.

Table 1. Correlation Between Posterior Fossa Measurements

Correlation Between Vermian Herniation and …	Pearson's R	2-Tailed p-Value
Non-herniated brainstem (Iter-FM)	− 0.639	0.008
Caudal displacement of SPN	0.590	0.043
Caudal displacement of IPN	0.510	0.031
Posterior fossa area	− 0.652	0.012
Correlation between posterior fossa area and …		
Non-herniated brainstem (Iter-FM)	0.745	0.002
Caudal displacement of IPN	0.554	0.31

Iter is the top of the brainstem and was identified as the rostral-most portion of the aqueduct of Sylvius, FM is the foramen magnum, SPN is the superior pontine notch, and IPN is the inferior pontine notch.

approach is based on a method first delineated by the Scottish zoologist D'Arcy Thompson in 1917 and later refined by Bookstein, for representing anatomic data as thin-plate splines, a method for plotting anatomic landmarks on a grid, adjusting for differences in overall size and analyzing landmark position variability statistically using partial-least-squares analysis (31). The method has been applied successfully for identifying abnormalities in corpus callosum shape in fetal alcohol syndrome (34,35). These shape differences also allow differentiation of those with fetal alcohol syndrome who have a characteristic neurocognitive impairment profile from those who do not (36). We believe this approach holds the same promise for Chiari malformation and possibly other malformations of the posterior fossa such as Dandy–Walker malformation.

To accomplish thin-plate spline analysis, images are imported into TPSDig, a program designed to collect landmark data for shape analysis [for details of techniques used see Tsai and Kinsman (11)]. For our Chiari 2 analysis, we chose six bony landmarks and six neural landmarks (Fig. 1). The data were then analyzed in Edgewarp, a program specifically designed for this type of shape analysis. The landmark datapoints are

Table 2. Comparison of Means: Chiari 2 Patients vs. Controls

Measure	Mean, Chiari 2	Mean, Controls	2-tailed p-value by t-test
Vermian herniation	1.986 cm	–	–
Medullary herniation	1.307 cm	– 0.196 cm	Essentially 0
Pons length	2.852 cm	2.686 cm	0.062
SPN herniation	– 0.149 cm	0.121 cm	0.067
IPN herniation	0.128 cm	1.071 cm	Essentially 0
Non-herniated brainstem	5.288 cm	5.783 cm	0.000017
Posterior fossa area	24.881 sq cm	28.717 sq cm	0.0042

Negative numbers refer to a distance above the line used for reference, e.g., the line perpendicular to the turcica sellae in the case of the SPN, or the foramen magnum in the case of medullary herniation. The mean for vermian herniation in controls is omitted since these subjects have no vermian peg.

converted into Procrustes shape coordinates. For each set of landmarks on a given image, the centroids—essentially the "center" of the shape the set of landmarks represent—is found and the shape is then scaled such that the sum of the squared distances to the shape's centroid is 1. The sets of scaled points can then be aligned to their centroids, and rotated in a way that minimizes the sum of the squared distances between landmarks. Applying this procedure to a set of control images thus yields an average or "consensus" shape independent of size—the same can be done for the set of cases with Chiari 2 malformation. This method yields an overall "consensus" shape for the data and eliminates the variable of size from analysis. Landmark variables can then be analyzed by several methods. When the number of landmarks is large, it is helpful to apply a statistical method, which will allow the reduction of complexity in the data. Principle components analysis has previously been used to reduce the dimensionality of morphometric data. (Indeed, the principle components of a distribution of shapes that satisfy particular criteria have a special name in the language of morphometrics—relative warps.) Once we analyzed the variability in our data, we found two major principal components that explain the differences in shape between the Chiari 2 group and the controls (Fig. 2). The other important finding from this analysis is that there is as much shape variation within the Chiari 2 group as there is between this group and unaffected controls.

A thin-plate spline generated from our data allows a graphic representation of group differences in shape, and helped us analyze patterns of malformation/deformation. The mathematics behind the generation of the thin-plate spline are complex, but may be conceptualized in the following way. Imagine placing the landmarks of one shape (the reference shape) on a very thin piece of sheet metal, and the landmarks of another different shape (the target shape) on another very thin piece of sheet metal. The thin-plate spline is a representation of the deformation or "bending" that the first shape would have to undergo to become the second shape. The effort one would need to expend to bend the first shape to the second shape is known as the bending energy. In our approach, the reference shape is taken to be the consensus shape for controls, and the shape defined by the sets of Chiari 2 landmarks is the target shape. It is possible to derive functions of the reference shape known as principal warps, which will provide the vectors by which one can multiply the reference shape to achieve the target shape. When the coefficients provided by these functions are multiplied by the difference between the Procrustes coordinates (which have already been scaled and rotated as mentioned above), representations of the deformation which needs to be applied to bring the reference to the target will result, and each of these is called a partial warp. Applying these partial warps to a grid drawn around the reference image produces the grid deformations shown in Figures 3A and 4A,B.

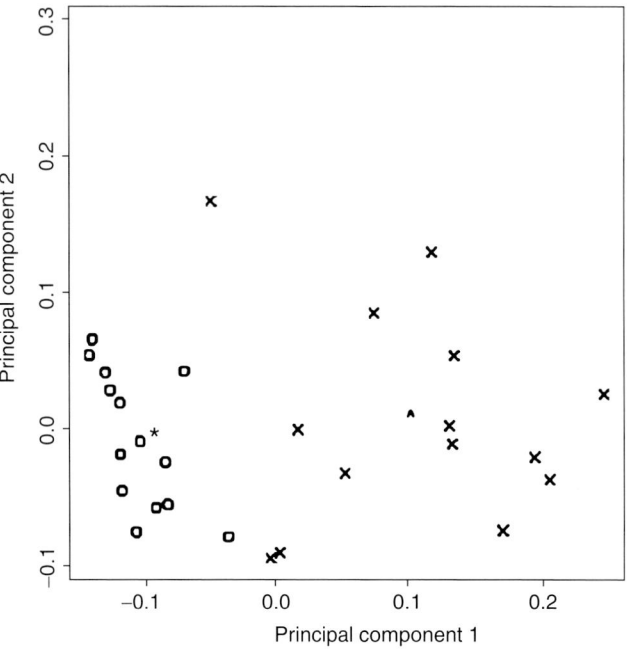

Figure 2. Principal component (relative warp) plot of Chiari 2 cases (x) and unaffected controls (o). Principal components are optimally-powerful explanatory factors of shape variability. The approximate position of the centroid of the Chiari 2 group is marked with a caret (^); that of the control group is marked with an asterisk (*).

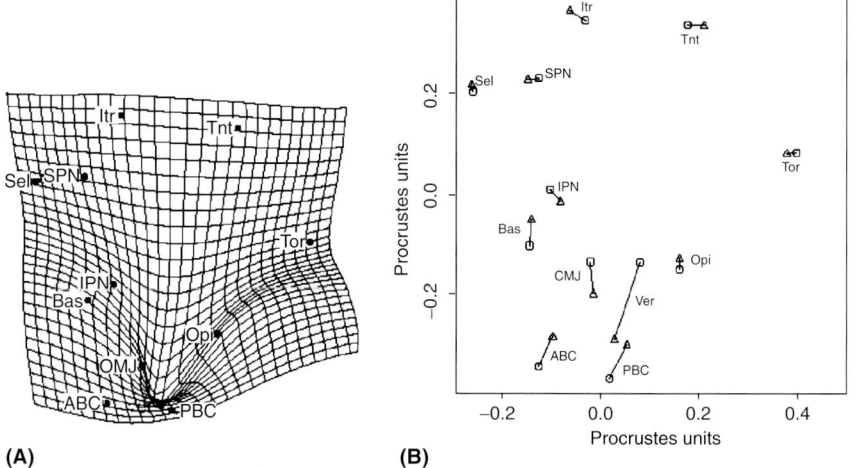

(A)   **(B)**

Figure 3. (**A**) Thin-plate spline generated from mean differences in shape coordinates between Chiari 2 patients and unaffected controls. Note the deformity of the grid centered on point Ver. (**B**) Crease plot demonstrating group means with reference to Procrustes coordinates. Chiari 2 patients are represented by triangles, controls by circles. The direction of greatest shape difference is largely vertical. *Abbreviations*: ABC, Anterior border of cervicospinal canal at the level of the C2 vertebrae; Bas, Basion; CMJ, Cervicomedullary junction; IPN, Inferior pontine notch; Itr, Iter (most rostral portion of sylvian aqueduct); Opi, Opisthion; PBC, Posterior border of cervicospinal canal at the level of the C2 vertebrae; Sel, Top of dorsum sellae; SPN, Superior pontine notch; Tor, Torcula; Tnt, Top of tentorium cerebelli; Ver, Caudalmost extent of midline cerebellar tissue (vermis ± tonsils).

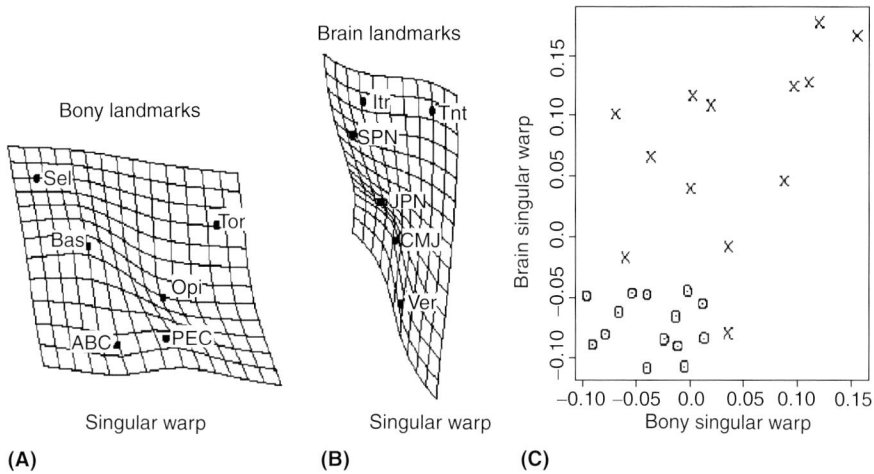

Figure 4. (**A**) is a deformation pattern on the six analyzed bony landmarks: Anterior border of the cervicospinal canal at the C2 vertebrae (ABC), Basion (Bas), opisthion (Opi), posterior border of the cervicospinal canal at the C2 vertebrae (PBC), top of dorsum sellae (Sel), and torcula (Tor, as a proxy for the internal occipital protuberance/internal inion, which can be difficult to visualize by MRI). Note the deformation at Opisthion. (**B**) is a deformation pattern on the six analyzed brain landmarks: Cervicomedullary junction (CMJ), inferior pontine notch (IPN), Iter (rostral portion of sylvian aqueduct), superior pontine notch (SPN), top of tentorium cerebelli (Tnt), and caudalmost extent of midline cerebellar tissue (vermis ± tonsils) (Ver). Note the deformation at landmark Ver. (**C**) is a scatterplot of the degree of brain rearrangement vs. the degree of bony rearrangement; the correlation is $r = 0.644$, significant at the 5% level. Each x represents a single Chiari 2 patient; each circle represents a single unaffected control.

Deformities in the grid allow a clear identification of group differences. The thin-plate spline in Figure 3A, which was generated from the mean differences between the Chiari 2 and control groups on the sets of coordinates, suggests that as expected, the vermian landmark is the point of greatest brain rearrangement. Less expected is the finding that the opisthion is the landmark where there is the greatest degree of bony rearrangement. Crease plots allow a depiction of group differences and their magnitude and direction. Figure 3B shows these group differences and a directionality that is roughly vertical. Degrees of warping can be statistically analyzed using scatterplots and by using the program Splus to do principle component plots (Fig. 2) and then partial least-squares analysis.

Further thin-plate spline analysis was done with all data and with the Chiari 2 data alone. Figures 4A,B and 5A,B show the thin-plate splines for bony and brain landmarks separately. These grids confirm the analysis of Figure 3, but the warp analyses allow an assessment of correlation between the principle components of brain and bone. As shown in Figure 5B, the correlation between the warps has an $r = 0.821$ with a p value of < 0.05. This confirms that posterior fossa shape change is also correlated with degree of vermian herniation. Figure 6 represents our analysis of the shape relationships between vermian herniation and brainstem herniation (as measured by the position of the cervicomedullary junction). Figure 6A shows the vertical vector component to be most important as expected. When the vertical Procrustes coordinates for the vermian and cervicomedullary landmarks are plotted it becomes clear that the shift in vermian landmark is largely independent of the shift of the CMJ landmark. This confirms our original analysis done with distances and areas.

The thin-plate spline analysis we accomplished with our data confirmed what we already knew about Chiari 2 malformation and added to our understanding of the tremendous variability present in individuals with the condition. It again points out

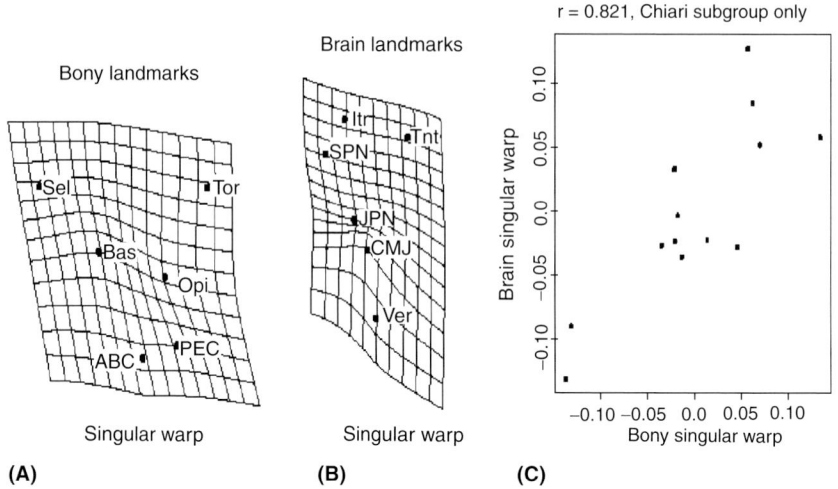

Figure 5. (**A**), (**B**), and (**C**) are similar to Fig. 4 (**A**), (**B**), and (**C**), respectively, except that Fig. 5 only considers Chiari 2 patients, not Chiari 2 patients and controls. Thus, in Fig. 5(**C**), each dot represents a single Chiari-2 patient. Abbreviations are the same as in Fig. 4. The correlation between the degree of brain rearrangement and the degree of bony rearrangement now increases to r = 0.821, which is statistically significant at the 5% level.

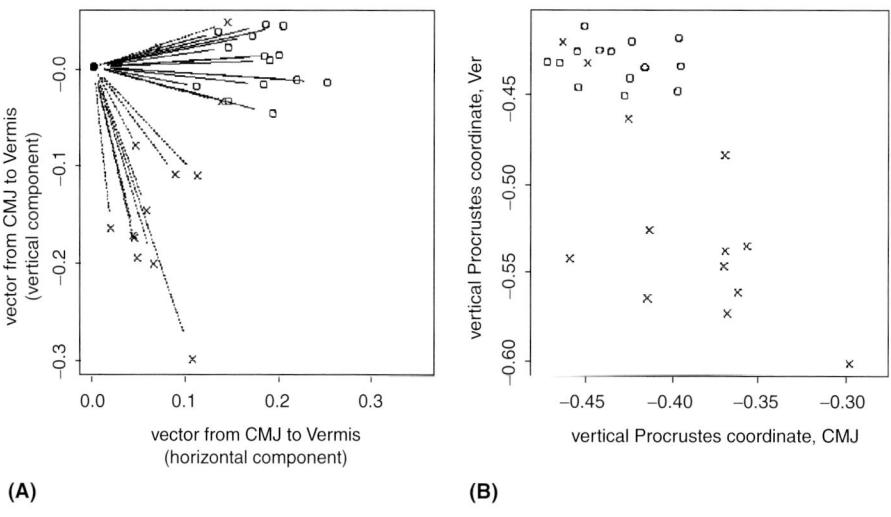

Figure 6. (**A**) is a plot showing the position of the vermian landmark vs. the position of the cervicomedullary junction landmark. Each Chiari 2 patient is represented by an x with a vector drawn with a dashed line; each control is represented by a circle with a vector drawn with a solid line. Note that the Chiari 2 cases are largely characterized by vectors running along the rostral-caudal axis. However, there are three Chiari 2 cases for which the vermian landmark is primarily horizontally displaced (that is, displaced along the antero-posterior axis) from the cervicome-dullary landmark; these cases more closely approach the morphological configuration of unaffected controls. (**B**) graphs the vertical Procrustes coordinate of the vermian landmark vs. the vertical Procrustes coordinate of the cervicomedullary landmark. The shift of the vermian landmark is largely independent of the shift of the cervicomedullary landmark; no correlation between vermian and cervicomedullary displacement can be seen, which is an observation consistent with the literature.

the interrelatedness between certain bony and neural abnormalities seen in the condition and the independence of other variables, thus reemphasizing the multi-factorial nature of the anatomic abnormalities seen in the condition, particularly differences in vermian herniation, brainstem herniation and combinations of the two. Our preliminary studies suggest age does not correlate well with any variable. We believe this points to a prenatal onset for most of the important aspects of the Chiari 2 malformation, a conclusion also made by a recent study of a 20-week fetus with MMC and Chiari 2 malformation using high-resolution MRI (37).

The work also confirms that with a little extra effort, much data and analysis can be accomplished from neuroimages obtained for clinical reasons in conditions where cases are limited in number. This approach, if used more systematically by several centers to test hypotheses about posterior fossa malformations, should quickly: (1) increase our understanding of these abnormalities, (2) aid in creating a better classification system for them and (3) hopefully improve outcomes through better management.

ACKNOWLEDGMENTS

We would like to thank Fred Bookstein for his help with data analysis. Eric Levey and Anthony Avellino provided helpful suggestions.

REFERENCES

1. Volpe JJ. 4th ed. Neurology of the Newborn. Philadelphia: W.B. Saunders Company, 2001.
2. Gray H. In: Williams PL, ed. Gray's Anatomy: The Anatomical Basis of Medicine and Surgery. 38th ed. New York: Churchill Livingstone 1995:1825–1861.
3. Griffiths PD, Wilkinson ID, Variend S, et al. Differential growth rates of the cerebellum and posterior fossa assessed by post mortem magnetic resonance imaging of the fetus: implications for the pathogenesis of the chiari 2 deformity. Acta Radiol 2004; 45:236–242.
4. Revel MP, Pons JC, Lelaidier C, et al. Magnetic resonance imaging of the fetus: a study of 20 cases performed without curarization. Prenat Diagn 1993; 13:775–799.
5. Chong BW, Babcook CJ, Pang D, Ellis W. A magnetic resonance template for normal cerebellar development in the human fetus. Neurosurgery 1997; 41:924–928; discussion 928-929.
6. Levine D, Barnes PD, Madsen JR, et al. Fetal fast MR imaging: reproducibility, technical quality, and conspicuity of anatomy. Radiology 1998; 206:549–554.
7. Nakayama T, Yamada R. MR imaging of the posterior fossa structures of human embryos and fetuses. Radiat Med 1999; 17:105–114.
8. Lan LM, Yamashita Y, Tang Y, et al. Normal fetal brain development: MR imaging with a half-Fourier rapid acquisition with relaxation enhancement sequence. Radiology 2000; 215:205–210.
9. Stazzone MM, Hubbard AM, Bilaniuk LT, et al. Ultrafast MR imaging of the normal posterior fossa in fetuses. AJR Am J Roentgenol 2000; 175:835–839.
10. Claude I, Daire JL, Sebag G. Fetal brain MRI: segmentation and biometric analysis of the posterior fossa. IEEE Trans Biomed Eng 2004; 51:617–626.
11. Tsai T, Bookstein FL, Levey E, Kinsman SL. Chiari-2 malformation: a biometric analysis. Eur J Pediatr Surg 2002; 12:S12–S18. 12 Suppl.
12. Peach B. The Arnold-Chiari Malformation; Morphogenesis. Arch Neurol 1965; 12:527–535.
13. Emery JL, MacKenzie N. Medullo-cervical dislocation deformity (Chiari 2 deformity) related to neurospinal dysraphism (meningomyelocele). Brain 1973; 96:155–162.
14. Naidich TP, McLone DG, Fulling KH. The Chiari 2 malformation: Part IV. The hindbrain deformity. Neuroradiology 1983; 25:179–197.
15. Roth M. Cranio-cervical growth collision: another explanation of the Arnold-Chiari malformation and of basilar impression. Neuroradiology 1986; 28:187–194.
16. McLone DG, Knepper PA. The cause of Chiari 2 malformation: a unified theory. Pediatr Neurosci 1989; 15:1–12.

17. McLone DG, Naidich TP. Developmental morphology of the subarachnoid space, brain vasculature, and contiguous structures, and the cause of the Chiari 2 malformation. AJNR Am J Neuroradiol 1992; 13:463–482.

18. Beuls E, Vanormelingen L, Van Aalst J, et al. The Arnold-Chiari type 2 malformation at midgestation. Pediatr Neurosurg 2003; 39:149–158.

19. McLone DG, Dias MS. The Chiari 2 malformation: cause and impact. Childs Nerv Syst 2003; 19:540–550.

20. Tubbs RS, Oakes WJ. Treatment and management of the Chiari 2 malformation: an evidence-based review of the literature. Childs Nerv Syst 2004; 20:375–381.

21. Wolpert SM, Scott RM, Platenberg C, Runge VM. The clinical significance of hindbrain herniation and deformity as shown on MR images of patients with Chiari 2 malformation. AJNR Am J Neuroradiol 1988; 9:1075–1078.

22. Gilbert JN, Jones KL, Rorke LB, et al. Central nervous system anomalies associated with meningomyelocele, hydrocephalus, and the Arnold-Chiari malformation: reappraisal of theories regarding the pathogenesis of posterior neural tube closure defects. Neurosurgery 1986; 18:559–564.

23. Tulipan N, Hernanz-Schulman M, Bruner JP. Reduced hindbrain herniation after intrauterine myelomeningocele repair: a report of four cases. Pediatr Neurosurg 1998; 29:274–278.

24. Tulipan N, Hernanz-Schulman M, Lowe LH, Bruner JP. Intrauterine myelomeningocele repair reverses preexisting hindbrain herniation. Pediatr Neurosurg 1999; 31:137–142.

25. Sutton LN, Adzick NS, Bilaniuk LT, et al. Improvement in hindbrain herniation demonstrated by serial fetal magnetic resonance imaging following fetal surgery for myelomeningocele. JAMA 1999; 282:1826–1831.

26. ClinicalTrials.gov, Management of Myelomeningocele Study.

27. Nishikawa M, Sakamoto H, Hukuba A, et al. Pathogenesis of Chiari malformation: a morphometric study of the posterior cranial fossa. J Neurosurg 1997; 86:40–47.

28. Christophe C, Dan B. Magnetic resonance imaging cranial and cerebral dimensions: is there a relationship with Chiari I malformation? A preliminary report in children. Eur J Paediatr Neurol 1999; 3:15–23.

29. DiMario FJ, Jr., Ramsby GR, Burleson JA. Brain morphometric analysis in neurofibromatosis 1. Arch Neurol 1999; 56:1343–1346.

30. Roth M. Reciprocity of the neural growth in the Arnold-Chiari malformation. Acta Radiol Suppl 1986; 369:260–261.

31. Bookstein FL. Linear methods for nonlinear maps: Procrustes fits, thin-plate splines, and the biometric analysis of shape variability. In: Toga A, ed. Brain Warping. New York: Academic Press, 1999:157–181.

32. Bookstein FL. Creases as local features of deformation grids. Med Image Anal 2000; 4:93–110.

33. Nestor PG, O'Donnell BF, McCarley RW, et al. A new statistical method for testing hypotheses of neuropsychological/MRI relationships in schizophrenia: partial least squares analysis. Schizophr Res 2002; 53:57–66.

34. Bookstein FL, Sampson PD, Streissguth AP, et al. Geometric morphometrics of corpus callosum and subcortical structures in the fetal-alcohol-affected brain. Teratology 2001; 64:4–32.

35. Bookstein FL, Sampson PD, Connor PD, et al. Midline corpus callosum is a neuroanatomical focus of fetal alcohol damage. Anat Rec 2002; 269:162–174.

36. Bookstein FL, Streissguth AP, Sampson PD, et al. Corpus callosum shape and neuropsychological deficits in adult males with heavy fetal alcohol exposure. Neuroimage 2002; 15:233–251.

37. Beuls EA, Vanormelingen L, Van Aalst J, et al. In vitro high-field magnetic resonance imaging-documented anatomy of a fetal myelomeningocele at 20 weeks' gestation. A contribution to the rationale of intrauterine surgical repair of spina bifida. J Neurosurg 2003; 98:210–214.

1.5

Imaging Developmental Brain Abnormalities in Children

Dan Connolly
Sheffield Children's Hospital, Royal Hallamshire Hospital, Sheffield, U.K.

Magnetic resonance imaging (MRI) is essential in assessment and identification of congenital brain malformations due to its capacity to produce detailed multi-planar imaging. A detailed understanding of normal brain development is essential in order to correctly identify and describe congenital brain abnormalities. Increasingly, congenital brain malformations are being identified in association with genetic abnormalities. MRI will therefore become increasingly important in providing information on the specific brain phenotypes with a view to later genetic counseling. While MRI has largely overtaken computed tomography (CT) in the assessment of congenital brain malformations in many centers, this remains an important first line investigation of the pediatric brain and continues to have important use particularly in the identification of intracranial calcification. CT also has the advantage, particularly with modern multi-slice scans, that imaging of the complete brain can be achieved in very short times. These very short times (a matter of a mere few seconds) can negate the requirement for sedation or anesthetic for scanning plus all the other considerations involved in monitoring and protecting a child in an MRI scanner. Multidetector CT also allows volume acquisitions of the brain to be obtained, thereby allowing mutliplanar reconstructions, thus reducing one of CT's main disadvantages when compared to MRI. Many of the new techniques evolving in MRI imaging of the pediatric brain attempt to reduce the problem of patient motion artefact. This includes the use of alternative k space acquisition, rapid scanner position techniques, and echo planar techniques. One must also consider the different chemical composition of developing brain from the fetus through the neonatal period from the first two years of life to the mature brain of the young child at 2–3 years of age. This alteration in composition of the brain requires alteration in the imaging parameters. In addition, alteration in scan parameters and techniques for improving diagnostic MRI scan quality are required depending on the degree of sedation of the patient. As the child matures we also have to consider whether the child is imaged in an MRI scanner designed for an adult in which coils are adapted and used to obtain best quality imaging or whether they may use an MRI-compatible incubator in order to provide better quality images. Ultrasound examination of the neonatal brain is discussed elsewhere in this text. However as the pediatric skull ossifies and the fontanelles close, ultrasound becomes less and less important in the assessment of these patients.

BRAIN MATURATION

The brain continues to undergo complex changes in appearance for the first two to three years of life after birth. Though these changes are not of the magnitude of the early in utero events they nevertheless are vitally important for the normal neurological and intellectual development of the child. The changes also are important for the radiologist to appreciate during the maturation of the brain to adapt the adult imaging appearances on both CT and MRI.

The brain increases in overall volume, though this by itself does not significantly affect interpretation of a brain scan if the brain is of normal size for age. At our center we routinely assess head circumference with reference centile charts before interpreting the scan.

The sulcation pattern alters, becoming more complex with age. Lack of progression of sulcation would suggest a congenital cortical abnormality or generalized brain insult.

The most important change affecting the brain in the first years of life and which can also be the most difficult to assess is the stage of myelination of the brain. As a rule of thumb, myelination progresses from the inferior part of the brain to the superior aspect, from central to peripheral white matter, and from posterior to anterior white matter (1–3). That is obviously a gross simplification of the process, but to illuminate further would merely invite replication of a current standard reference text.

When one attempts to define the stage of maturation of the pediatric brain one should have knowledge of the expected date of delivery of the child, the actual date of delivery of the child, the perinatal and pregnancy histories, the head circumference and an atlas of reference images for a normal child of that age having an MRI scan upon that scanner. In my experience, this constellation of happy coincidences rarely if ever happens, though radiologist experience and expertise can overcome many of these deficiencies.

THE STILL CHILD

A child must lie still for an MRI scan in an MRI scanner for some time. In older children they may achieve this with distraction and bribery. For children less than 5 or 6 years of age this becomes unfeasible. The scan length can be reduced or the child can be made to lie still by sedation or general anesthetic. In very small children the sedation may just be a post prandial sleep after a feed. Nevertheless, as the child is far from the parent/nurse/caregiver/radiographer within the scanner bore monitoring of vital signs is essential.

Monitoring of a sedated infant during an MRI scan is mandatory. MRI-compatible monitoring equipment normally allows monitoring of heart rate, respiratory rate, blood pressure and PaO_2. Any MRI scanner which is bought or installed with a view to conducting MRI upon sedated or anesthetised patients should have MRI compatible monitoring equipment as recommended by the manufacturers installed at the same time as the MRI scanner. Attempting to install this equipment at a later date after installing the magnet may be very disruptive. Following recovery from sedation or anesthetic the child may be discharged at the discretion of the supervising pediatrician/anesthetist if the child is an outpatient.

SEDATION

Adequate sedation is the most important factor in obtaining high quality MR images in children. All patients and accompanying persons entering the MRI scanner must be screened for contra-indications to MRI prior to the start of sedation. With modern multislice CT scanners due to the very short scan time, sedation is rarely required as small children can be restrained within the CT scanner long enough to obtain the CT imaging and older children can normally stay still for the few seconds required.

Many different drugs have been used for sedation of children. It is not possible in this text to fully describe the pros and cons of many of these different drugs. Any drugs used for sedation and the levels of appropriate monitoring should be discussed and approved in conjunction with local anesthetic and pediatric teams together with the degree of supervision required for this sedation. Suitable post-scanning monitoring and recovery must also be considered and agreed at a local level. Children who are to undergo sedation need to be given nothing by mouth for an agreed period of time before sedation is given. Sedation may be given orally, rectally, intravenously or by the intramuscular routes.

For children over 2 months of age, once the sedative drug has been administered the child should be moved to a quiet room but kept awake until entering the MRI scanner when the child should be reassured and allowed hopefully to start sleeping prior to the scan commencing. One important group who can often be scanned without drug administration are small infant's (less than 2 months old) who can often be scanned in a natural sleep period after a large feed. It is often helpful in these children to keep them relatively hungry just prior to the expected scan time so that they are more likely to take a large amount and sleep well during the scan.

GENERAL ANESTHETIC

In our institution children above 6 months of age and up to 5 years are routinely given general anesthetic. Although some of this patient group would have tolerated MRI scanning without sedation, it has been agreed in our institution that this would require anesthetic team supervision. There is no patient motion artifact in those who have general anesthetic. A significant proportion of sedated patients would have failed to obtain sufficient quality imaging with their sedation or would have required repeat attempts with general anaesthetic though the success of sedation is very dependent upon the nursing and general team support (4). If the scan is supervized by a pediatric neuroradiologist the chances of the patient requiring to return for repeat imaging are significantly reduced. The need to repeat a general anesthetic should be avoided and all lists should therefore be directly supervized by the reporting pediatric neuroradiologist.

ENTERTAINING THE OLDER CHILD

This is vital to keep them still and engaged long enough for a thorough evaluation to take place. Allowing them to bring their own music may be helpful but we find that a screen for DVDs of favorite movies or cartoons keeps them focussed and reduces motion artifact.

PREMATURE INFANT

Premature infants present further problems as they may require intensive care and ventilation prior to consideration of MRI scanning. Their very small size presents specific problems with coil selection and they also have very specific and significant problems with thermo regulation. Generally these premature infants are often initially imaged with ultrasound on the neonatal intensive care unit. Trans-fontanelle ultrasonography as will be discussed in later chapters is excellent for the examination of the deep areas of the brain and the localization of significant CNS pathology in the premature infant. If MRI scanning is required then consideration for maintaining the infant's body temperature must be taken including the use of heat-maintaining blankets, gloves, hats, and socks, and various other methods of maintaining the child's temperature.

CONTRAST AGENT

For the assessment of congenital cerebral malformation contrast is not routinely administered on either CT or MRI. In CT except for a congenital vascular malformation the use of iodinated contrast material is rare. Fortunately the pediatric population have very few reactions to contrast media (5).

Paramagnetic MRI contrast agents are used in the pediatric population for assessment of infection, tumors, and so forth. New research points to the use of contrast agents for perfusion imaging as being helpful. The standard dose is 0.1 mmol. per kg. Again, adverse reactions to MRI contrast agents are extremely rare particularly in the pediatric population. Some low grade tumors may be difficult to distinguish from cortical malformations and contrast may than be administered to try to assist in differentiation between the two pathologies.

CT Scanning

Standard axial planes parallel to the canthomeatal line are obtained. Thin 3 mm sections through the posterior fossa and 5 mm sections through the middle and anterior cranial fossae to the vertex are normally obtained. In younger children (under 2 years of age) some centers obtain 3 mm axials of the whole brain. New scanners allow multi-planar reconstruction of these images if required. The high water content of the neonatal brain means that slightly altered window levels can be used with a window level of 20 and a window width of 60 Hounsefield units. The optimal window levels and width change through the first three years of life until the child brain has fully matured and the normal adult window level and width can be used. Thinner sections can be obtained for assessment of cranio-synostosis and cranio-facial anomalies with 3D reconstructions if required (6). Alternatively, more limited studies can be obtained when simple clinical questions are asked, e.g., is there evidence of shunt malfunction or hydrocephalus?

MRI

Technical considerations include the following.

Coils

An improvement in the signal-to-nois ratio of an MR image is greatly assisted by using the closest-fitting surface receiver coil. This will of course vary as the child develops. Increasingly, manufacturers are producing specifically created pre-term and neonatal coils perhaps incorporated into MRI-compatible incubators (19). Alternatively, people have used coils created for other parts of the adult body which can be adapted to more closely fit the neonate such as an adult knee coil. Head coils with smaller internal diameters down to 24 cm can also be acquired from major manufacturers. Many units which routinely image neonates and other small children have often produced "home-made" coils through their MRI physics departments (7,20).

Sequence Choice and Imaging Protocol

Standard sequences of the adult brain are not appropriate in children less than 2 years old due to the increase in water content of the infant's brain compared to that of the adult. As myelination progresses during those first 2 years of life the appearance of the pediatric brain alters and becomes more like that of the adult brain as does the brain's constitution. This means that after 3 years of age more standard adult sequences can then be used. Short TR, short TE T1-weighted imaging is often more reliable and informative in this first 2 years than T2 imaging. Gradient echo T2 imaging is useful for assessment of susceptibility from previous hemorrhage or calcification. Diffusion weighted imaging is a particularly short sequence (often only taking in the region of 20–30 sec in the adult brain) which is extremely useful in assessing for regions of acute infarction. Proton density (long TR, short TE) and FLAIR sequences may be used but are not particularly useful in assessment of cerebral malformation. Proton density sequences in under 2 year olds normally have longer TR and TEs than in adults and older children in order to improve tissue contrast. Their main use is in assessment of cerebral surface collections and hematomas, particularly in the area of non-accidental head injury.

Vascular Imaging

For vascular imaging MRI angiography and MRI venography can be performed. It is important to know that the rate of flow particularly in the venous sinus is altered in the neonatal and early years of life and alterations in selected flow rate must be made in order to obtain good quality angiographic data if phase contrast angiography is used. Dynamic contrast enhanced subtracted MRI angiography is also a particularly useful sequence, restricted only by the small volume of contrast that can be administered to the pediatric age group (point 0.1 mmols per kg/check) (Griffiths and Chooi). Dynamic angiography has been validated in the pediatric age group and overcomes the problem of altered flow rate which may be very difficult to select particularly in the presence of vascular malformations. In order to overcome the altered water content of neonatal brain, the echo times, repetition times, and inversion times have to be increased in order to produce diagnostic quality images.

Of particular importance are fast imaging sequences which can be used in the sedated neonate. These include express, RF fast, and turbo prop type sequences, all of which seek to reduce scan times or to overcome patient movement (confirmed intravenous Gadolinium at 0.1 mmol per kg, Gadopentate Dimeglomene) (7–9).

CT Angiography

CT angiography and venography are increasingly being used in centers with multi-detector CT capability. They have the advantage of being potentially rapidly acquired in a scanner, which is much less likely to induce problems with claustrophobia. The disadvantage will of course be that there is radiation dose and iodinated contrast media dose. But with markedly reduced renal toxicity and reduced adverse reactions to iodinated contrast media, the obviation of the need for sedation makes CT angiography extremely attractive (10,11).

MRI Angiography

MRI angiography and venography have the advantage of a lack of iodinated contrast media and radiation dose to the neonatal or pediatric brain. MRI angiography time of flight studies such as MOTSA or SLINKY can produce exquisite angiographic images. When considering MRI venography, phased contrast rather than time of flight venography sequences may also be considered. Again the quality of imaging produced may be extremely high; 2D rather the 3D time of flight imaging is particularly useful in assessing for anomalies of the cervical carotid and vertebral arteries. They also have the advantage over 3D time of flight imaging in being less likely to be complicated by patient motion artifact. Overall however, contrast enhanced digitally subtracted MRI angiography is probably the most sensitive sequence for assessing the intracranial vasculature. It produces the highest quality images when looking at the cervical carotid and vertebral arteries and also allows flow assessment through vascular anomalies of the cranium. As the study is dynamic, there is capacity to assess flow through vascular anomalies or a lack of flow through other vascular anomalies such as cavernomas, thereby obviating the need for formal catheter angiography.

Our center has a large stereotactic radiosurgery practice for arterio-venous malformations including those in the pediatric population and we now routinely include contrast enhanced digitally subtracted MRI angiography as part of the pre-operative assessment and post procedural follow up of these patients in order to reduce the number of formal catheter angiograms required for pre-treatment and follow-up assessment of arterio-venous malformations. Later images in the contrast enhanced study also allow assessment of the intracranial venous system (12).

Routine MRI Sequences

Spine

Although in the neonate ultrasound may be used to assess for most spinal cord anomalies, as the child matures and the posterior elements ossify ultrasound becomes increasingly difficult. Ultrasound may also struggle to identify more subtle anomalies such as a fatty filum (13,21). Imaging of the spine will also become mandatory in conjunction with imaging of the brain if there is evidence of abnormality at the foramen magnum as may be demonstrated with some bony dysplasias such as achondrodysplasia, or there is a hind brain anomaly such as a Chiari 1 or 2 malformation.

Our center is a large tertiary referral MRI center for spine dysraphism surgery throughout the United Kingdom with a large scoliosis surgery service. Many children with a spine dysraphism may also have a scoliosis and scoliosis presents serious challenges to the imaging technician/radiographer and the radiologist attempting to interpret the images. We routinely obtain a coronal T2 sequence starting above the level of the initial spine curvature (Philips infinion 1.5 Tesla, Best, The Netherlands; TE 108, TR 4047, flip 90; slice thickness/gap 3.0/1.0, FOV 42, phase matrix 384, read matrix 512). This allows good assessment of the level of the conus, assessment for a split cord, assessment of the renal positions and configuration, and assessment of the vertebral bodies when looking for the failures of vertebral formation or segmentation. The coronal sequence will also allow good planning for oblique axial and sagittal images if significant scoliosis is present. If a split cord is identified then axial gradient echo T2 images should be obtained through this region to look for a bony spur/fibrous septum (alternatively CT or plain film myelography could be performed). We also obtain sagittal T1 and T2 images of the entire cord to include the entire posterior fossa and foramen magnum extending down to include the entirety of the sacrum (T1 sequence; TE 10.8, TR 483, flip 90, 3.0/1.0, fov 42, 256/512. T2 sequence; TE 108, TR 4138, flip 90, 3.0/1.0, FOV 42, 384/512). This allows full assessment for possible abnormalities including caudal regression. We also perform axial gradient echo T2 images through the level of the conus and extending for one vertebral body level below this level to assess for subtle susceptibility artifact, which may be the only clear demonstration of a small lipoma of the filum terminale (TE 14.0, TR 558, flip 35, 3.0/0.5, FOV 20, 200/256, 14 slices with 2 × sampling). A subtle lipoma may not be demonstrated on any of the other imaging sequences. We also perform wide block axial T1 spin echo images of the lower thoracic, lumbar, and sacral spine extending from T9 to S4 (TE 16.0, TR665, flip 90, 7.0/5.0, FOV 20. 192/256, 26 slices). This provides further useful information including clear assessment of the level of the conus, assessment of the posterior elements of the lumbar spine, and the presence of any possible fatty inclusion such as a lipoma, lipomyelomeningocele or dermoid. With this exhaustive set of images of the spine, subtle dysraphism is unlikely to be missed.

Brain

When starting to protocol a scan for a possible cerebral malformation, the scan protocol may of course be tailored and reduced if good clinical information is supplied. However, in reality, although the clinician may suggest that pathology may be suspected in a specific part of the cortex, for instance, extensive review of the entire brain is mandatory. Imaging in all three planes is also extremely useful and should routinely be included in the protocol. An FSE thin slice T2 of the entire cranium is our initial imaging sequence (TE 15/75, TR 8040, flip 90, FOV 23, 256/256, 60 slices). We also include a standard spin echo axial T1 (TE 16, TR 512, 4.0/2.0, FOV 20, 256/256) and sagittal T1 (TE 14, TR 493, 4.0/2.0, FOV 23, 256/256) of the brain together with a standard coronal T2 fast spin echo sequence (TE 100, TR 3000, 5.0/1.0, FOV 24, 352/512).

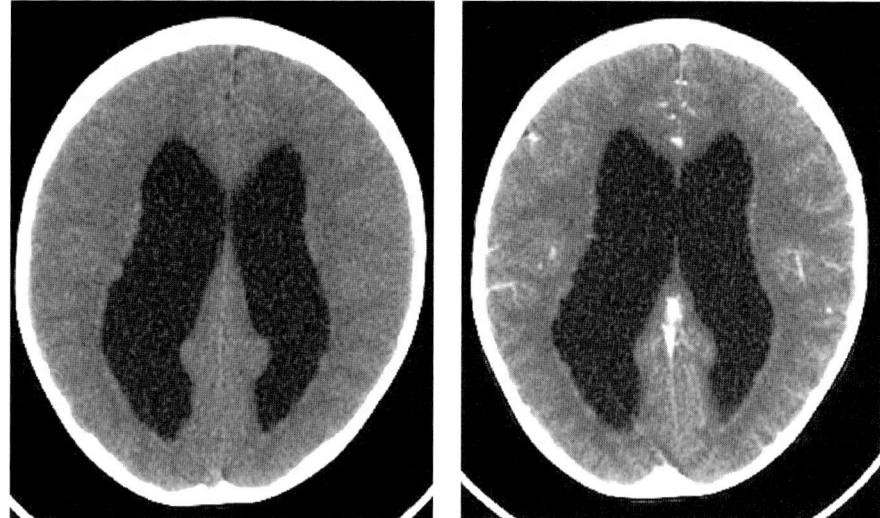

Figure 1. CT un-enhanced and enhanced demonstrating multi-focal sub-ependymal nodular heterotopia. This appearance is associated with a familial inheritance secondary to mutations of chromosome Xq28.

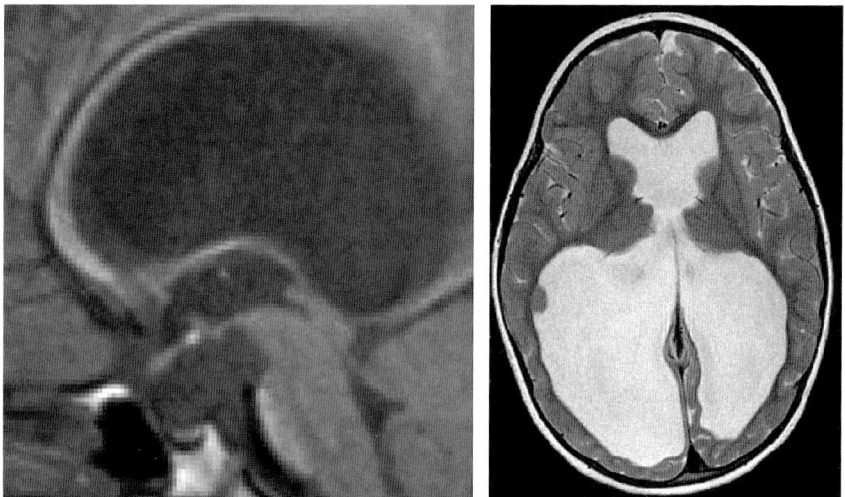

Figure 2. Sagittal SE T1 and axial FSE T2 images of a patient with nodular heterotopia, absent septum pellucidum and an ectopic posterior pituitary.

Standard imaging sequence however may not provide sufficient detail when one begins to assess for subtle focal areas of pachygyria or more likely polymicrogyria. Therefore, a volume T1 acquisition of the head (routinely we obtain the volume in the sagittal plane, therefore allowing a small overall volume to be acquired reducing scan times and secondarily improving image quality (TE 4.47, TR15, flip 25, 0.8/0.0, FOV 20.5, 256/256). Initially we produce coronal images though axial sagittal images may of course also be produced from the volume. We also routinely produce MPR reformat images in a curved plane parallel to the cortex particularly involving the frontal and peri Sylvian gray matter, though these reformats can be of any part of the cortex if there is radiological or clinical suspicion. Our imaging is routinely done on a 1.5 Tesla,

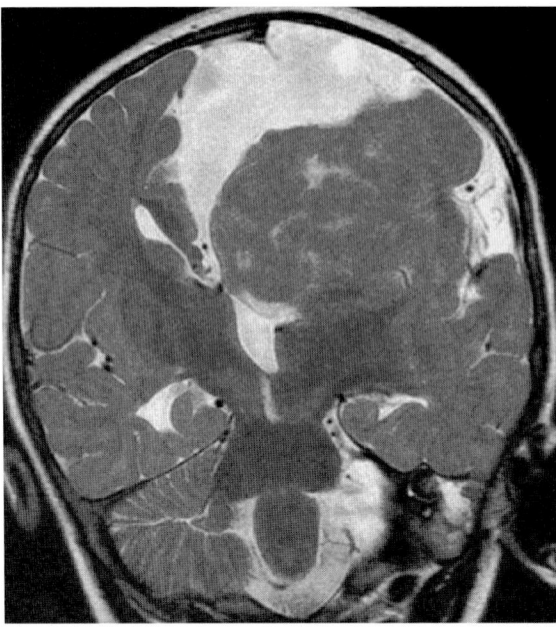

Figure 3. Coronal FSE T2 demonstrating agenesis of the corpus callosum and dysgenesis of the left cerebral hemisphere.

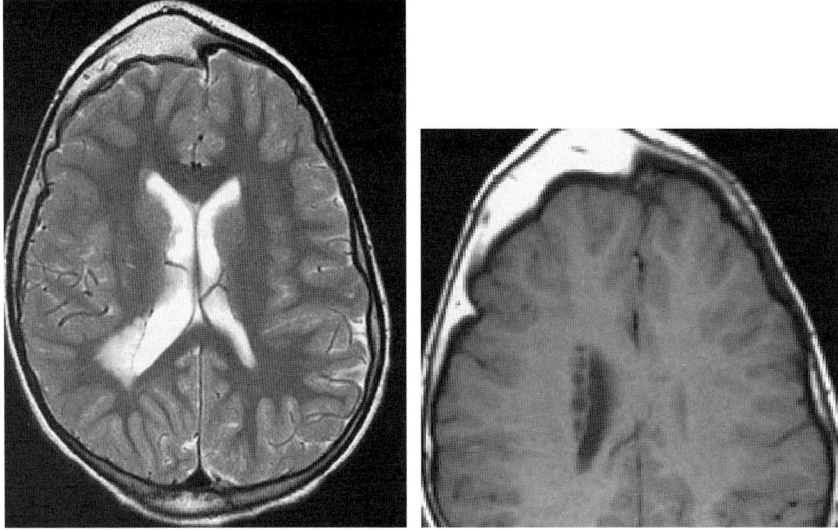

Figure 4. Axial FSE T2 and axial SE T1 of a patient with proteus syndrome demonstrating hemimegalencephaly with heterotopia, periventricular white matter astrogliosis, and a large subcutaneous lipoma.

Philips Infinion scanner (Best, The Netherlands). We do not routinely use inversion recovery sequences in the pediatric population despite their excellent T1 weighting and excellent depiction of the gray/white matter interface. We do acquire a DTI sequence (TE 60, TR 1400, 7.0/0.0, FOV 24, ETL 108, 108/108). FLAIR imaging is not part of our routine imaging of patients with potential cortical dysplasia or developmental anomaly. Although they are useful in older children to look for white matter signal abnormality, in our experience in the younger population they are of limited utility and rarely produce information which is not clearly demonstrable on a T2 sequence. Similarly proton density imaging, although very useful in the adult and

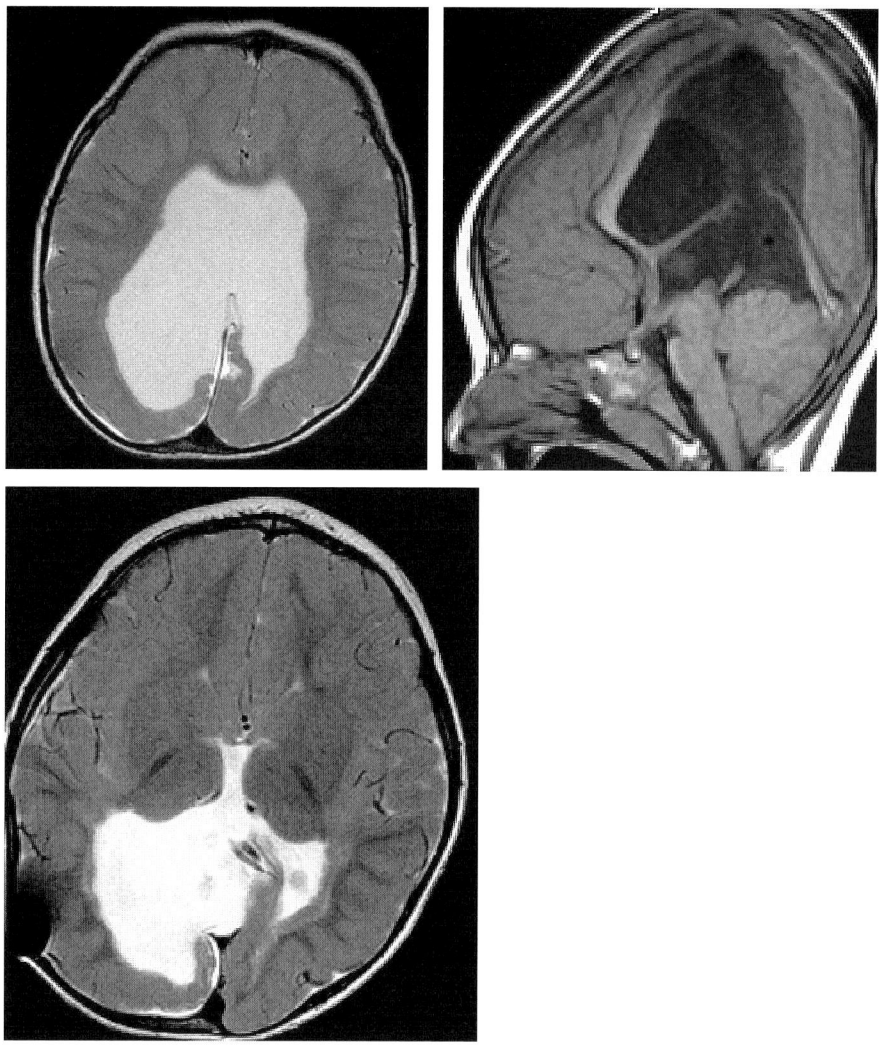

Figure 5. Axial FSE T2 and sagittal SE T1 images of a child with dysgensis of the corpus callosum, nodular heterotopia, and bilateral polymicrogyria.

mature adolescent brain, is of limited use in the area of imaging of developmental abnormalities. Again, proton density is useful in the pediatric population, specifically when looking for subdural hematomas in the area of possible non-accidental injury. Sagittal images are particularly useful when evaluating the pituitary region, foramen magnum, and vermis. Although in an older child they are also useful for looking at the corpus callosum, in a younger infant the corpus callosum is often poorly formed and thin due to the lack of myelinated white fiber tracts and can be falsely misleading. Coronal imaging is probably the best imaging plane for assessment of the corpus callosum, septum pellucidum, and optic chiasm. Coronal imaging is also particularly useful when looking for schizencephaly, holoprosencephaly, and periventricular leucomalacia. Gradient echo T2 star imaging is particularly useful when assessing for vascular abnormalities such as arterio-venous malformations, trauma, and calcification. Calcification may be subependymal in the case of tuberous sclerosis or cortical when associated with several cortical malformations. If gradient echo T2 imaging is negative when assessing for possible calcification, particularly in the case of tuberous sclerosis, we would then routinely do fine 1 mm CT axial sections through the lateral ventricles to assess for subtle subependymal calcification.

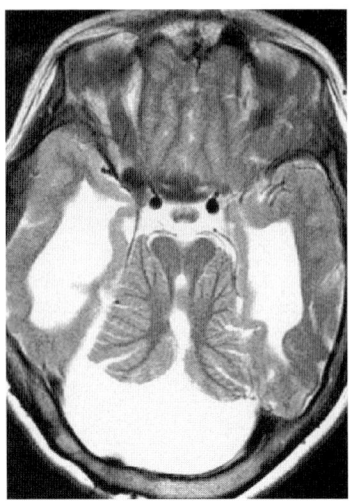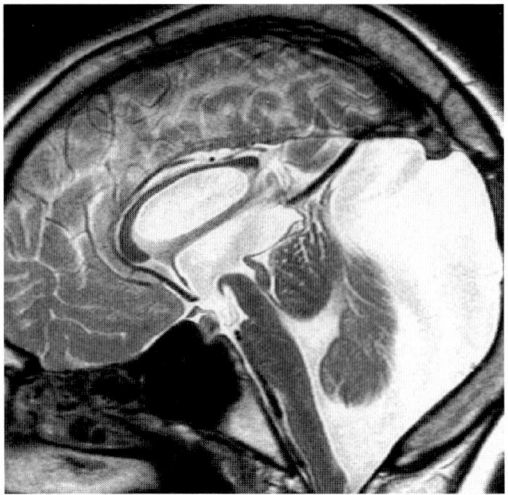

Figure 6. Axial and sagittal FSE T2 images of a child with hydrocephalus, vermian hypoplasia, and an enlarged posterior fossa in keeping with a Dandy–Walker malformation.

Fast Imaging Sequences of the Brain

Various rapid imaging sequences are increasingly used in the non-sedated or sedated pediatric population and these include; axial T1 RF fast (TE 3.35, TR 236, flip 70, 4.0/1.0, FOV 25, 192/256), axial T2 express (TE 75, TR 20 000, 7.0/0.0, FOV 25, 248/256) and Turbo prop sequences. We use the express and RF fast sequences in regular practice. Most of these techniques are based on single shot echo planar imaging. We now use this routinely in assessment of the fetus for in-utero malformations and in assessment of mobile neonates as discussed elsewhere in this book.

MRI Spectroscopy

This is of limited utility in assessment of the pediatric brain for developmental anomalies and spectroscopy is often within the normal range. However, it may aid differentiation from low grade cortical lesions in cases of suspected focal cortical malformation. The abnormality of the spectra, however, may be very limited compared to that which one might expect with a cortical malformation and therefore the utility again may be very limited. MRI spectroscopy may also be used to assess brain maturation of white matter and assessment of underlying leucodystrophies. Elevation of the lactate peak is particularly indicative of an underlying metabolic abnormality.

MRI Perfusion Imaging, Magnetization Transfer, and Diffusion Imaging

Perfusion imaging is useful in assessment of patients with vascular congenital brain malformations such as Sturge Weber where areas of relative hypo perfusion may be demonstrated, particularly in the region of the associated developmental venous anomalies seen in conjunction with the larger leptomeningeal vascular malformations. Perfusion imaging is also increasingly being used in the assessment of cortical malformations (14).

Diffusion imaging is increasingly used in the pediatric population and is particularly useful of course in stroke, trauma, and differentiation of tumor and abscess (22). Diffusion imaging may be very useful in the assessment of vascular congenital malformation and

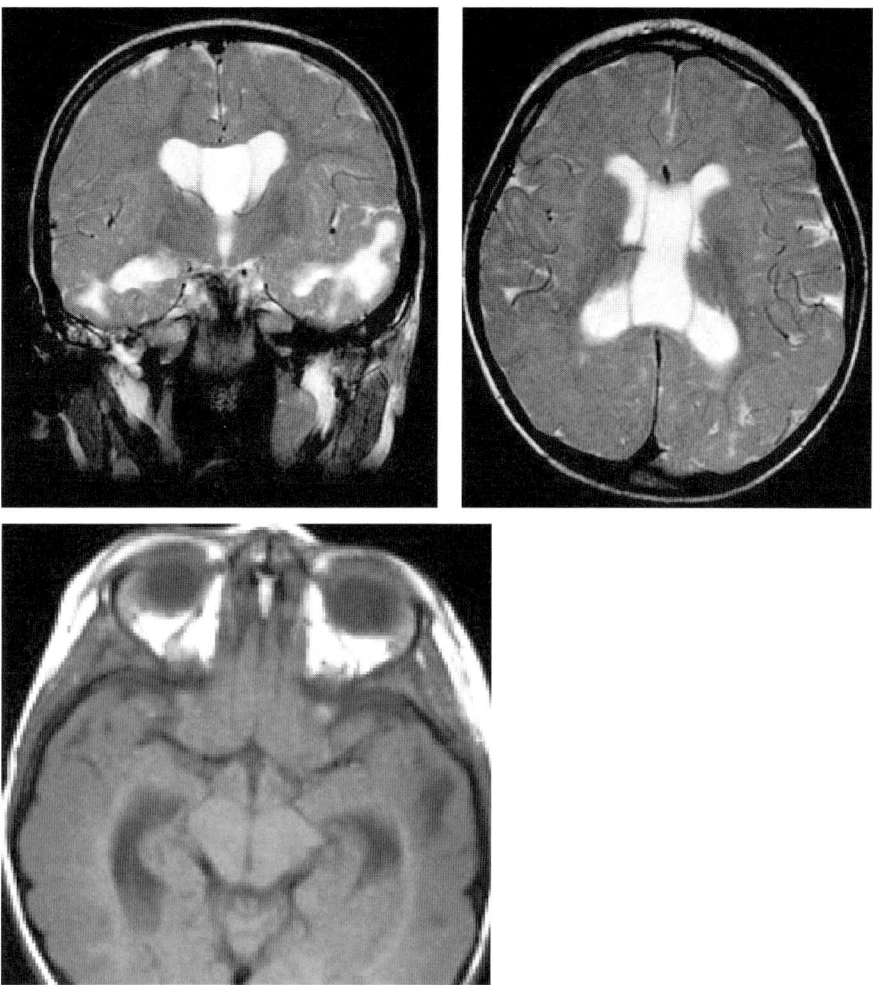

Figure 7. Axial and coronal FSE T2 images and axial SE T1 image of a 4 year old with bilateral pachygyria.

their impact on the brain. With more subtle small volume cortical abnormality, the utility of diffusion weighted imaging is less clearly demonstrated (7,15,16). Diffusion tensor imaging and brain maturation have started to be used to investigate the maturing child's brain and some investigators are already demonstrating an association between child development and evidence of white matter maturation on tensor imaging (17).

Magnetization transfer in different regions of the brain may reflect the state of myelination, but its use in assessment of congenital anomalies other than those related to vascular anomalies is largely still to be fully assessed (18).

Cerebrospinal Fluid Flow Imaging

Phased contrast studies such as used for MRI venography can be adapted to allow CSF flow studies to be performed. They are particularly useful when assessing for interuptions of normal flow pattern or for novel flow patterns. They are particularly useful in hind brain anomalies such as Chiari 1 and 2 malformation when people are being considered for foramen magnum decompressions; if only qualitative information rather than quantity of information is required about CSF flow, then other flow sensitive

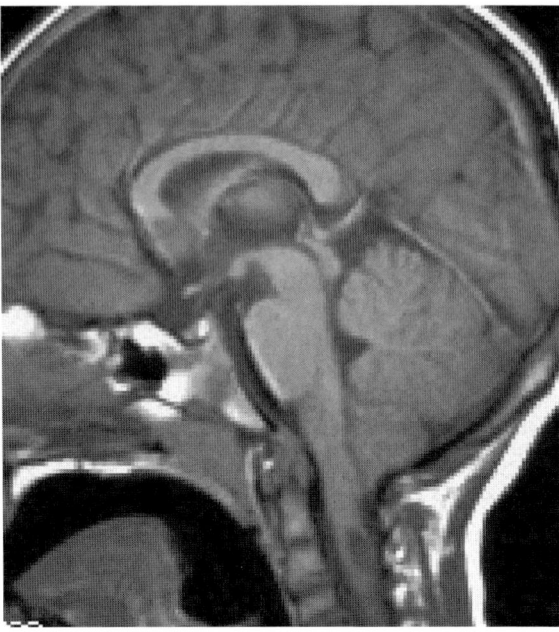

Figure 8. Sagittal T1 image showing a Chiari 1 malformation and small upper cervical cord syrinx.

sequences can be used such as steady state free procession sequences using 3D FT. Fast spin echo and FLAIR imaging sequences are also exquisitely motion-sensitive and may provide some qualitative information about CSF flow.

SUMMARY

The appearance of the brain alters drastically on both CT and MRI over the first 2–3 years of life post-delivery. This is primarily due to neuronal myelination.

A child up to at least 5 years of age must be kept still by one means or another in order to achieve maximal image quality and allow complete assessment for a congenital brain malformation. In small children up to 2 months of age a large feed prior to scanning may achieve this. In children from 2 months of age to at least 5 years of age sedation or general anesthesia will normally be required.

CT can be useful as a screening tool for gross abnormality, especially anywhere that calcification may be associated. Increasingly, modern CT scanners allow multi-planar reformats of the brain after volume acquisitions. CT is of course very useful in defining the bony anatomy of patients with plagiocephaly or craniosynostosis.

MRI is required for more complete demonstration of brain and spine congenital malformation.

Demonstration of one congenital brain abnormality makes the presence of another congenital brain abnormality more likely.

MRI allows brain imaging to be performed in three plane's rather than the one plane of standard CT. This can be achieved using standard MRI sequences.

Acquisition of an RF fast T1 weighted volume sequence allows multi planar reformatting to be achieved in any plane including curvilinear reformat. Such a sequence should always be considered to be part of a standard protocol when assessing children or adults for congenital brain malformations.

Newer imaging techniques, such as perfusion imaging, MRIDSA, and Spectroscopy are increasingly being used for characterization of lesions.

New rapid acquisition techniques may reduce the need for sedation and general anesthetic in the pediatric population as the image quality achieved with these sequences improves.

Some congenital brain malformations are associated with specific clinical presentations, for example, focal epilepsies such as gelastic seizures, hypopituitarism, and poor vision. For many other children the clinical presentation is far less specific. Indeed, some children with significant congenital brain malformation may have normal clinical development and no specific clinical problems.

Some congenital brain malformations are associated with other abnormalities including more generalized paediatric syndromes.

Some congenital brain malformations are associated with generic abnormalities. If proven, the presence of genetic abnormalities can be helpful to allow genetic counseling of affected families.

Ultrasound becomes increasingly less useful in imaging the pediatric neuraxis as skeletal maturation proceeds.

REFERENCES

1. Barkovich AJ. Congenital malformations of the brain and skull. In: Barkovich AJ, ed. Pediatric Neuroimaging. New York: Raven Press, 1995:177–275.
2. Barkovich AJ. Techniques and methods in pediatric neuroimaging. In: Barkovich AJ, ed. Pediatric Neuroimaging. New York: Raven Press, 1995:1–12.
3. Barkovich AJ. Normal development of the neonatal and ingant brain, skull, and spine. In: Barkovich AJ, ed. Pediatric Neuroimaging. New York: Raven Press, 1995:13–70.
4. Bluemke DA, Breiter SN. Sedation procedures in MR imaging: safety, effectiveness, and nursing effect on examinations. Radiology 2000; 216:633–634.
5. Mikkonen R, Kontkanen T, Kivisaari L. Late and acute adverse reactions to iohexol in a pediatric population. Pediatr Radiol 1995; 25:350–352.
6. Levi D, Rampa F, Barbieri C, Pricca P, Franzinin A, Pezzotta S. True 3D reconstruction for planning of surgery on malformed skulls. Childs Nerv Syst 2002; 18:705–706.
7. Rutherford M, Malamateniou C, Zeka J, Counsell S. MR imaging of the neonatal brain at 3 Tesla. Eur J Paediatr Neurol 2004; 8:281–289.
8. Forbes KP, Pipe JG, Bird CR, Heiserman JE. PROPELLER MRI: clinical testing of a novel technique for quantification and compensation of head motion. J Magn Reson Imaging 2001; 14:215–222.
9. Forbes KP, Pipe JG, Karis JP, Farthing V, Heiserman JE. Brain imaging in the unsedated pediatric patient: comparison of periodcically rotated overlapping parallel lines with enhanced reconstruction and single-shot fast spin-echo sequences. AJNR 2003; 24:794–798.
10. Alberico RA, Barnes P, Robertson RL, Burrows PE. Helical CT angiography: dynamic cerebrovascular imaging in children. AJNR 1999; 20:328–334.
11. Vassilyadi M, Jones BV, Ball WS, Jr. Identification of an arteriovenous fistula in a child. Case report and review of the literature. Childs Nerv Syst 2001; 17:685–688.
12. Husson B, Lasjaunias P. Radiological approach to disorders of arterial brain vessels associated with childhood arterial stroke—a comparison between MRIA and contrast angiography. Pediatr Radiol 2004; 34:2–4.
13. Hughes JA, De Bruyn R, Patel K, Thompson D. Evaluation of spinal ultrasound in spinal dysraphism. Clin Radiol 2003; 58:227–233.
14. Widjaja E, Griffiths PD. Intracranial MRI venography in children: normal anatomy and variations. AJNR 2004; 25:1557–1562.
15. Batra A, Tripathi RP. Diffusion-weighted magnetic resonance imaging and magnetic resonance spectroscopy in the evaluation of focal cerebral tubercular lesions. Acta Radiol 2004; 45:679–688.
16. Pillai JJ, Hessler RB, Allison JD, Park YD, Lee MR, Lavin T. Advanced MR imaging of cortical dysplasia with or without neoplasm: a report of two cases. AJNR 2002; 23:1686–1691.
17. Nagy Z, Westerberg H, Klingberg T. Maturation of white matter is associated with the development of cognitive functions during childhood. J Cogn Neurosci 2004; 16:1227–1233.
18. Tofts PS. Novel MR image contrast mechanisms in epilepsy. Magn Reson Imaging 1995; 13:1099–1106.

19. Whitby EH, Griffiths PD, Lonneker-Lammers T, et al. Ultrafast magnetic resonance imaging of the neonate in a magnetic resonance-compatible incubator with a built-in coil. Pediatrics 2004; 113:e150–e152.
20. Cowan FM. Magnetic resonance imaging of the normal infant brain: term to 2 years. In: Rutherford MA, ed. MRI of the Neonatal Brain. Edinburgh: WB Saunders, 2002:51–81.
21. Rohrschneider WK, Forsting M, Darge K, Troger J. Diagnostic value of spinal US: comparative study with MR imaging in pediatric patients. Radiology 1996; 200:383–388.
22. Medina LS, D'Souza B, Vasconcellos E. Adults and children with headache: evidence based diagnostic evaluation. Neuroimaging Clin N Am 2003; 13:225–235.

2.1

Ultrasound Methods and Anatomy

Pam Loughna
Academic Division of Obstetrics and Gynaecology, Nottingham City Hospital, Nottingham, U.K.

The introduction of high resolution ultrasound to routine obstetric practice has revolutionized prenatal diagnosis. Although anomaly scans in the mid-trimester are still not universally offered in the United Kingdom, the vast majority of obstetric units do provide a scan between 18 and 22 weeks when fetal anatomy is examined. The Royal College of Obstetricians and Gynaecologists first published guidelines for routine ultrasound in pregnancy including anomaly scans in 1997, and these were updated in 2000 (1,2). The central nervous system, one of the main organ systems to be examined, is the site of the first fetal abnormalities diagnosed by ultrasound: anencephaly and spina bifida (3,4).

It is possible, using high resolution ultrasound equipment, to obtain detailed anatomical information of the central nervous system from the first trimester, although the greatest number of malformations is detected at the mid-trimester anomaly scan. While the majority of scans are performed using a transabdominal approach with a 3.5 to 6 MHz transducer, transvaginal sonography can be of value particularly in the first trimester and the third, when the fetal head or lower end of the spine may be deep in the pelvis. Obstetric ultrasound examination of the fetal head usually utilizes transverse (axial) sections, with sagittal and coronal sections used less commonly (Figs. 1 and 2). However, the transvaginal approach may offer a trans-fontanelle view similar to that utilized in neonatology, particularly in the third trimester. Examination of the fetal spine uses transverse, sagittal, and longitudinal views (Figs. 3–5).

When scanning the fetal head, it is necessary to identify normal landmarks. The head shape is examined, and is normally ovoid. Care should be taken with the amount of pressure exerted by the sonographer, as it is possible to alter the fetal head shape by excess pressure. In the third trimester, the head of a breech presentation may appear long and thin (dolicocephalic) by virtue of intrauterine pressure effects. The integrity of the skull is also examined, to exclude encephalocoeles and general ossification defects such as osteogenesis imperfecta. In the normal fetal brain, certain anatomical structures are amenable to identification by ultrasound. The midline should be clearly visible, with the cavum septum pellucidum visible in the anterior third (Fig. 6). The lateral ventricles, being fluid filled, can be identified, with the choroid plexus occupying most of the posterior horn. The thalami, cerebellum and cisterna magna are also easily identified (Figs. 7 and 8).

The appearances of the intracranial anatomy alter with advancing gestation and the sonographer must be familiar with these developmental changes. The fluid filled lateral ventricles and the subarachnoid cisterns decrease in size with advancing gestation, causing dramatic changes in intracranial appearances (Fig. 9). In the first trimester, the choroid plexus and lateral ventricles are prominent (Fig. 10). It is usually possible to clearly identify the medial and lateral walls of the anterior and posterior horns of the lateral ventricles in the second trimester, with the choroid plexus appearing

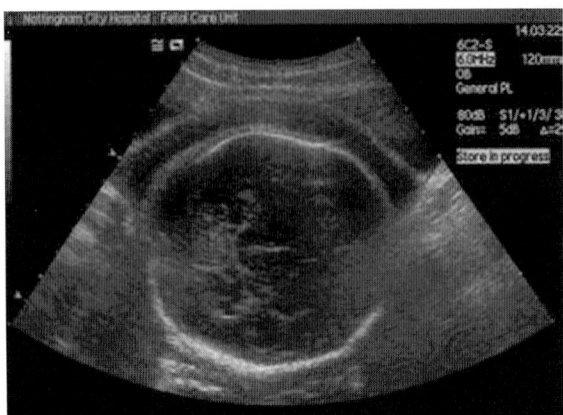

Figure 1. Transverse (axal) section of fetal head.

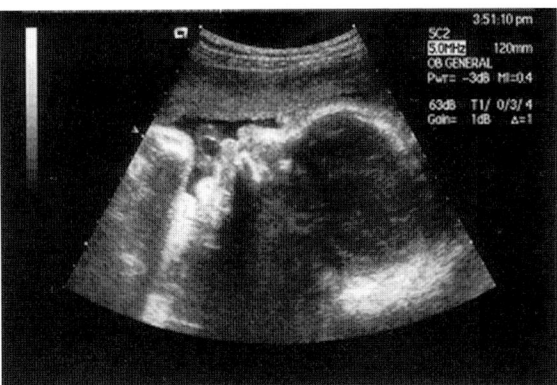

Figure 2. Sagittal section of fetal head.

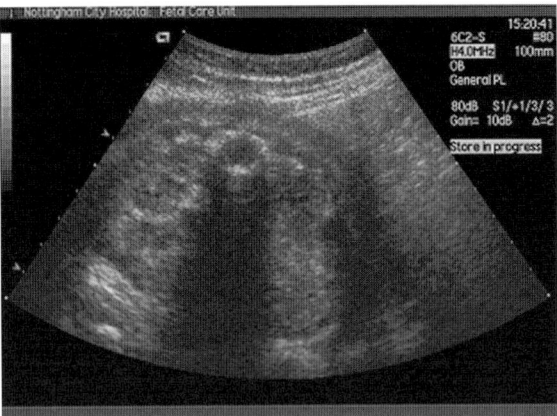

Figure 3. Transverse (axal) section of fetal spine.

to occupy most of the posterior horn. By the late third trimester, visualization of the intracranial contents becomes much more difficult, in part due to the ossification of the skull but also by virtue of fetal position when the head is deep within the mother's pelvis. It is usually only possible to identify the lateral wall of the anterior and posterior

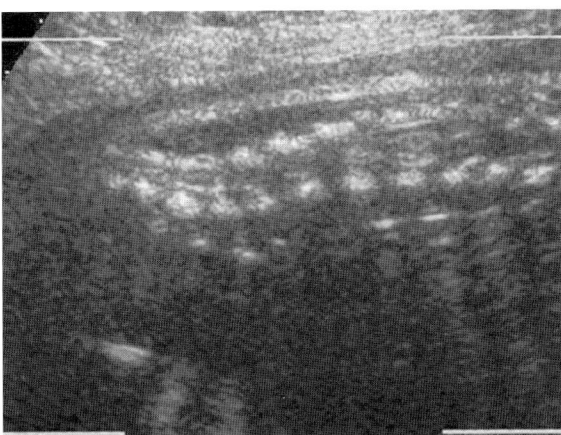

Figure 4. Sagittal view of fetal spine.

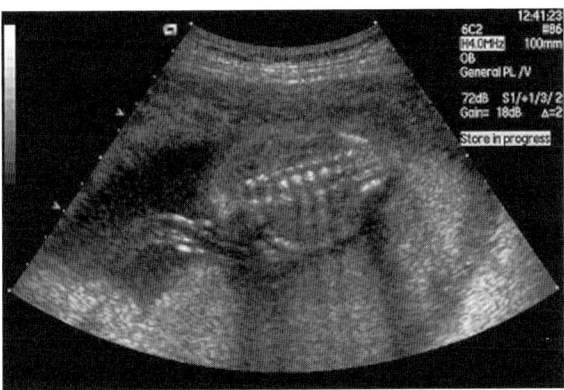

Figure 5. Coronal (longitudinal) view of fetal spine.

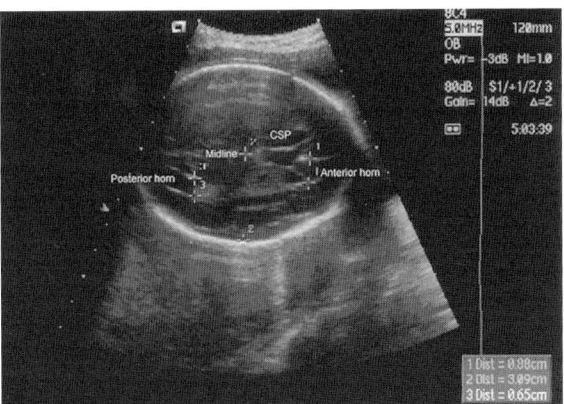

Figure 6. Normal midline demonstrating cavum septum pellucidum (CSP), anterior and posterior horns of the lateral ventricles.

horns, with the lateral ventricle occupying proportionally less of the cranial hemisphere than earlier in development. The ease with which the normal lateral ventricles can be identified, particularly in the second trimester, has permitted the derivation of reference ranges for size.

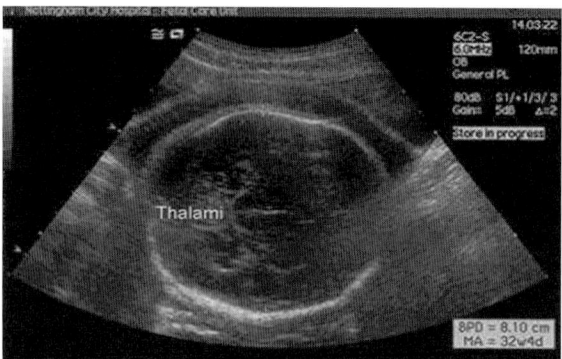

Figure 7. Thalami.

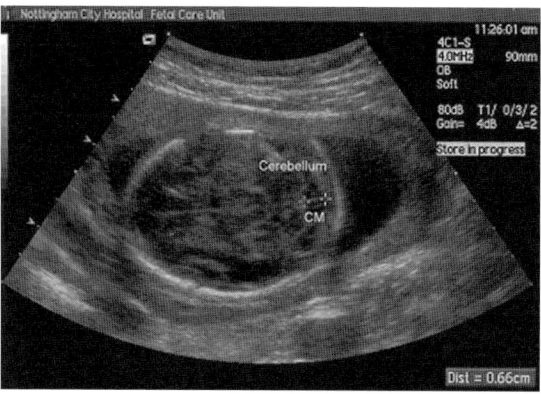

Figure 8. Cerebellum and cisterna magna.

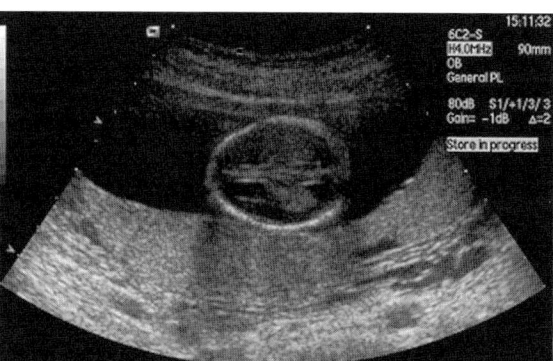

Figure 9. First trimester intracranial anatomy.

Many of the developmental changes within the cranium occur in the third trimester (cortical folding and myelination) and it is not possible to assess these changes using prenatal ultrasound.

The fetal spine is relatively easy to examine using ultrasound, although late third trimester assessment can be difficult by virtue of the fact that the spine may be posterior or immediately adjacent to the uterine wall rendering examination of the integrity of the overlying skin impossible. The spine should be examined along its entire length in transverse, sagittal and coronal planes identifying each vertebra and its skin covering.

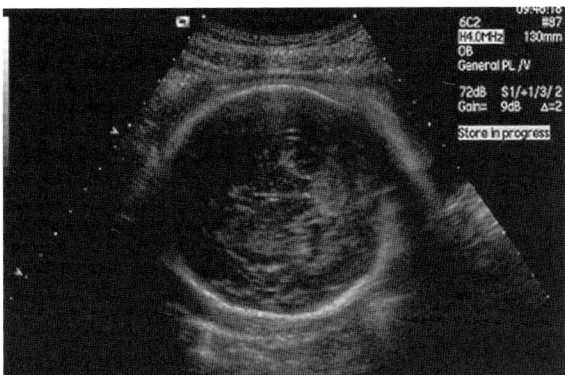

Figure 10. Third trimester intracranial anatomy.

In the sagittal plane, the spine and skin covering can be clearly seen, with the ossification centers in the vertebral bodies appearing as two parallel lines converging in the curved sacrum at the caudal end. In transverse views, the three ossification centers (body anteriorly and laminae posteriorly) can be seen, with the spinal cord lying within the closed neural canal. In coronal views, the spine can be seen as two or three parallel lines, again converging in the sacrum.

While considerable anatomical information may be gained from ultrasound in the first trimester, the most practical time for routine prenatal ultrasound in the screening for fetal anomalies is between 18 and 22 weeks. At this gestation, the intracranial anatomy is sufficiently developed to permit identification of many major malformations although it must be remembered that some significant anomalies may not be apparent at this stage, e.g., agenesis of the corpus callosum and Dandy–Walker malformation variants (5,6).

Thus, prenatal ultrasound is of great value in examining the integrity of the fetal central nervous system, but care is required in the diagnosis of anomalies which are not evident until after the routine anomaly scan in the mid-second trimester. In addition, it must be remembered that some structural anomalies involving myelination, migration, or cortical folding defects are not amenable to ultrasound detection before birth.

REFERENCES

1. RCOG. Ultrasound screening for fetal abnormalities. Report of the RCOG Working Party. London, Royal College of Obstetricians and Gynaecologists, 1997.
2. RCOG. Routine ultrasound screening in pregnancy. Protocols, standards and training. London, Royal College of Obstetricians and Gynaecologists. Bennett, 2000.
3. Campbell S, Johnstone F, Holt EM, May P. Anencephaly: early ultrasonic diagnosis and active management. Lancet 1972; 2:1226–1227.
4. Campbell S, Pryse-Davies J, Coltart TM, et al. Ultrasound in the diagnosis of spina bifida. Lancet 1975; 1:1065–1068.
5. Bennett GL, Bromley GB, Benacerraf BR. Agenesis of the corpus callosum: prenatal detection usually is not possible before 22 weeks of gestation. Radiology 1996; 199:447–450.
6. Malinger G, Lerman-Sagie T, et al. A normal second-trimester ultrasound does not exclude intracranial structural pathology. Ultrasound Obstet Gynecol 2002; 20:51–56.

2.2

Developmental Abnormalities of the Brain Shown by Ultrasound

Pam Loughna
Academic Division of Obstetrics and Gynaecology, Nottingham City Hospital, Nottingham, U.K.

The first diagnosis of fetal abnormality using ultrasound was the demonstration of anencephaly in 1972 by Campbell and Pearce, followed by the diagnosis of spina bifida three years later by the same team (1). Over the last thirty years, as it has become easier to examine fetal cranial anatomy using modern high resolution ultrasound equipment, the list of structural malformations correctly identified prenatally has increased. However, as outlined above (chap. 2.1), it is essential to bear in mind that some abnormalities will not be evident at the time of the routine fetal anomaly scan, and that others may not be amenable to ultrasound detection.

ANENCEPHALY

Anencephaly is defined as an absence of the cranial vault and cerebral hemispheres, and is caused by failure of fusion of the rostral neural tube. It represents a severe example of a neural tube defect, other examples being spina bifida and cephalocoeles. Neural tube defects have a multifactorial etiology, but may be associated with aneuploidy. There is considerable geographical variation in incidence.

Anencephaly can be diagnosed from 10–11 weeks gestation (Fig. 1), particularly if transvaginal ultrasound is used (2). However, the developing exposed brain can give the appearance of a normal cranium if care is not taken to identify the skull at such early gestations. In the mid-trimester, ultrasound appearances include the absent cranial vault, a short neck, and typical "frog-like" appearance of the exposed orbits (Fig. 2). The detection rate of anencephaly by ultrasound is high, being of the order of 96% with a sensitivity of 98% (3).

SPINA BIFIDA

The neural tube may fail to fuse at any stage along its length. However, the commonest site for neural tube defects to occur is the lower thoracic/lumbar and sacral part of the spinal column accounting for 85% of defects, with 10% being thoracic and 5% cervical (4). The etiology is multifactorial, as for all neural tube defects, but approximately 15% of cases are associated with aneuploidy (trisomy 13, trisomy 18, and triploidy).

Spina bifida can be classified by site and type [open (aperta) accounting for 85% and closed (occulta) the remaining 15%]. In open spina bifida (Fig. 3), the neural canal may be exposed or covered by a thin membrane. Most commonly, the lesion appears cystic. If the cystic component contains neural tissue, it is classified as a myelomeningocoele whereas if the cystic component is purely meninges, it is classified as a meningocoele.

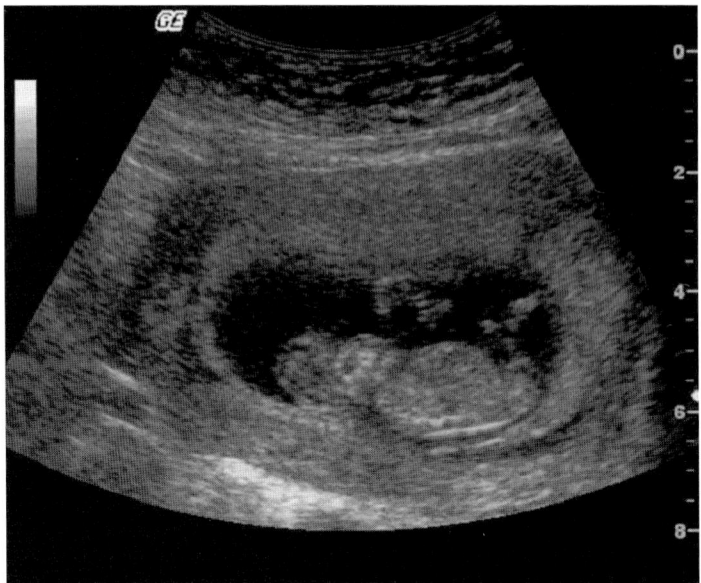

Figure 1. Anencephaly (1st trimester) showing absence of cranium.

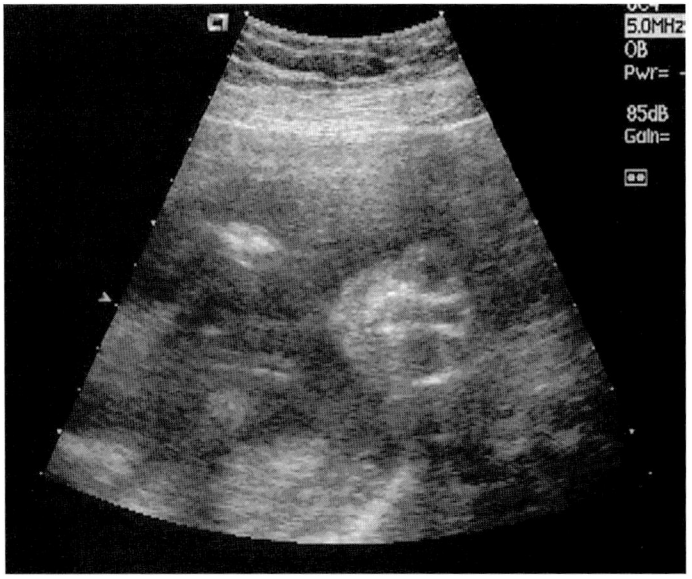

Figure 2. Facial appearance of anencephaly in 2nd trimester.

Associated anomalies can be found in the central nervous system. The most common association is with the Arnold-Chiari malformation which is caused by herniation of the cerebellar vermis giving rise to the so-called banana shaped cerebellum (Fig. 4) (5). This is present in at least 95% of cases of open spina bifida (6). In addition, there is commonly a deformity of the fetal skull giving rise to the so-called lemon sign, which is present in 98% of cases (Fig. 5) (6). Many cases will also demonstrate significant dilatation of the lateral ventricles which may progress to hydrocephalus

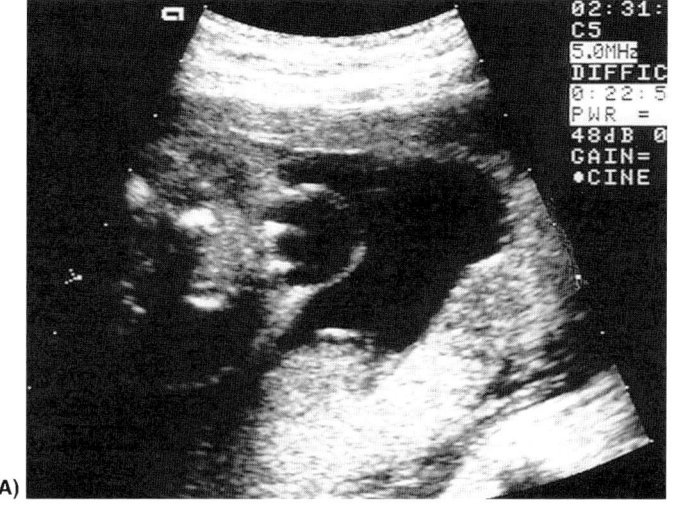

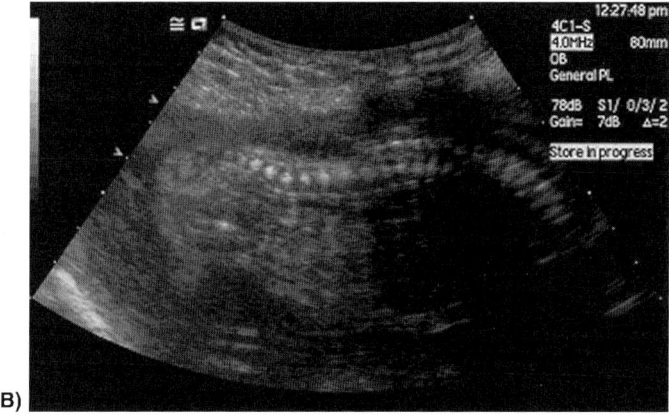

Figure 3. (A) Transverse (axial) view of neural tube defect with meningocoele. **(B)** Sagittal view of open neural tube defect, with membrane covering defect.

which is obstructive in origin. Other associated anomalies include deformities of the feet, both rocker bottom deformity, and talipes equinovarus being seen.

Mid-trimester obstetric ultrasound is very effective as a screening and diagnostic test for spina bifida, with detection rates approaching 100% in the United Kingdom (7) although they vary considerably across Europe (3). The most difficult cases to diagnose are those which include low sacral lesions, when intracranial signs may be absent. Careful examination of the fetal spine in three planes along its length, with attention paid to the integrity of the overlying skin, is required to maintain high detection rates.

ENCEPHALOCOELE

An encephalocoele, or cephalocoele, is a protrusion of the intracranial contents through a defect in the skull. They are rare, with occipital lesions being the most common. They may be isolated or be present as part of a syndrome. The diagnosis relies on the demonstration of a cystic mass arising from a defect in the fetal skull (Fig. 6). It is usually possible to identify the associated skull defect, although very small defects may be difficult to see with ultrasound. The differential diagnosis includes cystic hygroma, lesions of the scalp epidermis, and hemangiomas.

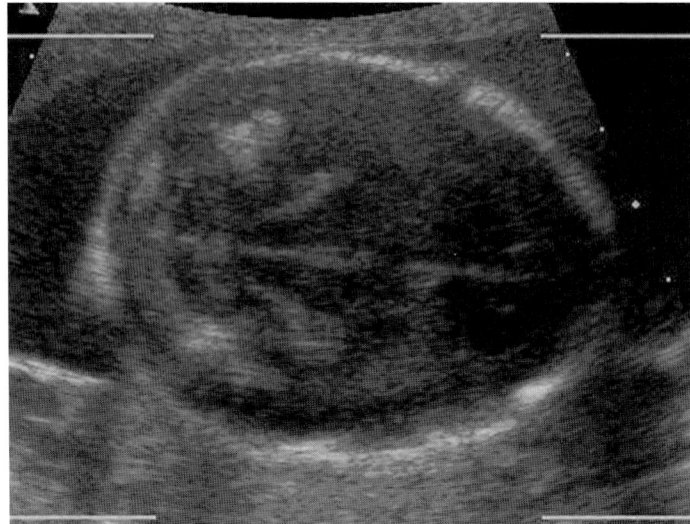

Figure 4. Banana-shaped cerebellum.

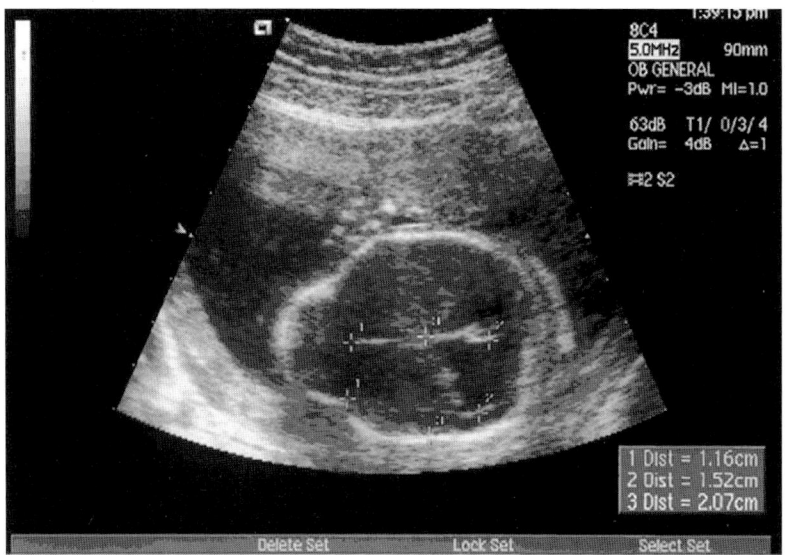

Figure 5. Lemon-shaped head with dilated lateral ventricles.

VENTRICULOMEGALY AND HYDROCEPHALUS

The anterior and posterior horns of the lateral ventricles are visible on fetal ultrasound examination, and the cisterna magna can also be identified. Dilatation of any part of the ventricular system, including the third ventricle, may be detected on ultrasound (Fig. 7). Ventriculomegaly refers to enlargement of the lateral ventricles alone, whereas hydrocephalus is defined as an increase in the intracranial content of cerebrospinal fluid. The anterior horn is measured from the midline to the lateral border, and the posterior horn is measured from the medial to lateral border of the atrium (8), which is normally virtually filled by the choroid plexus. The upper limit of normal is 10 mm.

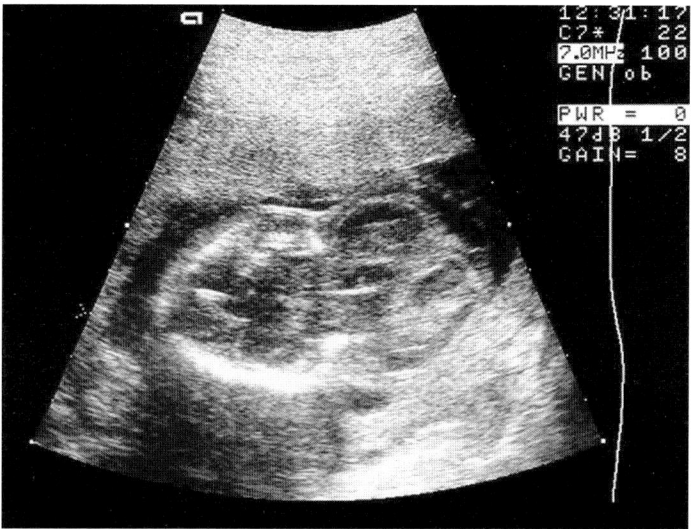

Figure 6. Occipital encephalocoele.

Ventriculomegaly can be caused by many factors, some of which are acquired, e.g., cytomegalovirus infection, and intracranial hemorrhage. Enlargement of the cerebral ventricles is associated with aneuploidy and other structural problems within the fetal brain and central nervous system. It is therefore necessary to perform a careful search for other anomalies whenever ventriculomegaly or hydrocephalus is detected by ultrasound. Some intracranial-associated anomalies may be difficult to confirm at the gestations at which routine anomaly scans are performed, e.g., agenesis of the corpus

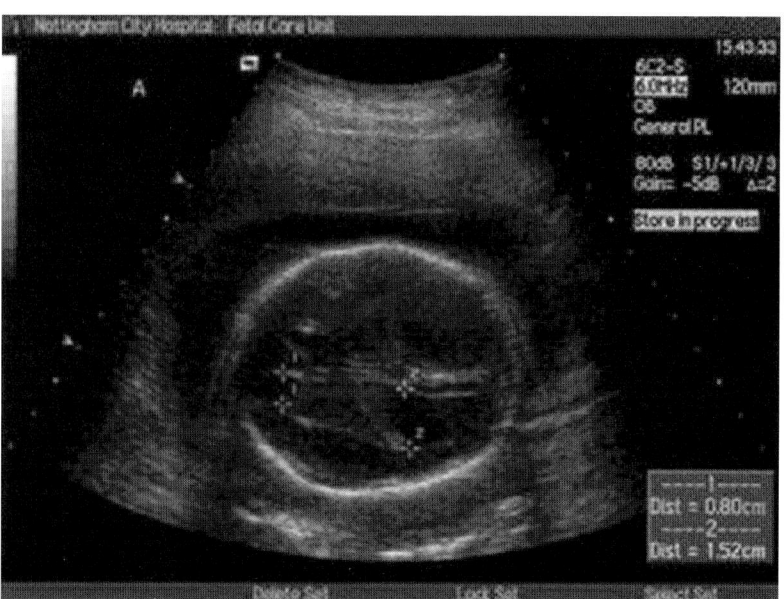

Figure 7. Ventriculomegaly, involving the lateral ventricles.

callosum (see below), and therefore additional imaging modalities such as MRI have a definite role to play in the investigation of this condition.

Hydrocephalus may be of three major types: aqueductal stenosis, communicating hydrocephalus, and Dandy–Walker malformation (see below). Aqueductal stenosis can be diagnosed by the finding of dilated lateral and third ventricles in the presence of a normal fourth ventricle. Communicating hydrocephalus arises when there is an obstruction to the flow of cerebrospinal fluid (CSF) outside the ventricular system or impairment of the reabsorption of CSF. All four ventricles are dilated, with concomitant enlargement of the subarachnoid space (so-called external hydrocephalus). Ultrasound is an effective mode for imaging the ventricular system, although external hydrocephalus may be difficult to demonstrate.

HOLOPROSENCEPHALY

This is a condition which arises from failure of fusion of the prosencephalon or forebrain. The left and right cerebral hemispheres and lateral ventricles are normally completely separated. In holoprosencephaly there is failure of this complete separation to a varying degree. As the embryological tissue responsible for the normal separation is also responsible for the development of facial midline structures, holoprosencephaly is associated with facial defects. There is a strong association with aneuploidy, particularly trisomies 13 and 18. Holoprosencephaly can be inherited in an autosomal dominant fashion with varied penetrance, anosmia sometimes being the only clinical finding in affected relatives, or as an autosomal recessive.

Alobar holoprosencephaly is the most severe form (Fig. 8). There is a single ventricle, which is sickle-shaped. No midline is visible. Facial features may include cyclopia or extreme hypotelorism with arhinia and proboscis, and median cleft lip. Microcephaly may also occur.

Semilobar holoprosencephaly has partial separation in the occipital region, but the lateral ventricles communicate anteriorly. Median cleft lip is an occasional association. Lobar holoprosencephaly has a well developed interhemispheric fissure although there is fusion anteriorly of the lateral ventricles and the cavum septum pellucidum is absent. This is the most challenging diagnosis to make using fetal ultrasound but may be

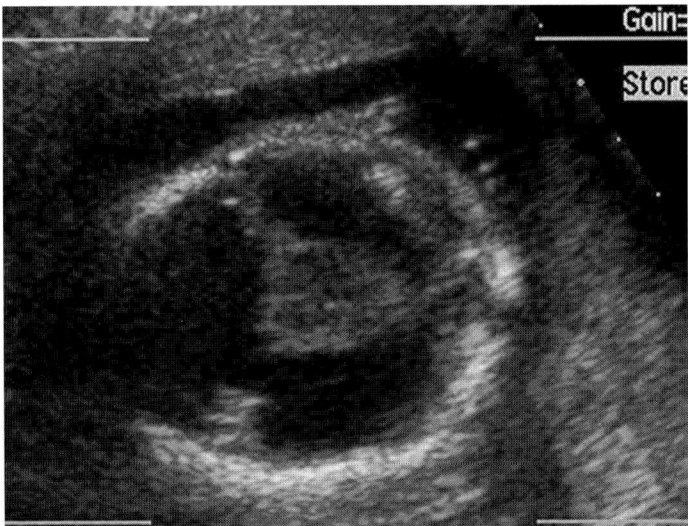

Figure 8. Holoprosencephaly.

suspected if the cavum septum pellucidum is absent, with communicating frontal horns of the lateral ventricles and an enlarged third ventricle (9). The presence of a normal cavum septum pellucidum excludes holoprosencephaly.

AGENESIS OF THE CORPUS CALLOSUM

The corpus callosum connects the two cerebral hemispheres and is important in exchange of sensory information between the left and right hemisphere. It makes up approximately 11% of the supratentorial brain. As there are other connections between the hemispheres, these non-callosal commissures can fulfil the function of the corpus callosum and therefore many individuals with isolated agenesis of the corpus callosum will be asymptomatic. However, approximately 80% of cases of ACC will have additional central nervous system anomalies including Dandy–Walker malformation, neural tube defects, and hydrocephalus (10). Other associated anomalies include aneuploidy (particularly trisomy 13 and 18). The prognosis is dependent on the presence or absence of associated anomalies.

As the corpus callosum is not fully formed until approximately 20 weeks gestation, diagnosis of agenesis by ultrasound before that time is challenging. The diagnosis is suspected by the finding of separation of the anterior horn of the lateral ventricles and dilatation of the posterior horns with dilatation and upward displacement of the third ventricle. There is associated ventriculomegaly in most cases, and 10% of all cases of mild ventriculomegaly will have ACC (11). Coronal views of the fetal head permit identification of the corpus callosum, which appears as a hypoechoic structure. The pericallosal artery can be identified sweeping over it, using color Doppler on sagittal views (Fig. 9).

As the rostral portion of the corpus callosum is the last part to develop, partial agenesis involving this part can occur. In this situation, the anterior part is normal, with a normal cavum septum pellucidum and the frontal horns are normal. However, there will be mild dilatation of the posterior horns of the lateral ventricle.

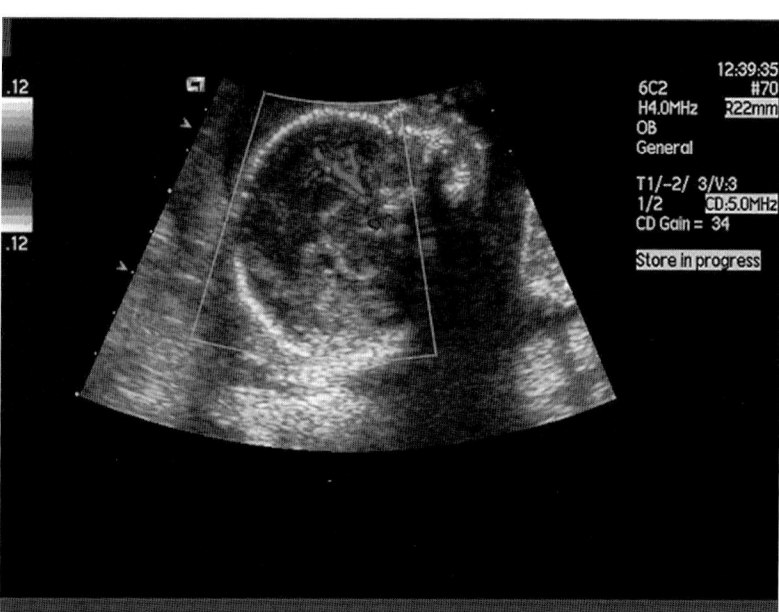

Figure 9. Normal corpus callosum with callosal artery.

Ultrasound demonstration of agenesis of the corpus callosum is not possible before 18 weeks, as the corpus callosum is not fully formed until that gestation. Partial agenesis may present with very subtle changes in appearance particularly at the time of the routine fetal anomaly scan, and many cases will not be diagnosed (12).

DANDY–WALKER MALFORMATION

The initial term Dandy–Walker syndrome was used to describe the association of ventriculomegaly, a large cisterna magna, and defect of the cerebellar vermis (Fig. 10). Changes in imaging technology, particularly CT scanning and MRI, have lead to refinement of the terminology used to describe posterior fossa anomalies.

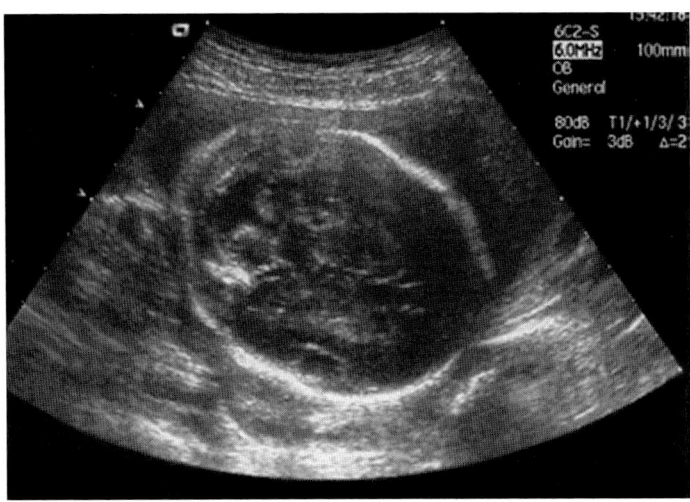

Figure 10. Dandy–Walker variant, showing defect in inferior cerebellar vermis.

Using ultrasound, the appearances of the classic Dandy–Walker malformation (complete agenesis of the cerebellar vermis with enlargement of the cisterna magna) are straightforward from mid-pregnancy, and the diagnosis has been made at 14 weeks gestation using transvaginal sonography (13). However, partial defects are much more difficult to detect using prenatal ultrasound, with the appearances changing with advancing gestation so that a normal looking posterior fossa and cerebellum may be shown to be abnormal in the third trimester or on postnatal imaging (12). As Dandy-Walker malformation may be familial, repeated ultrasound or MRI should be considered before excluding a recurrence. Postnatal cranial imaging can identify partial Dandy-Walker malformation in asymptomatic individuals with no enlargement of the cerebral ventricles, and such defects are presumably rarely identified by prenatal ultrasound. Many other cerebral malformations are associated with Dandy–Walker malformation, but a significant number of these are not identifiable using prenatal ultrasound, e.g., polymicrogyria.

There is a well-recognised association between agenesis of the corpus callosum and the Dandy–Walker malformation. Therefore, if either condition is suspected on prenatal ultrasound, a careful examination of the cerebral anatomy must be performed.

ARTERIO-VENOUS MALFORMATIONS

The commonest congenital arterio-venous malformation involves the vein of Galen. The diagnosis may be suspected when a mid-line cystic structure is identified which has evidence of high blood flow when color Doppler is applied. The use of color Doppler permits accurate diagnosis and ultrasound follow up is necessary to monitor the cardiovascular status of the fetus, as high output failure (hydrops) may occur.

ARACHNOID CYSTS

The differential diagnosis of intracranial cysts includes arachnoid cysts. These may be difficult to differentiate from porencephalic cysts, Dandy–Walker malformation (if within the posterior fossa), and agenesis of the corpus callosum (if midline). Hemorrhage may be seen within the cysts, but application of color Doppler will not demonstrate high flow.

LISSENCEPHALY

Cellular migration defects, such as lissencephaly, are not detectable by prenatal ultrasound unless there are associated malformations, such as ventriculomegaly or agenesis of the corpus callosum.

DESTRUCTIVE (ACQUIRED) LESIONS

Intracranial tumors are rare, with teratomas being the most common group. They may arise during the second half of gestation, a routine anomaly scan having normal intracranial appearances.

Intracranial hemorrhage may arise from a number of causes. The extent of the damage caused depends on the location of the hemorrhage. Porencephalic cysts represent areas of destruction of cerebral tissue which may be related to infection, trauma or hemorrhage.

Hydranencephaly, which results form the secondary destruction of the developing brain enveloped in meninges and skull, should be suspected when there is an intact falx with no obvious cerebral tissue. Schizencephaly, in which there are gray matter-lined clefts within the substance of the brain, is rarely detected by ultrasound, unless the clefts are very deep or there is associated ventriculomegaly.

The interpretation of prenatal ultrasound of the fetal central nervous system requires understanding of both the developmental changes which occur with advancing gestation and the limitations of the imaging technique being applied.

REFERENCES

1. Campbell S, Pryse-Davies J, Coltart TM, et al. Ultrasound in the diagnosis of spina bifida. Lancet 1975; 1:1065–1068.
2. Goldstein R, Filly R, Callen PW. Sonography of anencephaly: pitfalls of early diagnosis. J Clin Ultrasound 1989; 17:397–402.
3. Boyd P, Wellesley D, De Walle HE. Evaluation of the prenatal diagnosis of neural tube defects by fetal ultrasonographic examination in different centres across Europe. J Med Screen 2000; 7:169–174.
4. Holmes L, Driscoll S, Atkins L. Etiologic heterogeneity of neural-tube defects. New Eng J Med 1976.
5. Niolaides K, Campbell S, Gabbe SG, Guidetti R. Ultrasound screening for spina bifida: cranial and cerebellar signs. Lancet 1986; 2:72–74.
6. Van den Hof M, Nicolaides K, Campbell J, Campbell S. Evaluation of the lemon and banana signs in one hundred thirty fetuses with open spina bifida. Am J Obstet Gynecol 1990; 162:322–327.
7. Chitty L, Hunt G, Moore J, Lobbe MO. Effectiveness of routine ultrasonography in detecting fetal structural abnormalities in a low risk population. BMJ 1991; 303:1165–1169.
8. Campbell S, Pearce J. Ultrasound visualization of congenital malformations. Br Med Bull 1983; 39:322–331.

9. Pilu G, Sandri F, Perolo A. Prenatal diagnosis of lobar holoprosencephaly. Ultrasound Obstet Gynecol 1992; 2:88–94.

10. Comstock C, Culp D, et al. Agenesis of the corpus callosum in the fetus: its evolution and significance. J Ultrasound Med 1985; 4:613–616.

11. Goldstein R, LaPidus A, et al. Mild lateral ventricolmegaly: clinical course and outcome. Am J Obstet Gynecol 1990; 164:863–867.

12. Pilu G, Hobbins J. Sonography of fetal cerebrospinal anomalies. Prenat Diagn 2002; 22:321–330.

13. Achiron R, Achiron A. Transvaginal ultrasonic assessment of the early fetal brain. Ultrasound Obstet Gynecol 1991; 1:336–342.

2.3

Magnetic Resonance Imaging Methods and Anatomy

Elspeth H. Whitby and Martyn N. J. Paley
Academic Unit of Radiology, University of Sheffield, Sheffield, U.K.

IMAGING THE DEVELOPING FETUS

Magnetic Resonance Imaging (MRI) Methods and Anatomy

MRI Technique

MRI of the fetus was initially restricted by motion artifact (Fig. 1A). This was overcome by the use of pancuronium bromide injected into the umbilical vessels or fetal musculature (1). This restricted the procedure to patients undergoing fetal sedation for other therapeutic or interventional procedures and the in utero MRI was performed while the paralysis lasted (about 2 hours). Another approach was to give the mother intravenous benzodiazepines in order to sedate her and the fetus (2), again this was used for other diagnostic or therapeutic procedures and not routinely used for the purpose of fetal MRI. The initial studies under such conditions allowed assessment of the scope and likely value of fetal MRI if motion artifacts could be overcome. Those studies used T1 weighted images.

The advent of ultrafast imaging techniques allowed a rapid increase in the use of MRI to image the fetus. Single Shot Fast Spin Echo (SSFSE) produces a slice every second, effectively freezing fetal motion and producing a heavily T2 weighted image (Fig. 1B) (3).

SSFSE or Rapid Acquisition Recalled Echo (RARE) as it was originally named by its developer Jurgen Hennig (4) uses a train of 180 degree pulses following an initial 90 degree pulse. The spin echoes collected after each 180-degree pulse are separately phase-encoded to collect all of k-space within a single T2 signal decay. The images tend to be very T2 weighted and were originally used to produce MRI myelograms of the spine to highlight the cerebrospinal fluid.

The degree of T2 weighting achieved can be varied by locating the center of k-space at different times within the T2 decay by altering the way the phase encode gradients are applied. The echo spacing is important in determining filtering effects (blurring) on the image due to T2 decay. Motion during data collection can also cause complex artifacts in SSFSE. Ideally short echo spacing is used to minimize artifacts although this requires increased bandwidth which affects the signal-to-noise ratio. Susceptibility artifacts are not prominent on SSFSE sequences, which make them insensitive for hemorrhage.

Significant magnetization transfer effects may be seen between mobile and bound proton pools when performing multi-slice SSFSE, which can give rise to variable contrast effects between slices. There have been concerns about using MR imaging in pregnant women and guidelines are set out by the National Radiation Protection Board

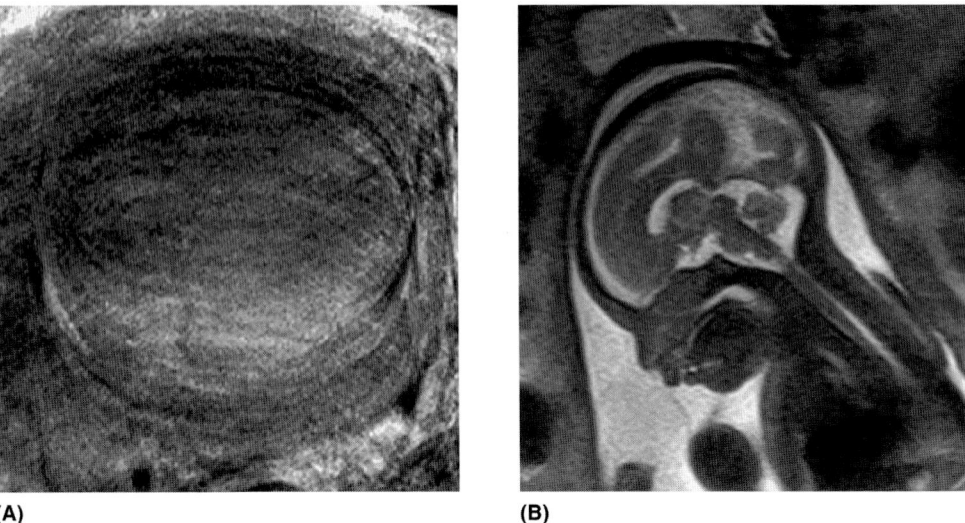

(A)   (B)

Figure 1. (A) T2W axial image obtained using standard MRI sequences. No detail is seen due to the large amount of movement. **(B)** T2W sagittal MRI of the fetal brain obtained using ultrafast sequences. The brain and CSF spaces are seen in detail.

(NRPB) as to the amount of heat [termed specific absorption rate (SAR)] that can be generated while conducting the examination (see chap. 2.5).

All our MRI examinations are performed on the same standard 1.5 T clinical system (Eclipse or Infinion — Philips Medical Systems, with 27 mT/m gradients) using Single Shot Fast Spin Echo (SSFSE) sequences to produce high resolution, T2 weighted images obtained in short scan times. The procedure is explained to the patient and informed consent obtained (this is standard practice in most institutions now). The protocol consists of 20 5 mm-thick SSFSE images [TR 24,000 ms, TE 75 ms, Echo Train Length 132, field of view (FOV) 25 cm, matrix 212×256, acquisition time 20 s] obtained in the three natural, orthogonal planes. These images are supplemented by twenty 3 mm-thick SSFSE images (TR 38,000 ms, TE 156 ms, Echo Train Length 140, FOV 25 cm, matrix 256×256, acquisition time 30 s) acquired in the axial, coronal, and sagittal planes if clinically indicated. T1weighted scans are used at the discretion of the radiologist. Neither maternal sedation nor muscular blockade of the fetus is used. We have noticed that the fetus is often very mobile during the first few images, which makes acquisition difficult, but the fetus soon settles. We believe that the fetus accommodates to the noise so it is worth doing all the same sequence types together, as a change in the acoustic noise pattern often results in more fetal movement. Each slice sequence is started manually and planned from the previous slices to allow adjustment for a change in fetal position.

Gadolinium is not used and not advised for fetal imaging (5) as it circulates in the fetal amniotic fluid and may dechelate, but there are no reports stating it is detrimental.

Other Sequences

Many other MRI methods are hampered by the presence of fetal motion at earlier gestational ages. However, a number of research centers are now investigating the role of more advanced imaging sequences in utero.

T1 Weighted Imaging

Although T1 weighted imaging is not really an advanced imaging sequence, it has been more difficult to establish a robust ultrafast method for in utero MRI than T2 weighted imaging. This is due to the very long T1 times found in the fetal brain

(2–3 seconds), lack of significant T1 contrast between parenchyma and CSF due to the water-like nature of the fetal brain (6), and the presence of significant T2 coherence signal which must be effectively spoiled to retain T1 contrast on fast imaging sequences (Fig. 2A). Absolute relaxation time measurements have been difficult to measure in utero due to the long times required to acquire equilibrium signals. Inversion recovery (IR) or Turbo-IR sequences tend to have longer acquisition times than the simpler FLASH-based fast imaging methods and so have not been as successful due to motion artifacts. In our experience the most successful T1 weighted sequence for in utero imaging to date has been the RF spoiled FAST sequence which can be completed in a few seconds, compatible with in utero imaging, and which uses phase scrambling rather than gradient spoiling to remove the large coherent T2 signal which confounds T1 contrast on normal T1 sequences. T1 weighted images are useful to look at myelination in the third trimester and to distinguish fluid from fat. It is possible that areas of cortical dysplasia can be detected on T1 images in late pregnancy. In cases such as tuberous sclerosis, the brain lesions associated with the conditions (multiple tubers and subependymal nodules) are low signal on T2 and high on T1 (7). We have also found it useful in cases where there has been brain damage due to TORCH infections. The microcalcifications and earlier microhemorrhages are seen as bright areas.

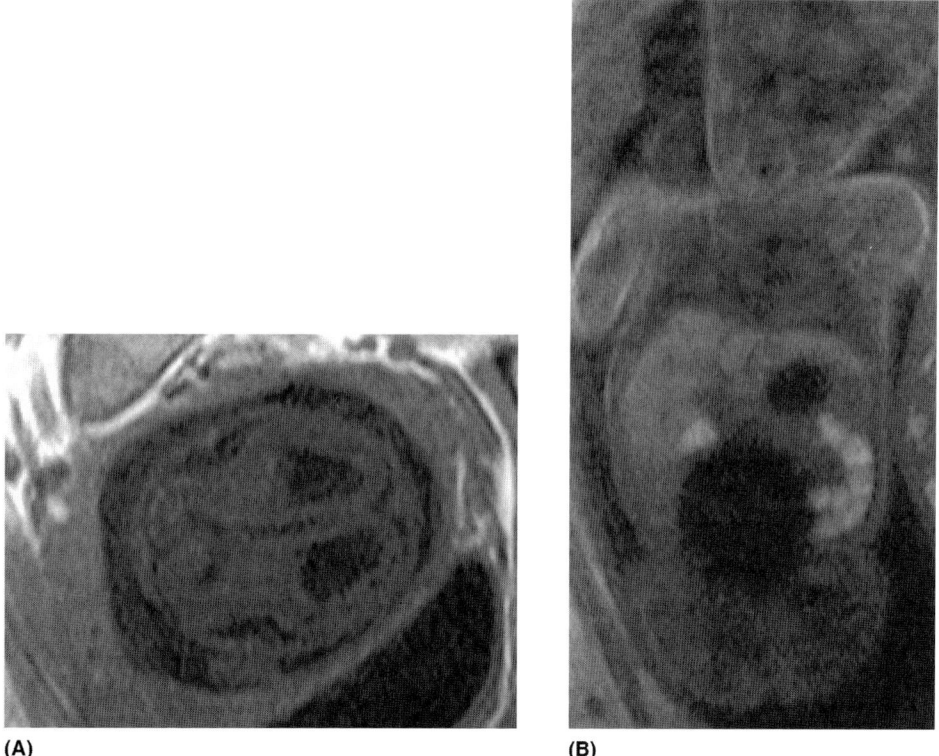

(A)   **(B)**

Figure 2. (A) T1W axial image of the fetal brain at 24 weeks gestational age; the sylvian fissure is open and square shaped. **(B)** T1W coronal image of the fetal body. The lungs are low signal, liver intermediate signal, and large bowel high signal.

T1 images are very useful to delineate the liver, diaphragm, and lungs in cases with diaphragmatic hernias (8) and to image the terminal large bowel as this contains meconium and is high signal on T1 weighted images (Fig. 2B) (9).

Spectroscopy

In-utero proton MRI spectroscopy is difficult in early gestational age fetuses due to the extended acquisition time required and the increased chance of fetal motion (10–13). Despite this, in utero spectroscopy holds great promise for monitoring the developing brain due to the presence of the neuronal marker N-acetyl aspartate (NAA). The appearance of lactate in cases of serious brain pathology has already been used successfully as an antenatal prognostic marker (14). Studies of fetuses close to term when the head is engaged in the maternal birth canal are generally more successful. However, little is yet known about the absolute concentrations or relaxation times of metabolites in the fetal brain as a function of gestational age, and so interpretation of spectra must be approached with great care. A number of studies have produced good quality spectra during development of premature infants (15) but only a few studies have been performed in utero (12). In utero spectroscopy studies are usually performed using a single voxel technique (Fig. 3), either PRESS with a long echo time (TE = 135 ms) to look for inverted lactate doublets or STEAM with a short echo time (TE = 20 ms) to assess the presence of short T2* metabolites. A detailed long term study is required to establish normative data for in utero spectroscopy in normal pregnancies and in pathology. However, this will present a formidable challenge.

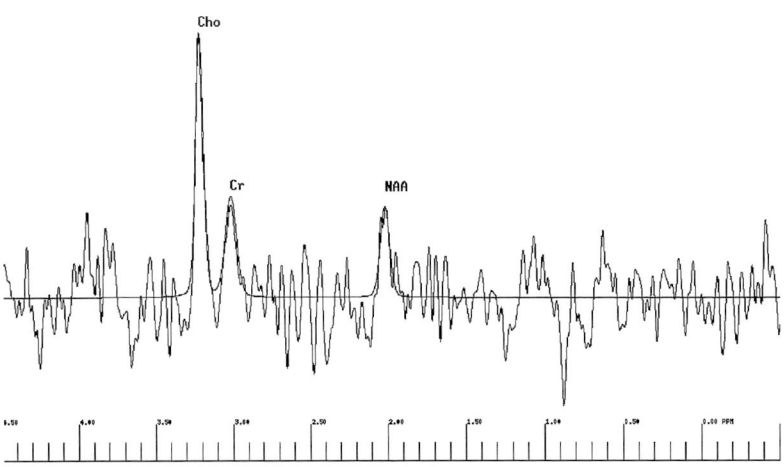

Figure 3. Spectrum from the fetal brain at 32 weeks gestational age, obtained with a PRESS sequence.

3D MRI

3D imaging would appear to be a good choice for imaging small fetal structures and for assessing volumetric changes over time. Use of 3D fetal MRI has been limited to some extent by the long acquisition times required and the possible presence of slice aliasing from the maternal body (16). Newer MRI systems with improved gradient performance allow 3D sequences to be performed within just a few seconds, providing the possibility of contiguous thin slice imaging of the fetal brain. Use of pre-saturation or outer volume suppression methods can help reduce slice aliasing effects for 3D sequences but may prolong the acquisition time further. Another drawback of high resolution 3D imaging in utero is the high acoustic noise often associated with these imaging sequences. Future combination of 3D acquisitions with parallel imaging promises to dramatically reduce the time required for in utero studies, and the use of 3D for fetal imaging is likely to increase rapidly if this is successful. Thin slice 3D imaging can be used to reduce the number of scan planes required, as the data can be reformatted to any plane using post-processing. Post processing techniques have allowed calculation of the ventricular volume and obtained information not available from the 2D images (17).

Functional MRI

Several investigators have attempted to perform functional MRI (fMRI) in utero (13,18–20). This is complicated by the fact that it is not clear whether the fetus has received or is capable of responding to a particular functional stimulus at a particular age. It is well known that fetuses often respond to sound external to the mother as judged by fetal motion, although the high noise environment of the MRI scanner is not the ideal environment for attempting auditory fMRI studies. Attempts to elicit visual stimulation by shining a bright light on the maternal abdomen have also been reported (18). Again, it is not clear exactly what stimulus the fetus actually receives within the womb. From initial studies, it has been claimed that the BOLD response may be negative in the fetus due to lack of a rapid hemodynamic response as found in adults. This would result in increased levels of paramagnetic deoxy-hemoglobin in the venous system, reducing the MRI BOLD signal as opposed to the usual increase in BOLD signal due to inflow of additional oxy-hemoglobin at the activated site as found in the developed adult brain. This was based on the assumption that the fetus would behave in a similar fashion to the neonate. The recent work by the group in Nottingham has shown a BOLD response greater than in adults. Auditiory stimuli activated the temporal lobe while visual stimuli activated the frontal lobes (20). Of course slight motion of the fetus over the extended functional stimulus paradigm can play a significant role in confounding attempts to measure function. The details of functional processes in the developing brain will require many further carefully controlled in utero studies to be fully understood and for fMRI to play a useful role in the clinical environment.

Diffusion Weighted Imaging

Diffusion weighted imaging (DWI) plays an increasingly important role in neurological studies due to its high sensitivity to ischemic changes as proven in many cases of adult ischemic stroke. As DWI is very sensitive to changes in the ability of water to move directionally, it is anticipated that DWI would provide useful information in the developing brain as structures gradually differentiate and attain directionality, e.g., myelination of white matter. Most diffusion weighted imaging is currently performed using a pair of Stejskal-Tanner gradients located around the 180 degree pulse in a spin echo echo planar imaging sequence (SE-EPI) which reduces fetal motion artifacts. However, EPI is often difficult to perform in the abdomen due to the large FOV required and fetal tissue sometimes appears near the edge of the uniform region of the magnet where artifacts may occur, so care must be taken in assessing DWI in utero. Diffusion weighting is adjusted by altering the strength, width, and spacing of the pair of gradients and a so called b-factor is used to characterize the degree of exponential diffusion weighting used. The diffusion is not always equal in all directions but often exhibits distinct directionality (anisotropic motion). To describe this more fully a tensor (a form of multi-dimensional vector) is used resulting in DTI (Diffusion Tensor Imaging). The tensor is measured by applying the pairs of diffusion gradients along many different spatial directions. The diffusion data is then used to solve for a series of eigenvalues and eigenvectors which characterize the diffusion tensor in a rotationally invariant way so that it is independent of the patient position within the magnet. The most significant eigenvalue components then yield an estimate of the directionality of the diffusive properties of the tissue. Sophisticated post-processing by following the direction of the tensor along streamlines enables the routes of bundles of fibers to be extracted and overlaid on the 3D anatomy.

For routine clinical studies the diffusion tensor is not usually measured; instead, maps of apparent diffusion coefficient (ADC) along three orthogonal directions and the "trace" of the diffusion tensor (sum of three orthogonal components) is used to assess regions where water diffuses rapidly (high ADC, low intensity diffusion weighted images) and where water diffusion is more restricted (low ADC, high intensity diffusion weighted images). Most in utero studies to date have focused on this more rapid assessment of diffusion in the fetal brain, although several fetal DTI measurements and fiber tracking studies have recently been reported. Currently we use DWI in cases of possible ischemia to assess the cerebral grey and white matter (Fig. 4A).

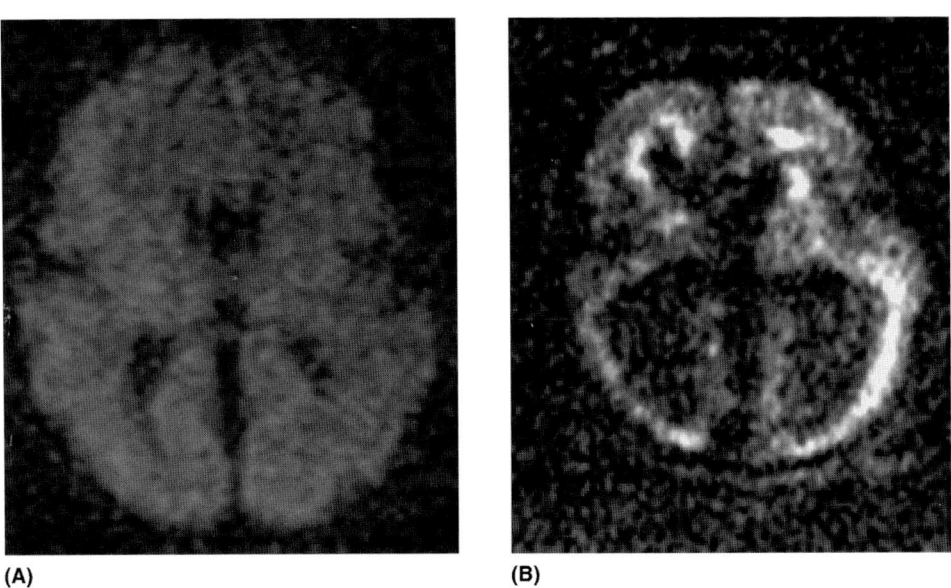

(A)   **(B)**

Figure 4. (A) DWI at 32 weeks gestational age showing normal appearances. **(B)** DWI at 26 weeks gestational age. There is ventriculomegaly and high signal surrounding the ventricles due to tissue damage from cytomegalovirus infection.

Abnormalities are seen on the DWI following infective processes in some cases (Fig. 4B); changes are also seen on the T2 and T1 images.

FLAIR

FLAIR has not been used extensively for in utero imaging as both brain and CSF signal are suppressed in a similar way by the fluid nulling, due to the long T1 relaxation time of the fetal brain which is quite similar to the T1 of CSF. Also the long inversion time required prolongs the acquisition time making FLAIR sequences very prone to motion artifact.

SENSE/Zoom/Interactive Pilot

Parallel imaging is expected to play a major role in fetal imaging over coming years. Most parallel imaging methods use information from multiple receiver coils to substitute for phase encoding data. This enables scans to be acquired with fewer phase encode steps and thus in a proportionally shorter time. However, to do this it is vital to know the sensitivity maps of the RF coils used, which are measured using a prior reference scan. Significant challenges exist for methods that use prior reference scans due to the risk of fetal motion between acquisition of the reference and acquisition of the undersampled data. An alternative or an adjunct to reducing the number of phase encode steps is to excite several slices simultaneously. Simultaneous slice methods such as the SPIRIT and simultaneous multi-slice imaging with slice-multiplexed RF pulses recently introduced by our group (21,22) may help to reduce the time required to image the fetus by factors in the range 8–16, which will obviously be of great benefit for reducing motion artifacts. Use of SENSE with 3D sequences also promises to produce significant time savings for fetal scanning.

Use of zoomed fields of view with outer volume suppression to suppress signal from maternal tissues may also play an important role in increasing spatial resolution for fetal imaging, although corresponding improvements in coil technology will be required to achieve the increased signal-to-noise ratio (SNR) required to support this.

Improved interactive pilot capability developed originally for use in cardiac imaging is now available on modern MRI systems and can be used to reduce the time needed to localize the standard axial, sagittal, and coronal 2D planes. However, use of interactive pilots may be obviated in future if rapid parallel 3D methods currently in development are successful. Our group is working on a new parallel method which combines simultaneous multi-slab thin slice 3D acquisition with two directions of SENSE encoding to produce very short volumetric acquisition times. In combination with multi-planar reformatting of the acquired volume, this may prove to be an optimal method for whole body fetal screening without the need for aligning scan planes with the fetal anatomy.

Safety

The initial in utero MRI studies where the fetus was sedated or paralysed use T1 weighted sequences. However with the ultrafast technique the images are heavily T2 weighted.

There is no evidence to suggest that exposure of the fetus to electromagnetic radiation is detrimental but the current advice, from the NRPB, is to avoid MRI in the first trimester, only image with field strengths less than 2.5 T, and keep the specific absorption rate (SAR) as low as possible. Intravenous contrast is not advised due to the dechelation of the Gadolinium across the placenta and the recirculation of the Gadolinium in the amniotic fluid, thus increasing its half life. The SAR is maximal at the surface of the maternal body so the risk to the fetus is minimal due to the efficient heat-dissipating action of the amniotic fluid.

There is also concern about the acoustic noise as the SSFSE technique has a noise level of almost 100 decibels. The mother is provided with ear protection but this is not possible for the fetus. The noise level of the fast sequences has the potential to damage hearing, although amniotic fluid may reduce the acoustic noise by 30 dB – 50 dB (28). The most recent information comes from a prospective study that followed up children who had been imaged in utero in the third trimester. Thirty-five children who were between one and three years of age and nine children who were between eight and nine years of age at assessment were studied. These children had all undergone clinical scans in utero at 1.5 T and in some cases the study also included PRESS and STEAM spectroscopy sequences in addition to T2 weighted imaging. Detailed follow-up was obtained together with a detailed neurological examination at three months of age. In all but two cases findings were normal. The abnormalities in these two cases may or may not be related to the MR imaging, but no problems were detected with hearing (23–26). Animal studies have not been conclusive although some suggest that there are hazardous effects of repeated exposure to static mevissen, fluctuating magnetic fields, peeling, prolonged exposure, or in utero exposure at high field (4.7 T) (27). These studies do not accurately reflect the events of a single or repeated in utero examination in the clinical setting in the second or third trimester. The total safety of the MRI technique can never be fully established. Further larger studies are required, especially when children reach reproductive age to assess if the reproductive tissues are affected by MRI. Currently it is advisable to keep the field strength to 1.5 T, use low SAR, keep scan times as short as possible and avoid scanning in the first trimester.

For NRPB current guidelines, see chap. 2.5.

ANATOMY

CNS

Brain—Supratentorial and Infratentorial

For normal development of the brain see previous chapters.

With the advent of the ultrafast SSFSE imaging method, initial studies concentrated on the ability of the technique to demonstrate the anatomy of the fetal brain. These studies established that the technique is both reliable and accurate for fetuses beyond 20 weeks gestational age (29). Several groups had obtained experience using fetal sedation and these groups soon moved to using the ultrafast technique. Several new groups started to work in this field including our own group.

Supratentorial Structures

CEREBRAL VENTRICLES. This is probably the most important structure to assess on the in utero MR images. Our experience, and that of others, suggests that in utero MRI may increase the detection rate of abnormalities associated with ventriculomegaly compared to ultrasound. It is reported that ultrasound detects other abnormalities in 15% of cases. In our experience, isolated ventriculomegaly referred from ultrasound has associated abnormalities in around 50% of unselected cases.

The ventricle is a monoventricle until 10 weeks gestational age. The third ventricle is 1 mm wide until 28 weeks gestational age. After this it enlarges up to a maximum of 1.9 mm (30).

SULCATION. MRI knowledge of sulcation and gyration is expanding and the addition of a recent MRI atlas has helped (31), as prior to this, comparison was made to histological atlases where the fetal brain had been fixed. There have also been several recent papers on development of the brain which provide essential information for anyone wanting to perform and interpret fetal MRI. It is important to realize that there is individual variation for the pattern and time of development (32) and that co-existing pathology may influence development (29,33). The primary sulci: interhemispheric, calcarine, sylvian, parieto-occipital fissures, and the cingulate sulcus have developed by 22 weeks gestational age (Fig. 5) and all the main sulci are visible by 28 weeks. Opercularization of the insula starts at 20 weeks and continues until term. The secondary and tertiary sulci develop after 28 weeks.

PARENCHYMA. At 23 to 28 weeks the multilayered pattern of the cerebral parenchyma is seen (Fig. 6). On T2 weighted images these are:

Innermost low signal germinal matrix in a periventricular distribution
High signal deep intermediate zone
Low signal migrating cells
High signal superficial intermediate zone
Outermost low signal cortical ribbon.

These layers are clearly seen on post-mortem fetal images (see chap. 4.5). The low signal layers are reported to be due to the high cellularity and gradual reduction in thickness with increasing gestational age until 28 weeks (34). Low signal is seen in areas that start to myelinate, e.g., thalami and pallidi by 27 weeks and caudate and putamen by 34 weeks (Fig. 7) (35), brain stem at 23 weeks, posterior limb internal capsule by 31 weeks optic radiations by 35 weeks (35). The corpus callosum has been reported to develop by 20 weeks (36) but this has not always been seen in our experience and we would be reluctant to report partial agenesis of the corpus callosum before 24 weeks.

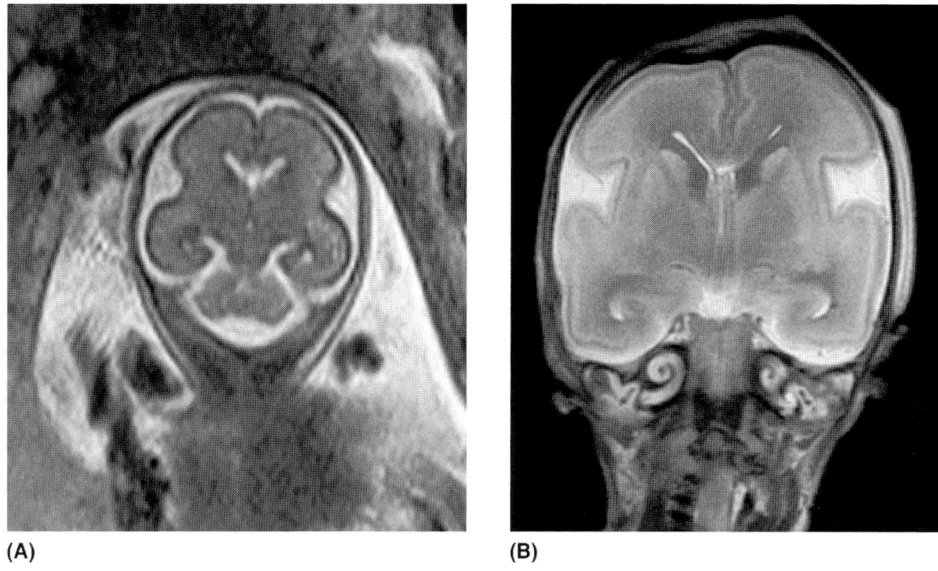

(A)   (B)

Figure 5. (**A**) T2W coronal image at 26 weeks gestational age. The sylvian fissure is open and square-shaped, interhemispheric fissure is seen. (**B**) T2W post-mortem image (coronal), the sylvian fissure and interhemispheric fissure are clearly seen. The cingulate fissure is seen as a small indentation.

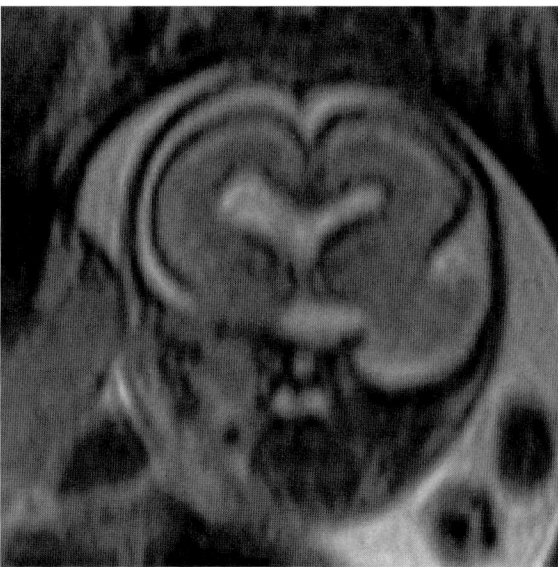

Figure 6. Coronal in utero image demonstrating the layers of the migrating neurons.

The trigone of the cerebral ventricles is normally less than 10 mm throughout pregnancy. There is a physiological hydrocephalus until 25 weeks, where the trigone is less than 10 mm, but due to the small cerebral size the ventricles appear large. This may persist at the level of the occipital horns until 30 weeks (35).

SAGITTAL SECTION. Midline. This clearly demonstrates the anatomy of the midline structures and is particularly useful for the corpus callosum. It also shows the central, calcarine, and cingulated sulci (Fig. 8).

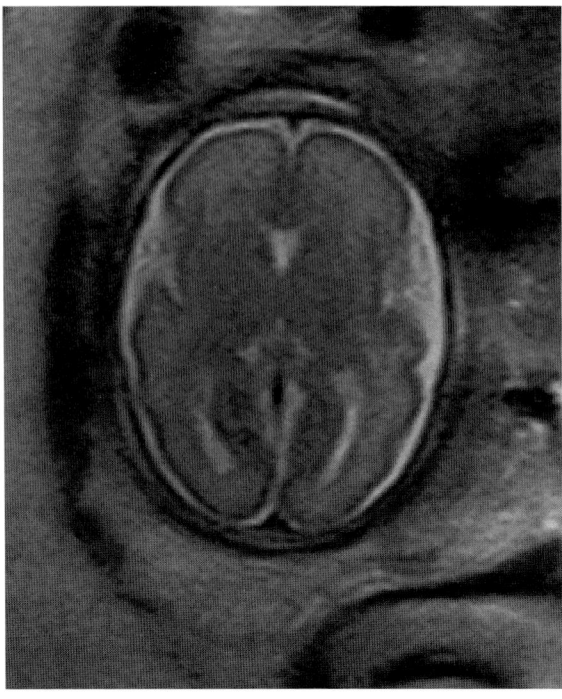

Figure 7. Axial T2W image. There is low signal in the thalami and pallidi due to myelination here.

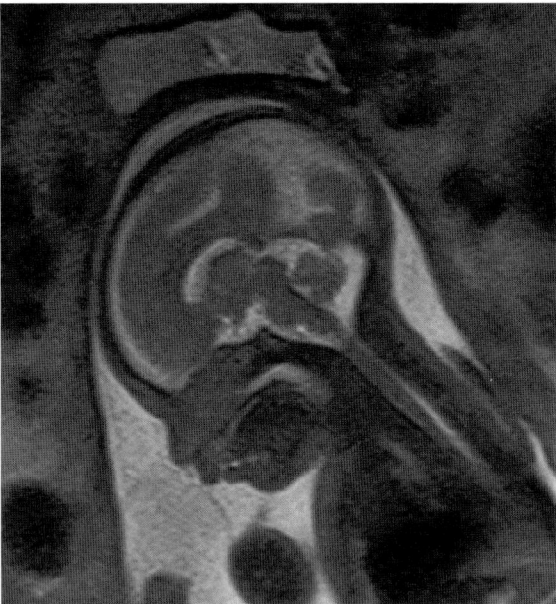

Figure 8. T2W sagittal image. The central sulcus, calcarine sulcus, and cingulate sulcus can all be seen.

RIGHT AND LEFT OF MIDLINE. These slices allow detection and assessment of the ventricles, the periventricular regions and the choroid plexus. They also provide information on the sulci and gyri as they develop (Fig. 9).

CORONAL SECTION. This is useful for the corpus callosum and cavum septum pellucidum as they can be seen clearly on each slice and followed throughout their length.

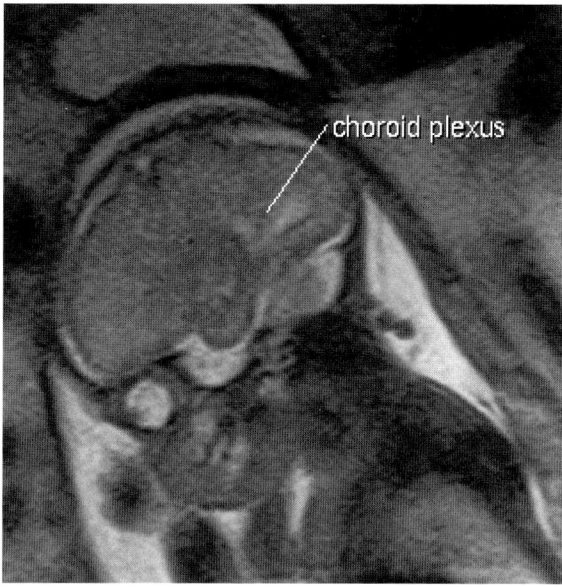

Figure 9. Parasagittal section T2W: the choroid plexus is seen within the posterior horn of the lateral ventricle.

The diameter of the ventricles can be measured at the level of the trigones and this should be done on both the coronal and the axial slices. The position of the choroid plexi can be clearly seen. The coronal section is also useful to assess the developing sulci and gyri especially the sylvian fissure, which is wide and open in the second trimester (Fig. 10A,B).

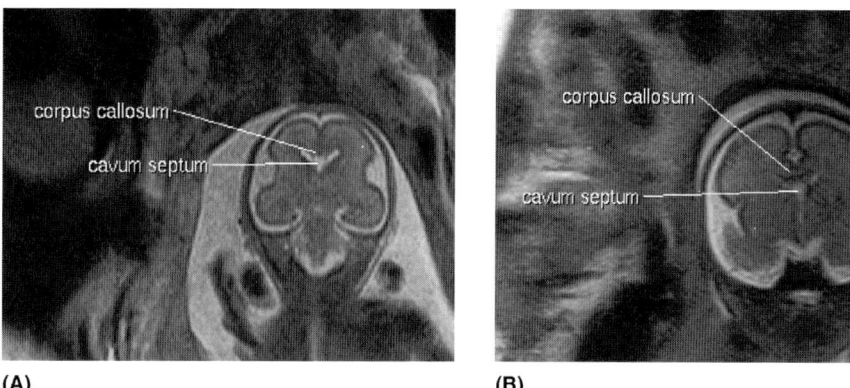

(A)   **(B)**

Figure 10. (A) T2W at 22 weeks gestational age. Note the square and open sylvian fissure and the corpus callosum. **(B)** T2W 34 weeks gestational age fetus. The sylvian fissure is closing and the corpus callosum and cavum septum pellucidum are clearly seen.

These slices show the developing germinal matrix and its migration out towards the periphery with increasing gestational age. The five layers can be identified and consist of outer, intermediate, and inner high signal with intervening low signal on the T2 weighted image.

AXIAL. The rostrum and splenium of the corpus callosum can be identified, the ventricles can be seen and their size measured at the level of the trigone, providing a useful second measurement to that one taken in the coronal plane. The periventricular regions and the germinal matrix can be identified and the layers of the developing cerebral parenchyma seen (Fig. 11A,B).

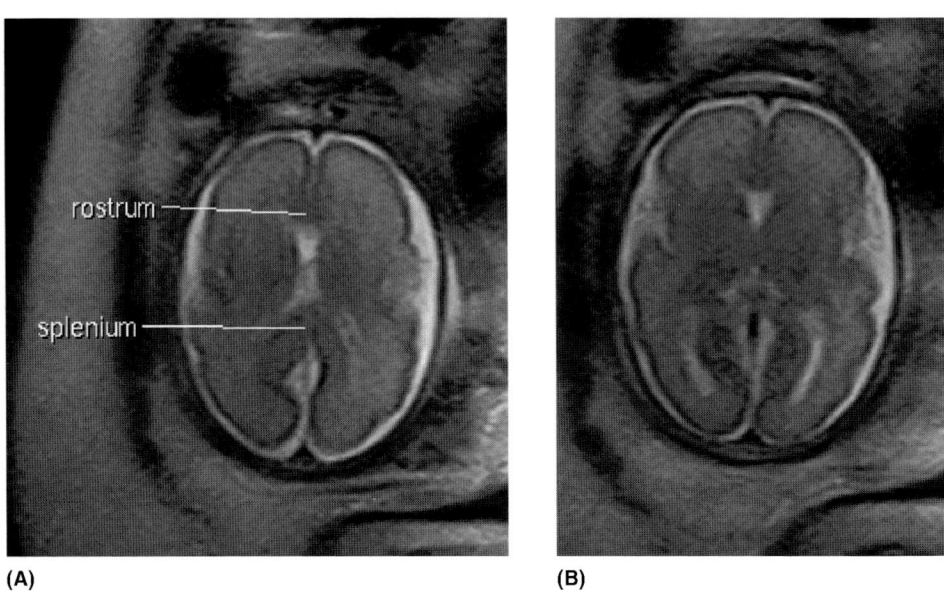

(A)   **(B)**

Figure 11. (A) Axial T2W section demonstrating the splenium and rostrum of the corpus callosum. **(B)** Axial T2W image. There are layers of different shades of gray from the periventricular region outwards that are bands of migrating neurons from the germinal matrix.

The optimal time for sulcal gyral delineation appears to be 28–32 weeks. Prior to this there is little development and after this the subarachnoid space is small and differentiation of the sulci can be difficult.

INFRATENTORIAL. The development of the cerebellum is dealt with in chap. 1.4.

The cerebellum develops after the bony posterior fossa. The theory of its development was put forward by McLone et al. (37). This was based on observations of the development of Chiari 2 malformations in fetuses with an open myelomeningocele. He suggested that a build-up of CSF pressure was required to expand the bony posterior fossa and that if this did not occur, as in cases where the CSF could leak out continuously, the posterior fossa did not expand and the growth of the cerebellum that followed was normal but squashed into too small a space, hence the tonsillar herniation. Recent work on both in utero images and post-mortem fetal images showed that this is most likely the case, as fetuses with open myelomeningoceles have small posterior fossas (38).

When measuring the posterior fossa to assess size we use anatomical landmarks. The venous confluence internally corresponds with the insertion of the neck muscles externally. If the venous confluence is elevated the posterior fossa is often enlarged. A line drawn from the venous confluence usually runs along the hard palate (Fig. 12) and provides a useful way to assess the size of the posterior fossa in clinical practice.

Spine

Normal Anatomy

It is difficult to see the verterbrae on in utero MRI and until additional image sequences are available, this is better visualized with ultrasound. However the spinal cord,

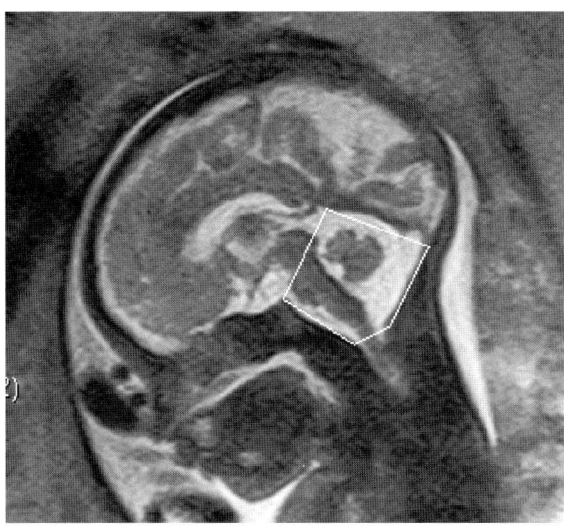

Figure 12. Normal posterior fossa. The venous confluence internally is at the same level as the insertion of the neck muscles externally.

surrounding CSF and musculature are seen clearly with MRI. The role of MRI is becoming increasingly important with the increase in in utero spinal surgery. Selection criteria for in utero spinal surgery in cases of spinabifida include a gestational age less than 26 weeks, Chiari 2 malformation, normal foot movements and no deformities of the feet, and a level of the lesion above S1. Despite over 200 cases worldwide, the indications and utility are not yet fully evaluated. There is evidence to suggest that the fetuses operated on in utero have a reversal of the Chiari 2 malformation and better foot movements post-natally than would be predicted from the prenatal imaging studies. Also a smaller percentage require shunting than expected. The Chiari 2 malformation is a developmental lesion that occurs later in pregnancy than the primary defect so that in utero surgery should prevent this. In addition, the surgical procedure prevents the neural placode getting contaminated in later pregnancy by amniotic fluid metabolites and possibly even meconium. It also reduces direct trauma against the uterine wall, etc. The majority of the initial patients who had in utero surgery have gone on to develop tethered cords and some have developed inclusion cysts requiring further surgery. Assessment prior to surgery is essential. The initial assessment is done with ultrasound and this is vital to establish the presence of normal leg movements. The spinal defect can be seen with ultrasound, but T2 weighted MR imaging gives detail on the site and state of the spinal cord and ideal visualization of the cerebellum and any Chiari formation both pre- and post-treatment. It is vital to assess all available information including alpha feto protein (AFP) levels.

A consortium of three American institutions has proposed a randomized unblinded controlled trial of in utero treatment of spina bifida. This should establish if the in utero surgery is of benefit or not. In utero MRI of the spine has also been reported to be useful in cases of diastomatomyelia where the diagnosis is made from ultrasound on direct and indirect signs but can be confirmed on MRI. MRI will directly demonstrate the split cord, provide detailed anatomical information, and is useful to detect other somatic malformations. Postnatal MRI allows accurate detection of all aspects of the lumbasacral dysraphism.

Yet another situation where in utero MRI of the spine has been suggested but not proven as yet is in cases where there is thought to be a lipoma of the spinal cord. Occasionally on ultrasound these may have lower echogenicity than expected and could be confused with a myelomeningocele. In utero MRI would provide a second line imaging modality to reduce such a misdiagnosis. It also allows additional imaging of the fetal genitourinary system.

Sagittal Section

With increasing gestational age it is difficult to obtain a complete spine on a single sagittal section, but the fetus should be imaged such that the entire spine is seen, even if this requires serial images. The termination of the spinal cord should be identified and its anatomical level assessed. The position of the cord and its width should be assessed throughout its length. There is a normal increase in width of the cord at the level of the cevical spine and filum. The position of the increase in width is dependent on fetal position to some extent, but a cord that is persistently pulled towards the ventral surface may be tethered or split. The entire cord should also be imaged in the coronal section to assess the position, width, and termination point. Any areas of concern should be imaged in the axial section.

Images produced do not show the vertebra, but abnormalities of the vertebrae resulting in abnormal positioning of the spinal cord and fetus will be identified.

Figures 13–16 demonstrate the utility of in utero MRI to demonstrate the spinal canal and cord. The normal appearances are shown on Figure 13 (sagittal section) and Figure 14 (axial) section. Figure 15A,B demonstrate a lumbar myelomeningocele. The defect in the back is seen best on the axial image (Fig. 15B) where there is a lack of bone and muscle covering the spinal canal. On the sagittal image (Fig. 15A) a gray line can be seen in the fluid filled "cyst" at the level of the bony defect and this is neural tissue.

In cases with an open myelomeningocele it has been noticed that the extra axial CSF space seen in normal fetuses is lost (Fig. 16A,B). This is seen prior to the development of a Chiari 2 malformation and is only seen in cases with an axial myelomeningocele or meningocele. At present it is uncertain whether this represents a stage prior to the development of a Chiari 2 malformation or a different subgroup of patients. Some patients have myelomeningocele and normal extra axial CSF space but this is the minority in our experience. Prospective studies are required to assess this further.

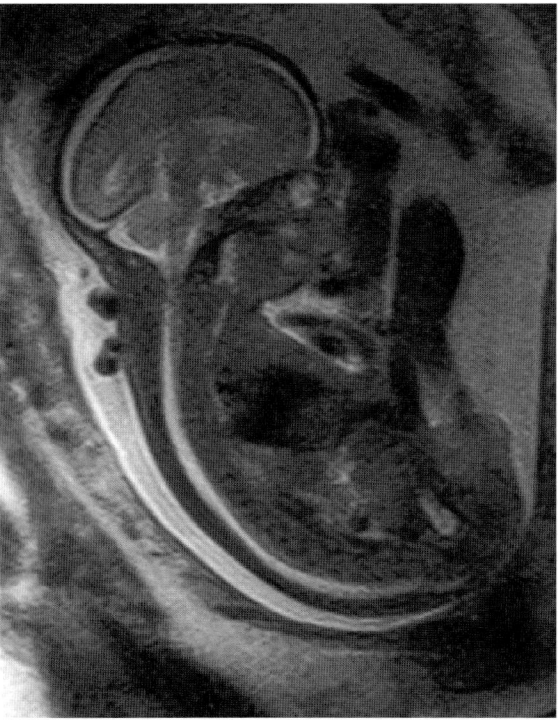

Figure 13. Sagittal spine T2W. The spinal cord is dark, the CSF bright. The vertebral bodies can be seen but in limited detail. The continuity of the covering muscles and skin is easily seen.

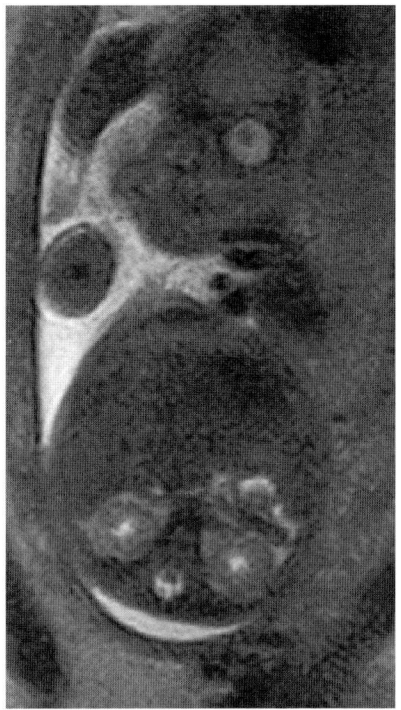

Figure 14. Axial section through the spinal cord. Only small sections can be imaged at a time due to the normal curved position of the baby. The spinal cord is seen as a central dark area surrounded by "bright" CSF.

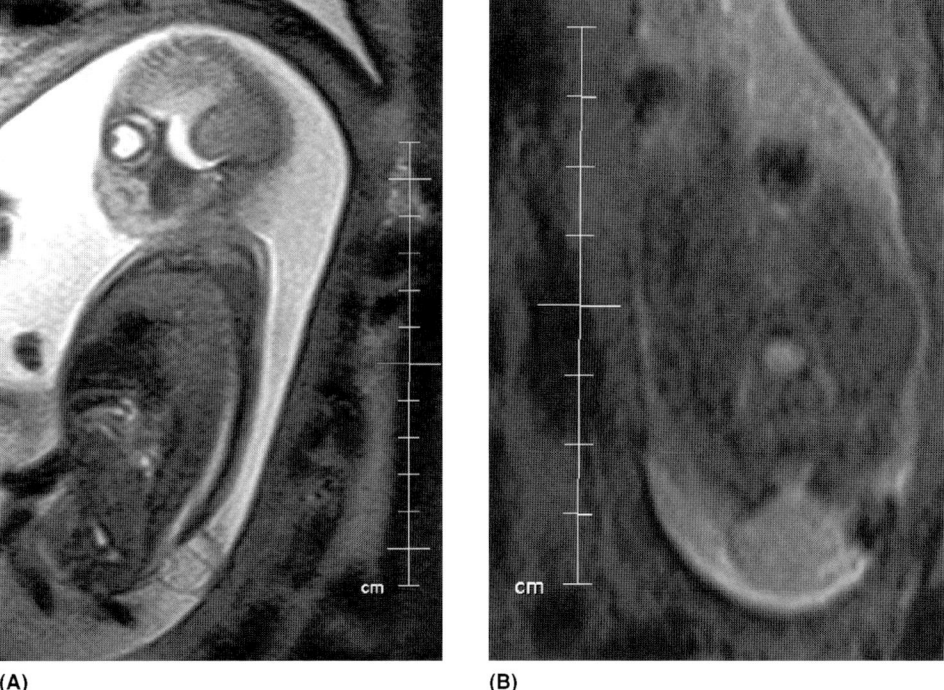

(A)   (B)

Figure 15. (**A**) Sagittal section through a 20-week fetus with a lower lumbar open myelomeningocele. The strand of dark signal seen in the fluid filled myelomeningocele is neural tissue. (**B**) Axial section through the defect: The spinal canal axial section through the spine. The spinal cord is seen as a central dark circle surrounded by bright CSF.

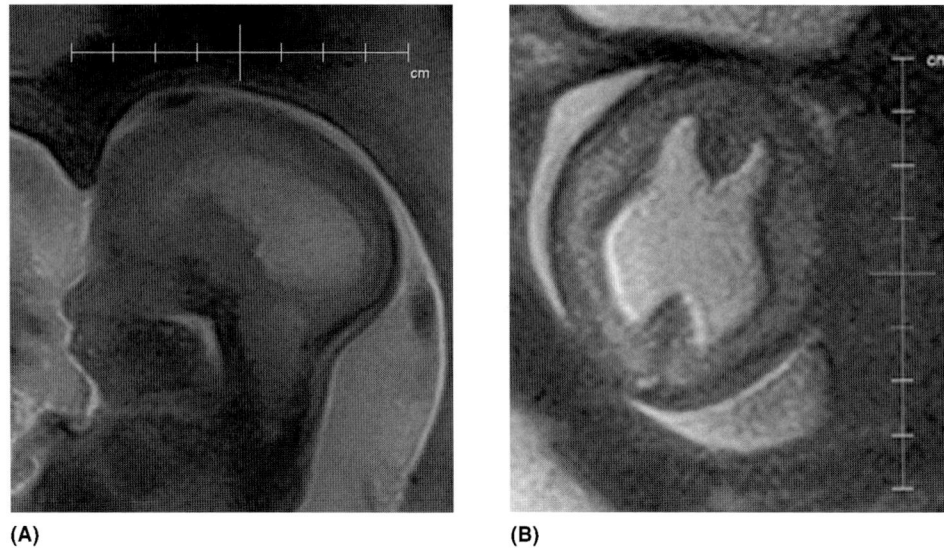

(A)　　　　　　　　　　　　　　　　　**(B)**

Figure 16. (**A**) Sagittal section Chiari 2 malformation and no extraaxial CSF space. (**B**) Axial section. Note the complete lack of extraaxial CSF.

At present there is little evidence to suggest that fetal MRI of the spinal cord provides any additional diagnostic information over that available from ultrasound. However, most authors who have looked at using in utero MRI in spinal cases agree that it provides additional anatomical detail and reassurance of the diagnosis made from ultrasound that allows counseling of the patient. It also helps reduce the likelihood of an erroneous diagnosis, especially if termination of pregnancy is considered.

Some workers advocate that the in utero MRI should not only image the body region requested by the ultrasonographic staff but should include a whole body scan. We do not routinely do this for several reasons. It would be difficult to cover the entire body in a safe time and without exposing the patient to high SAR levels. If a limited body scan were performed it would be unlikely to detect additional pathology unseen at ultrasound. Our group works as a team assessing as many relevant clinical factors as possible as well as the MRI and find that, unless the condition detected has associated pathologies, a whole body scan is unlikely to detect additional unexpected lesions. However, the development or rapid parallel MRI techniques may in future make the possibility of fetal whole body screening a reality.

REFERENCES

1. Weinreb JC, Lowe TW, Santos-Ramos R, Cunningham FG, Parkey R. Magnetic resonance imaging in obstetric diagnosis. Radiology 1985; 154:157–161.
2. Williamson RA, Weiner CP, Yuh WT, Abu-Yousef MM. Magnetic resonance imaging of anomalous fetuses. Obstet Gynecol 1989; 73:952–956.
3. Stehling MK, Mansfield P, Ordidge RJ, et al. Echo-planar imaging of the human fetus in utero. Magn Reson Med 1990; 13:314–318.
4. Hennig J, Nauerth A, Friedburg H. RARE imaging: a fast imaging method for clinical MRI. Magn Reson Med 1986; 3:823–833.
5. Rofsky NM, Pizzarello DJ, Weinreb JC, Ambrosino MM, Rosenberg C. Effect on fetal mouse development of exposure to MR imaging and gadopentetate dimeglumine. J Magn Reson Imaging 1994; 4:805–807.
6. Stazzone MM, Hubbard AM, Bilaniuk LT, et al. Ultrafast MR imaging of the normal posterior fossa in fetuses. AJR Am J Roentgenol 2000; 175:835–839.

7. Fogliarini C, Chaumoitre K, Chapon F, et al. Assessment of cortical maturation with prenatal MRI Part II: abnormalities of cortical maturation. Eur Radiol 2005.

8. Hubbard AM, Adzick NS, Crombleholme TM, et al. Congenital chest lesions: diagnosis and characterization with prenatal MR imaging. Radiology 1999; 212:43–48.

9. Garel C, Mizouni L, Menez F, et al. Prenatal diagnosis of a cystic type IV sacrococcygeal teratoma mimicking a cloacal anomaly: contribution of MRI. Prenat Diagn 2005; 25:216–219.

10. Heerschap A, Kok RD, van den Berg PP. Antenatal proton MRI spectroscopy of the human brain in vivo. Childs Nerv Syst 2003; 19:418–421.

11. Fenton BW, Lin CS, Macedonia C, Schellinger D, Ascher S. The fetus at term: in utero volume-selected proton MRI spectroscopy with a breath-hold technique—a feasibility study. Radiology 2001; 219:563–566.

12. Kok RD, van den Bergh AJ, Heerschap A, Nijland R, van den Berg PP. Metabolic information from the human fetal brain obtained with proton magnetic resonance spectroscopy. Am J Obstet Gynecol 2001; 185:1011–1015.

13. Hykin J, Moore R, Duncan K, et al. Fetal brain activity demonstrated by functional magnetic resonance imaging. Lancet 1999; 354:645–646.

14. Roelants-van Rijn AM, Groenendaal F, Stoutenbeek P, van der Grond J. Lactate in the foetal brain: detection and implications. Acta Paediatr 2004; 93:937–940.

15. Kreis R, Ernst T, Ross BD. Development of the human brain: in vivo quantification of metabolite and water content with proton magnetic resonance spectroscopy. Magn Reson Med 1993; 30:424–437.

16. Kubik-Huch RA, Wildermuth S, Cettuzzi L, et al. Fetus and uteroplacental unit: fast MR imaging with three-dimensional reconstruction and volumetry—feasibility study. Radiology 2001; 219:567–573.

17. Schierlitz L, Dumanli H, Robinson JN, et al. Three-dimensional magnetic resonance imaging of fetal brains. Lancet 2001; 357:1177–1178.

18. Fulford J, Vadeyar SH, Dodampahala SH, et al. Fetal brain activity in response to a visual stimulus. Hum Brain Mapp 2003; 20:239–245.

19. Fulford J, Vadeyar SH, Dodampahala SH, et al. Fetal brain activity and hemodynamic response to a vibroacoustic stimulus. Hum Brain Mapp 2004; 22:116–121.

20. Gowland P, Fulford J. Initial experiences of performing fetal MRI. Exp Neurol 2004; 1:S22–S27. 190 Suppl.

21. Paley MNJ, Lee KJ, Wild JM, Fichele S. Simultaneous parallel inclined readout image technique. British Chapter ISMRIM. Edinburgh 2004 p. 26.

22. Lee KJ, Wild JM, Griffiths PD, Paley MN. Simultaneous multi-slice imaging with slice-multiplexed RF pulses. Magnetic resonance in medicine, 2005; 54:755–760.

23. Kok RD, de Vries MM, Heerschap A, van den Berg PP. Absence of harmful effects of magnetic resonance exposure at 1.5 T in utero during the third trimester of pregnancy: a follow-up study. Magn Reson Imaging 2004; 22:851–854.

24. Myers C, Duncan KR, Gowland PA, Johnson IR, Baker PN. Failure to detect intrauterine growth restriction following in utero exposure to MRI. Br J Radiol 1998; 71:549–551.

25. Clements H, Duncan KR, Fielding K, Gowland PA, Johnson IR, Baker PN. Infants exposed to MRI in utero have a normal pediatric assessment at 9 months of age. Br J Radiol 2000; 73:190–194.

26. Baker PN, Johnson IR, Harvey PR, Gowland PA, Mansfield P. A three-year follow-up of children imaged in utero with echo-planar magnetic resonance. Am J Obstet Gynecol 1994; 170:32–33.

27. Carnes KI, Magin RL. Effects of in utero exposure to 4.7 T MR imaging conditions on fetal growth and testicular development in the mouse. Magn Reson Imaging 1996; 14:263–274.

28. Glover P, Hykin J, Gowland P, Wright J, Johnson I, Mansfield P. An assessment of the intrauterine sound intensity level during obstetric echo-planar magnetic resonance imaging. Br J Radiol 1995; 68:1090–1094.

29. Levine D, Barnes PD, Sher S, et al. Fetal fast MR imaging: reproducibility, technical quality, and conspicuity of anatomy. Radiology 1998; 206:549–554.

30. Hertzberg BS, Kliewer MA, Freed KS, et al. Third ventricle: size and appearance in normal fetuses through gestation. Radiology 1997; 203:641–644.

31. Garel C. MRI of the Fetal Brain. Heidelberg: Springer, 2004.

32. Chong BW, Babcook CJ, Pang D, Ellis WG. A magnetic resonance template for normal cerebellar development in the human fetus. Neurosurgery 1997; 41:924–928 discussion 928–929.
33. Levine D, Barnes PD. Cortical maturation in normal and abnormal fetuses as assessed with prenatal MR imaging. Radiology 1999; 210:751–758.
34. Brisse H, Fallet C, Sebag G, Nessmann C, Blot P, Hassan M. Supratentorial parenchyma in the developing fetal brain: in vitro MRI study with histologic comparison. AJNR Am J Neuroradiol 1997; 18:1491–1497.
35. Girard N, Raybaud C, Poncet M. In vivo MRI study of brain maturation in normal fetuses. AJNR Am J Neuroradiol 1995; 16:407–413.
36. Hansen PE, Ballesteros MC, Soila K, Garcia L, Howard JM. MR imaging of the developing human brain. Part 1. Prenatal development. Radiographics 1993; 13:21–36.
37. McLone DG, Dias MS. The Chiari 2 malformation: cause and impact. Childs Nerv Syst 2003; 19:540–550.
38. Griffiths PD, Wilkinson ID, Variend S, Jones A, Paley MN, Whitby E. Differential growth rates of the cerebellum and posterior fossa assessed by post mortem magnetic resonance imaging of the fetus: implications for the pathogenesis of the chiari 2 deformity. Acta Radiol 2004; 45:236–242.

2.4

In Utero Magnetic Resonance Imaging of Developmental Abnormalities of the Fetal CNS

Elspeth H. Whitby
Academic Unit of Radiology, University of Sheffield, Sheffield, U.K.

Abnormalities can be classified in several ways but here we will use the classification based on embryological stages explained in chap. 1.2 and confine this to supratentorial structures as cerebellar abnormalities are dealt with in chap. 1.4.

PRIMARY NEURALATION

Cases of anencephaly are detected accurately on booking ultrasound examinations and do not get referred for in utero magnetic resonance imaging (MRI).

Cephaloceles are less easily defined by ultrasound and the contents of the lesion are best defined by in utero MRI. Cephaloceles occur predominantly in the occipital (70%) (Figs. 1 and 2) or frontal regions (15%). In North American and European countries these are rarely basil or sphenoidal (Fig. 3) but these are more frequent in Asia and Latin America, Africa, and Australia. They contain meninges, cerebrospinal fluid (CSF) and sometimes cerebral parenchyma. The prognosis depends on the contents of the sac (parenchyma or not) and the amount of tissue within the sac, the development of hydrocephalus, the state of the development of the brain and the effects of distortion and destruction of the adjacent brain within the skull vault, and any co-existing abnormalities. These include chromosomal disorders, e.g., trisomy 13, 18, and 13q, or 16q deletions and syndromes (1–3). Other associated malformations include Dandy–Walker and Klippel-Feil syndrome (4). Renal, respiratory, and cardiac abnormalities are also seen. 60–80% of babies with a cephalocoele and no brain tissue in the sac develop normally whilst this figure is reduced to 10–20% when there is brain tissue within the sac. Babies with hydrocephalus do less well than those without.

In utero MRI will clearly define the contents of the cephalocoele detected on ultrasound whilst it may be difficult to distinguish an encephalocele from a meningocele by ultrasound. Ultrasound relies on the detection of a skull defect to make the diagnosis and this may be difficult in cases with for example a cephalic presentation or oligohydramnios. The differential diagnosis on ultrasound would include an epidermoid cyst, vascular malformation, teratoma or hygroma.

VENTRAL INDUCTION

Abnormal ventral induction results in holoprosencephaly due to abnormal expansion and cleavage. There is a wide spectrum of abnormalities that fall into this category as described by DeMyer (5). In the severest form, alobar holoprosencephaly, there is

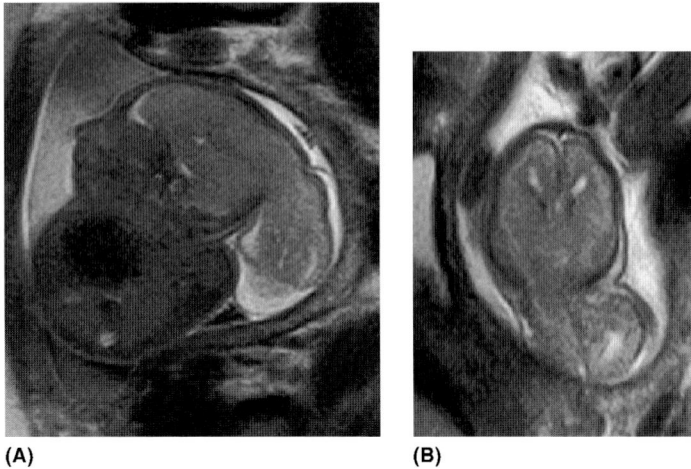

(A)   (B)

Figure 1. Large occipital cephalocele containing meninges, CSF and parenchyma (occipital encephalocele) at 23 weeks gestational age. (**A**) Sagittal section; (**B**) axial section.

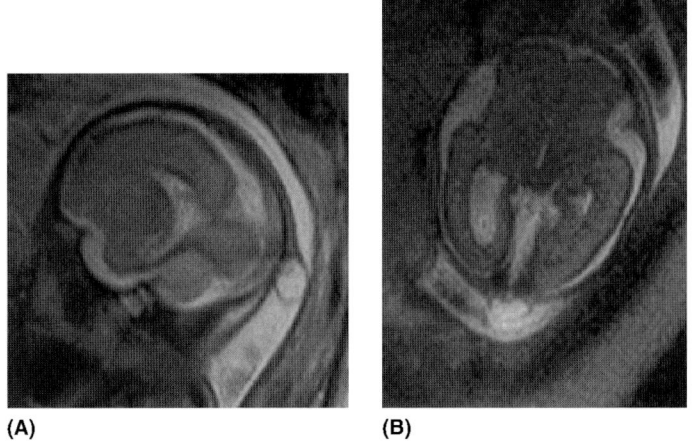

(A)   (B)

Figure 2. Small occipital cephalocele containing meninges and CSF only. The brain looks normal (occipital meningocele). Images are at 24 weeks gestational age. Further images were obtained at 32 weeks gestational age. The diagnosis was confirmed after delivery. (**A**) Sagittal section: The continuity with the CSF is difficult to see on this image and the defect in the skull was small. (**B**) Axial section: The small defect in the skull can be seen.

virtually no sagittal cleavage of the forebrain. The thalami consist of a fused mass, the lateral ventricles form a monoventricle and there is no interhemispheric fissure or falx. The third ventricle is absent (Fig. 4). Many of these fetuses are aborted, those that go to delivery are frequently stillborn and long-term survival is not possible. At the less severe end of the DeMyer classification is lobar holoprosencephaly. The typical features of this disorder are poorly formed frontal lobes, frontal horns of lateral ventricles and anterior falx. These can produce comparatively subtle radiological findings but the septum pellucidum is always absent. Disorders that fall between the ends of the spectrum are called semilobar holoprosencephaly. The interhemispheric fissure and falx cerebri are partly present. The front of the brain is fused and

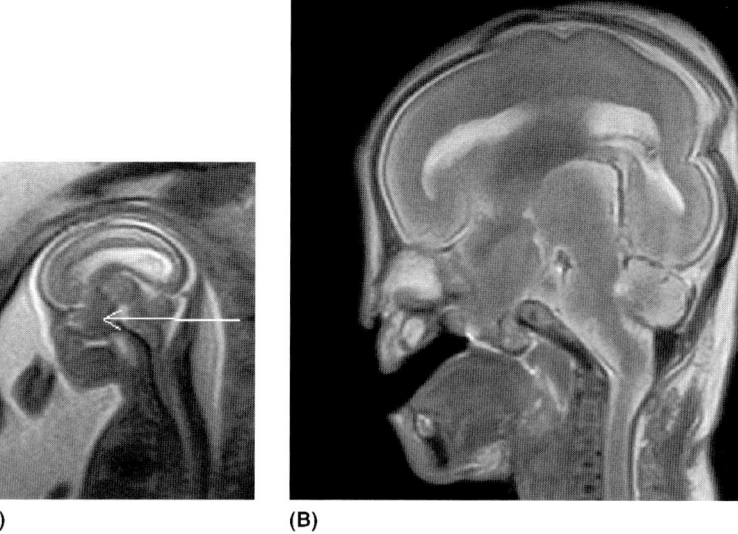

(A)   (B)

Figure 3. (**A**) Sphenoidal encephalocele (arrow) in a fetus with multiple developmental abnormalities at 20 weeks gestational age. The diagnosis was confirmed by post-mortem MRI. (**B**) Post-mortem MRI of (**A**), confirming the sphenoidal encephalocele and other complex abnormalities.

underdeveloped and the thalami are partly fused (Fig. 5). It is important to obtain good quality coronal images.

All forms of holoprosencephaly have an absence of the fornix and septum pellucidum. It can occur in numerous genetic conditions and is seen in 1–2% of children of diabetic mothers.

Ultrasound can detect the alobar form relatively easily at the 20 week anomaly scan but some cases have been mistaken for ventriculomegaly. Distinguishing between semilobar and alobar holoprosencephaly can be difficult and the lobar form is often not detected on ultrasound (6).

In our experience in utero MRI has detected numerous different types of holoprosencephaly when the referring ultrasound has detected ventriculomegaly, intracerebral cysts, abnormal facial features or absent septum pellucidum.

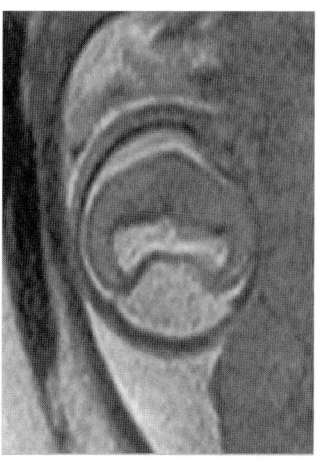

Figure 4. Alobar holoprosencephaly at 20 weeks gestational age. Confirmed at autopsy.

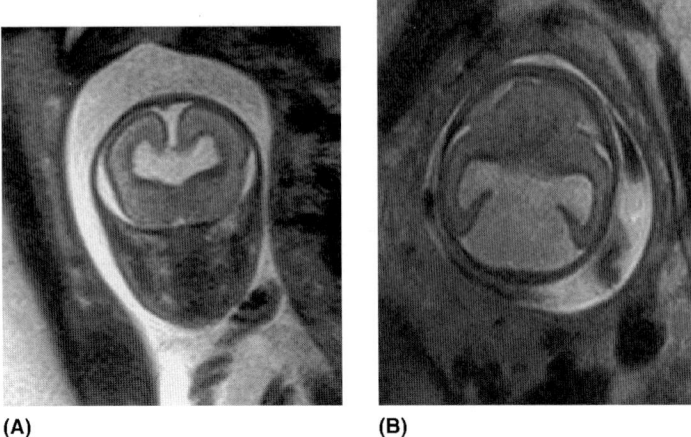

(A)   **(B)**

Figure 5. Semilobar holoprosencephaly at 23 weeks gestational age. (**A**) Coronal image. Note the attempt to form an interhemispheric fissure, the fused thalami, the absence of the septum pellucidum. (**B**) Axial image.

The prognosis is poor in all forms, even those not associated with genetic syndromes.

A variant of holoprosencephaly associated with the absence of the septum pellucidum is septo-optic dysplasia. It is difficult to define the optic nerves on in-utero MRI so even in the absence of the septum pellucidum there should be an air of caution to making this diagnosis although it should feature in the differential. Isolated absence of the septum pellucidum is rare but it is seen with other malformations most commonly agenesis of the corpus callosum, and basal encephaloceles or is ruptured due to severe hydrocephalus. Its absence has also been reported associated with hypoxic ischaemic lesions, e.g., schizencephaly (Fig. 6).

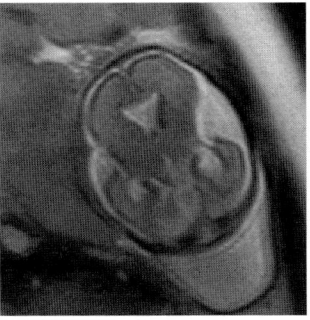

Figure 6. Septo optic dysplasia and schizencephaly at 20 weeks gestational age. Note the absence of the cavum septum pellucidum but the presence of the corpus callosum.

FAILURE OF COMMISSURATION

The largest commissural tract connecting the cerebral hemispheres is the corpus callosum. This genu develops first then the body then the splenium (posterior) and finally the rostrum (anterior), failure of development results in agenesis of the corpus callosum. The classical appearance of this is wide space lateral ventricles with straightening of the ventricular contours and in some cases dilatation of the posterior horns of the lateral ventricle to form the classic colpocephaly (Fig. 7). This does not

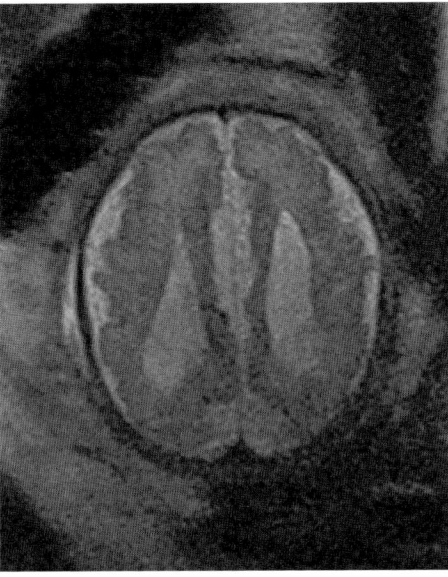

Figure 7. Axial section with dilated posterior horns of the lateral ventricles (colpocephaly).

always occur and isolated mild ventriculomegaly with normal configuration of the ventricles diagnosed on ultrasound may be associated with partial or complete agenesis. The corpus callosum should be fully formed by 20 weeks gestational age but in the authors experience it is difficult to make a diagnosis of complete or partial agenesis before 24 weeks gestational age as there can be a physiological delay in complete formation. In utero MR allows direct visualization of the corpus callosum, or its absence, in the sagittal section (Figs. 8 and 9) but the coronal and axial sections are also important to check the entirety of the structure. The coronal sections often demonstrate the Bundles of Probst (Fig. 10). Figures 8–10 are from a set of twins at 28 weeks gestational age. Hypertrophy of the hippocampal commisure may mimic the splenium of the corpus callosum but the attachment into the cerebral hemispheres is more lateral than a corpus callosum and connects to the fornices (Fig. 11). The typical lateral ventricle morphology of widespread ventricles and high-riding third ventricle is maintained. This is more easily demonstrated on MRI than ultrasound. In utero MRI allows direct visualization of the corpus callosum or it's absence and most authors agree that this appears easier and more accurate than with ultrasound. In utero MRI is

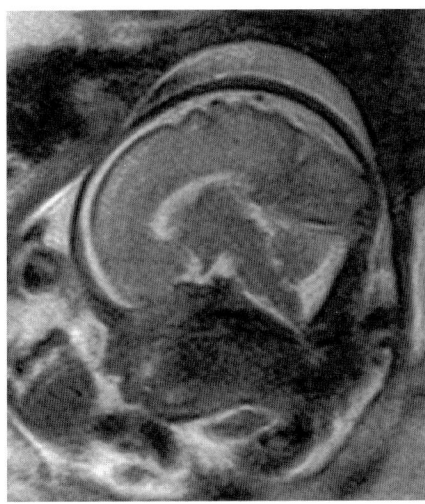

Figure 8. Sagittal section of normal corpus callosum.

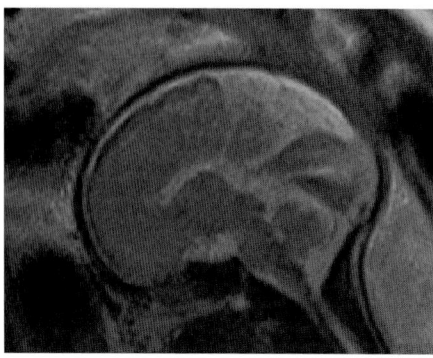

Figure 9. Sagittal section of the twin in Fig. 8 with complete agenesis of the corpus callosum. Note how the sulci enter the third ventricle.

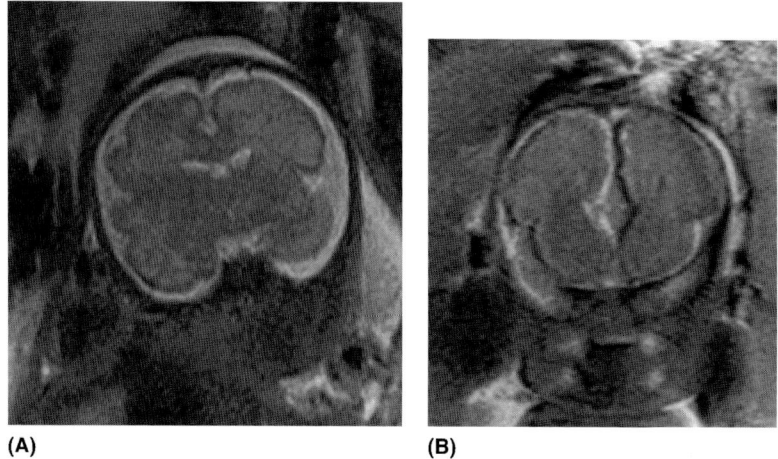

(A)   **(B)**

Figure 10. (**A**) Sagittal section of a normal twin at 28 weeks gestational age. (**B**) Coronal section with agenesis of the corpus callosum, twin of (**A**).

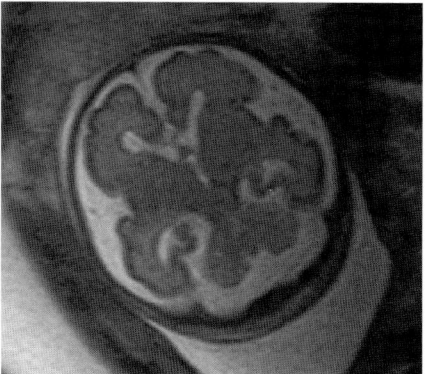

Figure 11. Coronal section. Absence of the corpus callosum, hypertrophy of the hippocampal commissure that connects to the fornices (arrow) and can be mistaken for the splenium of the corpus callosum.

valuable in cases where there is partial absence of the corpus callosum, which is a difficult diagnosis by ultrasound. In all cases there should be a careful search for associated abnormalities and MRI is especially useful for abnormalities of gyration not easily detected with ultrasound, although often only detectable in the thirds trimester. It is also associated with lipomas, interhemispheric cysts and syndromes such as Dandy–Walker.

The prognosis depends on the presence or absence of associated abnormalities but as mentioned above these may only be detectable in late gestation and decisions may need to be made prior to this. In cases of isolated agenesis of the corpus callosum there is still debate over the prognosis. The studies available are on small numbers and do not follow up the children for long. It is likely that there will be detectable abnormalities in all cases but these may be mild.

ABNORMALITIES ASSOCIATED WITH FAILURE OF COMMISSURATION

Dandy–Walker Malformation

This is a cerebellar abnormality and is dealt with in more detail in chap. 1.4. The classical Dandy–Walker malformation comprises of vermian agenesis, cystic enlargement of the fourth ventricle, enlargement of the posterior fossa and an elevated tentorium. Dandy–Walker variant comprises of some of the above, often a hypoplastic inferior cerebellar vermis. It is often associated with other malformations such as callosal dysgenesis, cephaloceles, and cortical migrational abnormalities (7–9).

Lipomas

Lipomas of the corpus callosum are rare and are usually associated with hypogenesis or agenesis of the corpus callosum (10). It is a hyper echoic mass on ultrasound, a high signal mass on T1 weighted MRI images and low signal on T2 weighted images. In utero MRI is useful to detect associated abnormalities especially those of gyration. The prognosis depends on the existence and type of associated abnormalities; in 50% of cases they are asymptomatic.

Abnormal Cortical Formation

Neurons migrate from the germinal matrix adjacent to the lateral ventricles outward to the cortex where they organize themselves into discrete layers and form their synaptic connections. Abnormal migration results in a range of cortical abnormalities including the following:

Microcephaly

This is defined as a head circumference greater than 2 standard deviations below the mean for gestational age. This is usually because of inadequate growth and development of the brain. It is usually associated with below average intelligence but not always (11,12). In some cases it is familial but most cases are sporadic (13).

A form of microcephaly is associated with normal sulcal and gyral formation and normal cortical thickness is termed radial microbrain. The total volume of the brain is approximately 30% of normal.

Microcephaly is often associated with other abnormalities including lissencephaly (Fig. 12A,B), porencephaly, holoprosencephaly, agenesis of the corpus callosum and ventriculomegaly.

Megalencephaly

This is a disorder of neuronal proliferation which results in increased size and weight of the brain, traditionally greater than two standard deviations above the mean. Hemimegalencephaly is when half of the brain is involved. This is often seen as unilateral ventriculomegaly on ultrasound. The ability of in utero MR to show the parenchyma clearly allows subtle cases of hemimegalencephaly to be detected. It occurs in a wide variety of disorders and syndromes (Klippel Trenaunay Weber, epidermal nevus and proteus syndromes) (14–16) and produces a broad spectrum of clinical abnormalities in

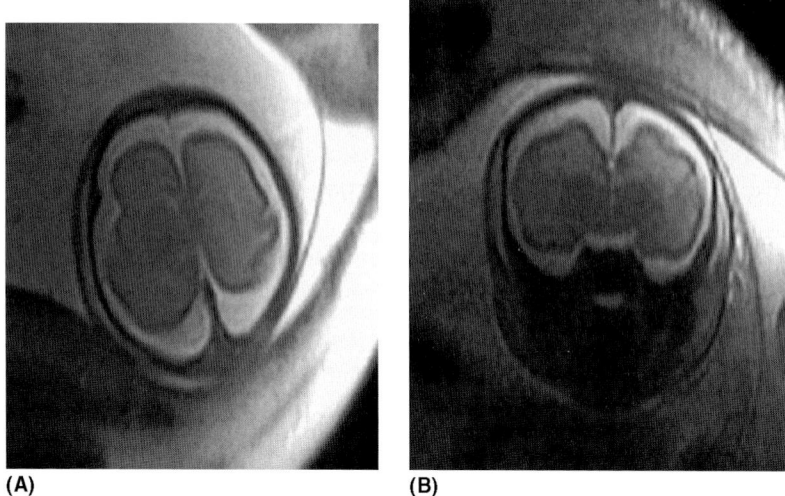

(A)   (B)

Figure 12. (A) and **(B)**. This fetus was 28 weeks gestational age. Both the skull size and the brain size were well below the 10th percentile but the body was normal in size. The brain development is also delayed and there is little evidence of migration compatible with a diagnosis of microcephaly and simplified gyral pattern (microlissencephaly).

motor and cognitive behavior. It is usually associated with migrational abnormalities including heterotopic parenchyma (Fig. 13A,B) and arrested migration (Fig. 14). In utero MR allows more accurate depiction of the asymmetry especially if the affected hemisphere is the one closest to the ultrasound transducer and not easily visualized. MR is also superior in detecting any polymicrogyria and potential heterotopias and gliosis.

Polymicrogyria

Subtle heterotopias may be missed on antenatal imaging. MRI has been shown to be more sensitive than ultrasound.

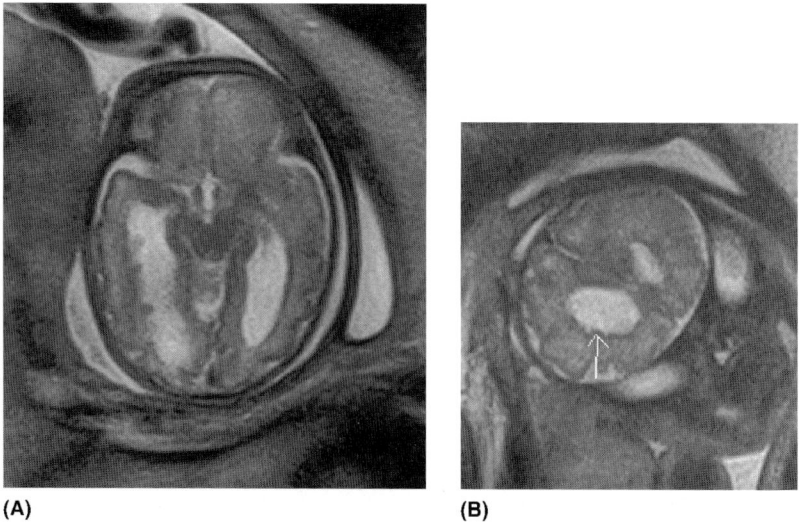

(A)   (B)

Figure 13. (A) and **(B)**. Hemimegalencephaly and heterotopic parenchyma—initially seen as an irregular ventricular margin on ultrasound (axial and coronal sections).

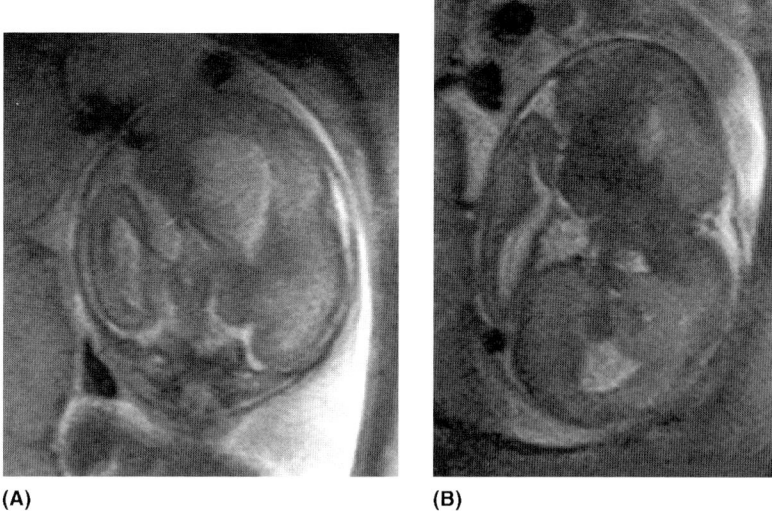

(A)   **(B)**

Figure 14. (**A**) Coronal section: the left hemisphere is grossly enlarged. The sagittal sinus can be seen as a low signal "dot" displaced to the right of the midline. Note the overgrowth of the skull. (**B**) Axial section.

Polymicrogyria may be present with or without laminar necrosis. It is a heterogeneous group of conditions due to over folding of the cortical ribbon with or without fusion of adjacent sulci. The form without laminar necrosis is thought to occur earlier than that with (12–17 weeks compared with 18–24 weeks). The distinction is made at the histological level, both appear the same on imaging. The cerebral cortex is poorly visualized by ultrasound making the diagnosis of polymicrogyria impossible. MRI however can directly visualize the developing cortex but care must be taken to ensure that the normal for each gestational age is known. Ideally the MRI should be done prior to the extra axial space becoming too small to allow detailed visualization of the sulci (this occurs around 34 weeks gestational age).

Polymicrogyria may occur anywhere but is most frequent around the sylvian fissure (17–19).

Lissencephaly

At present it is difficult to accurately detect lissencephaly in anything earlier than the third trimester. Partly this is due to the absence of a large database of normal variation in sulcal and gyral development and the knowledge that in utero MRI appears to lag behind histological knowledge of development by up to 8 weeks. This is thought to be due to the fact that thin sections are possible at autopsy and a small dimple is classed as evidence of sulcal formation. These are easily missed with MR imaging as the slices are 3 mm to 5 mm thick. The lissencephaly may affect the entire cortical surface or may be partial. The affected children almost always present with developmental retardation and seizures. The developing sulci are often abnormally orientated and the sylvian fissures lack opercularization (Figs. 15A,B and 16 A,B) (20).

Heterotopias

These are either subependymal or subcortical.

Subependymal heterotopias are better visualized with MRI than ultrasound. They may be focal or diffuse, unilateral or bilateral. They can be an isolated finding but are often associated with abnormalities, e.g., agenesis of the corpus callosum. They may be sporadic or hereditary with autosomal dominant, recessive or X-linked modes of

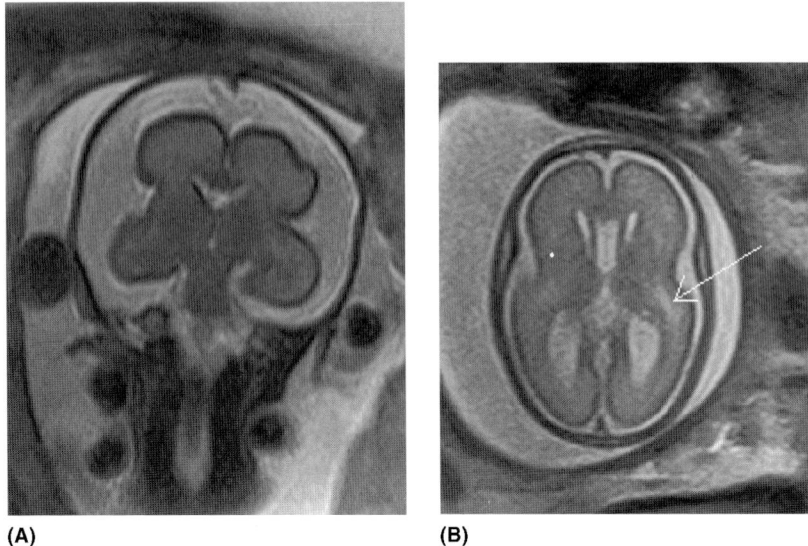

(A)   **(B)**

Figure 15. (**A**) and (**B**) 26 weeks gestational age by dates and scan but developmentally delayed with little sulcal and gyral formation. In addition there is an area of high signal (arrow) suggesting abnormal migration.

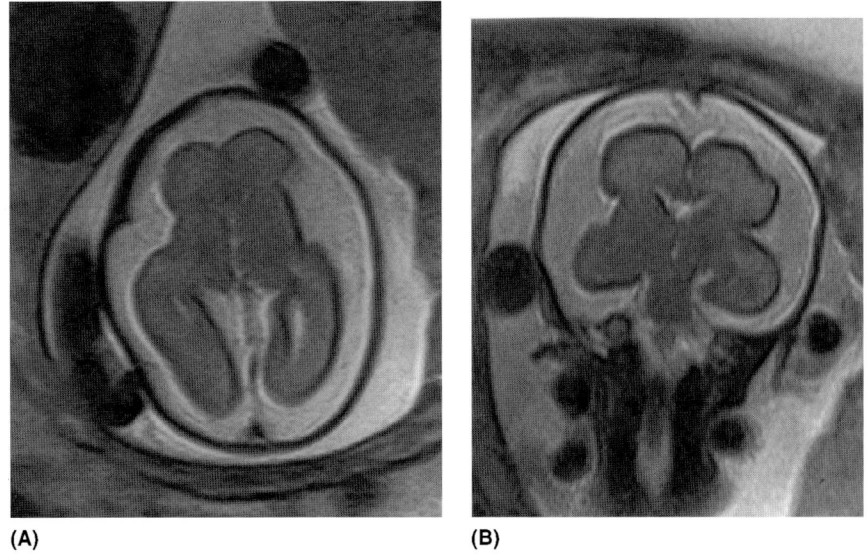

(A)   **(B)**

Figure 16. (**A**) and (**B**) 28 weeks gestational age. Delayed development of the sulci and gyri, only the sylvian fissure is seen to be developing. The overall head size is normal but the brain is small for gestational age resulting in a large extra-axial space.

inheritance. They are neurons which have failed to migrate normally. They can be seen as: Irregular walls of the ventricles (Fig. 13B), large nodules on the ventricular walls (Fig. 13A) or a periventricular band that is bright on ultrasound and high signal on T1 MRI (16,21).

Subcortical Heterotopias

These are thought to be due to interrupted migration and are sporadic in nature. It has been reported that the corpus callosum is dysgenic in 70% of cases (22). They are

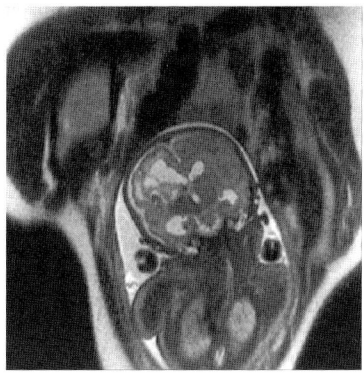

Figure 17. A 32-week gestational age fetus. There are cysts in the periventrilcular parenchyma in the right parietal region. There had previously been a large intraventricular-bleed with periventricular extension resulting in damage to the parenchyma.

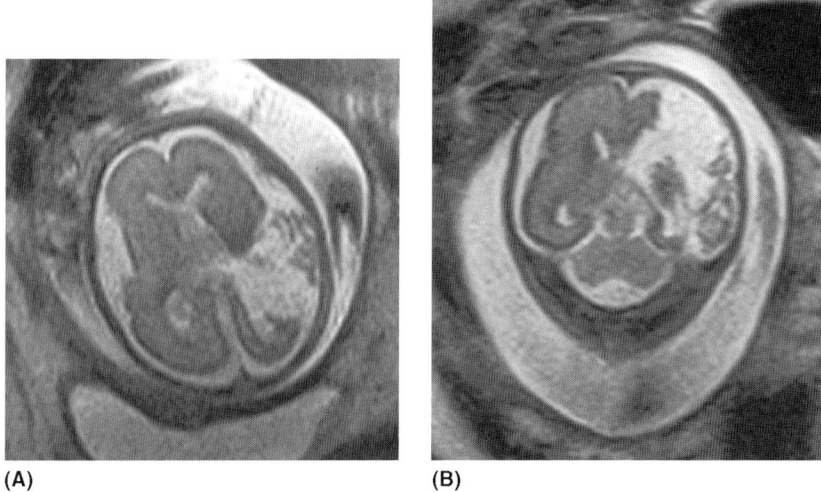

(A)   (B)

Figure 18. 26-week gestational age fetus with a destruction of the left parietal region following vascular infarction. (**A**) Axial section; (**B**) coronal section.

not common and difficult to visualize antenatally. MRI should be more accurate than ultrasound due to its ability to image the cortex in detail and visualize the different signal intensity bands formed by the migrating neurons.

ACQUIRED ABNORMALITIES

The majority of the work has been done on developmental abnormalities but the same techniques can be used to image acquired abnormalities. In our experience these tend to present later in gestation, often in the third trimester. Examples include periventricular leucomalacia following haemorrhage (Fig. 17), and vascular infarction (Fig. 18).

REFERENCES

1. Cohen MM, Jr., Lemire RJ. Syndromes with cephaloceles. Teratology 1982; 25:161–172.
2. Robson CD, Barnewolt CE. MR imaging of fetal head and neck anomalies. Neuroimaging Clin N Am 2004; 14:273–291.
3. Wininger SJ, Donnenfeld AE. Syndromes identified in fetuses with prenatally diagnosed cephaloceles. Prenat Diagn 1994; 14:839–843.

4. Bindal AK, Storrs BB, McLone DG. Occipital meningoceles in patients with the Dandy–Walker syndrome. Neurosurgery 1991; 28:844–847.

5. DeMyer W. Median facial malformations and their implications for brain malformations. Birth Defects Orig Artic Ser 1975; 11:155–181.

6. Peebles DM. Holoprosencephaly. Prenat Diagn 1998; 18:477–480.

7. Klein O. Dandy Walker. J Neurosurg 2005; 102:353–354.

8. Klein O, Pierre-Kahn A, Boddaert N, Parisot D, Brunelle F. Dandy–Walker malformation: prenatal diagnosis and prognosis. Childs Nerv Syst 2003; 19:484–489.

9. Adamsbaum C, Moutard ML, Andre C, et al. MRI of the fetal posterior fossa. Pediatr Radiol 2005; 35:124–140.

10. Ickowitz V, Eurin D, Rypens F, et al. Prenatal diagnosis and postnatal follow-up of pericallosal lipoma: report of seven new cases. AJNR Am J Neuroradiol 2001; 22:767–772.

11. Martin HP. Microcephaly and mental retardation. Am J Dis Child 1970; 119:128–131.

12. Sells CJ. Microcephaly in a normal school population. Pediatrics 1977; 59:262–265.

13. Cohen T, Zeitune M, McGillivray BC, et al. Segregation analysis of microcephaly. Am J Med Genet 1996; 65:226–234.

14. Tinkle BT, Schorry EK, Franz DN, Crone KR, Saal HM. Epidemiology of hemimegalencephaly: a case series and review. Am J Med Genet A 2005; 139:204–211.

15. Flores-Sarnat L. Hemimegalencephaly: part 1. Genetic, clinical, and imaging aspects. J Child Neurol 2002; 17:373–384; discussion 384.

16. Kuzniecky RI. Magnetic resonance imaging in developmental disorders of the cerebral cortex. Epilepsia 1994; 35:S44–S56.

17. Levine D, Barnes PD, Madsen JR, Li W, Edelman RR. Fetal central nervous system anomalies: MR imaging augments sonographic diagnosis. Radiology 1997; 204:635–642.

18. Glenn OA, Norton ME, Goldstein RB, Barkovich AJ. Prenatal diagnosis of polymicrogyria by fetal magnetic resonance imaging in monochorionic cotwin death. J Ultrasound Med 2005; 24:711–716.

19. Soussotte C, Maugey-Laulom B, Carles D, Diard F. Contribution of transvaginal ultrasonography and fetal cerebral MRI in a case of congenital cytomegalovirus infection. Fetal Diagn Ther 2000; 15:219–223.

20. Kojima K, Suzuki Y, Seki K, et al. Prenatal diagnosis of lissencephaly (type II) by ultrasound and fast magnetic resonance imaging. Fetal Diagn Ther 2002; 17:34–36.

21. Osborn RE, Byrd SE, Naidich TP, Bohan TP, Friedman H. MR imaging of neuronal migrational disorders. AJNR Am J Neuroradiol 1988; 9:1101–1106.

22. Billette de Villemeur T, Chiron C, Robain O. Unlayered polymicrogyria and agenesis of the corpus callosum: a relevant association? Acta Neuropathol (Berl) 1992; 83:265–270.

2.5

The Balance Between Magnetic Resonance Imaging and Ultrasound

Elspeth H. Whitby
Academic Unit of Radiology, University of Sheffield, Sheffield, U.K.

Ultrasound is an inexpensive high resolution flexible technique that has revolutionized prenatal diagnosis of fetal abnormalities. Alternative techniques may be used for cases where there is doubt over the diagnosis or additional detail is required for a definitive diagnosis to aid patient management. Computed tomography (CT) and x-ray techniques use ionizing radiation. Magnetic resonance imaging (MRI) is non-ionising and multiplanar.

There has been an exponential increase in the number of papers published on in utero MRI since the introduction of fast MRI techniques. However a lot of these are still case reports or small series and few have detailed follow-up data.

Ultrasound is highly observer dependent but there are plenty of specialist centers or tertiary referral centers where an expert opinion can be obtained. While the MRI scans are considered to be less operator dependent, in our experience, the more experienced the radiographer in performing in utero MRI the faster and better quality the MRI scan obtained. Our first scan had an on-table time of 83 minutes, while we routinely do a single area scan in 15–20 minutes now (1,2). The more experienced the radiologists the more likely they are to detect subtle abnormalities.

Although MRI produces images that are easily transferred to other centers or are readily available for doctors involved at all stages in the patient care, the interpretation of the images is not straightforward and this is the main problem at present. Interpretation requires an understanding of normal and abnormal findings and the types of pathology at each gestational age.

In our experience it is easiest to start with the third trimester pregnancies as radiologists likely to become involved in this type of work will have had experience in neonatal and/ or pediatric radiology. Prior to this stage the developing fetus is different from anything encountered and the pathologies are unique. It is also essential to build up a database of knowledge of normal at each gestational age. There have been two recent publications that provide essential data on normal fetal development and include some pathologies. These are ideal bench books for a department undertaking this kind of work (3).

In utero MRI should be seen as an adjuvant to the antenatal ultrasound in cases where there is diagnostic doubt or difficulty. MRI is poor for fast moving body parts and produces a shadow for the fetal heart due to its rapid movement. MRI can be used for limbs but this is technically difficult and usually much better visualized by ultrasound. MRI of the fetal brain provides detailed anatomical information due to the high contrast between the brain matter and the surrounding CSF. Certain pathological changes are better visualised on MRI, e.g., hemorrhage, posterior fossa abnormalities, cortical dysplasia, and heterotopias.

Acquired disorders are more challenging on both ultrasound and MRI. White matter damage may show initially as a loss of the normal layered pattern seen (especially the intermediate layer). Isolated germinal matrix insults result in an irregular ventricular wall and nodularity, although this is also seen with heterotopic gray matter. Ventricular dilatation often indicates the existence of associated lesions. Antenatal ultrasound has been reported to detect associated conditions in 15% of cases, in utero MRI detects associated abnormalities in 50% of cases.

Ultrasound and MRI should be used together along with other information to obtain a full picture for the patient and management team. In many cases this would include some or all of the following: genetic testing, virology, and bacteriology imaging, etc., and involvement of geneticists, pediatricians, pathologists, pediatric surgeons, radiologists, obstetricians etc.

SAFETY OF ULTRASOUND AND MRI

MRI Safety

The initial in utero MRI studies where the fetus was sedated or paralyzed use T1 weighted sequences. However, with the ultrafast technique the images are heavily T2 weighted. There is no evidence to suggest that exposure of the fetus to electromagnetic radiation is detrimental, but the current advice is to avoid MRI in the first trimester, only image with field strengths less than 2.5T, and keep the SAR as low as possible. Intravenous contrast is not advised due to the dechelation of the Gadolinium across the placenta and the recirculation of the Gadolinium in the amniotic fluid, thus increasing its half life. The SAR is maximal at the surface of the maternal body so the risk to the fetus is minimal due to the efficient heat-dissipating action of the amniotic fluid. There is also concern about the acoustic noise as the SSFSE technique has a noise level of almost 100 decibels. The mother is provided with ear protection but this is not possible for the fetus. However there have been no documented effects on follow-up studies but further studies with larger numbers are required to prove this (4–7). Animal studies have not been conclusive although some suggest that there are hazardous effects of repeated exposure to static (8) or fluctuating magnetic fields (9), prolonged exposure (10), or in utero exposure at high field (4.7T) (11). These studies do not accurately reflect the events of a single or repeated in utero examination in the clinical setting in the second or third trimester. The major concern is to detect intrauterine growth retardation. In addition, the noise level of the fast sequences has the potential to damage hearing, although amniotic fluid may reduce the acoustic noise by 30dB–50dB (12). The most recent information comes from a prospective study that followed up children who had been imaged in utero in the third trimester. Thirty-five children who were between one and three years age and nine children who were between eight and nine years of age at assessment were studied. These children had all undergone clinical scans in utero at 1.5T and in some cases the study also included PRESS and STEAM spectroscopy sequences in addition to T2 weighted imaging. Detailed follow-up was obtained together with a detailed neurological examination at three months of age. In all but two cases findings were normal. The abnormalities in these two cases may or may not be related to the MR imaging. No problems were detected with hearing (4). Although in this study no harmful effects were detected, total safety of the MRI technique can never be fully established. Further larger studies are required, especially when children reach reproductive age to assess if the reproductive tissues are affected by MR. Currently it is advisable to keep the field strength to 1.5T, use low SAR, keep scan times as short as possible and avoid scanning in the first trimester.

The medical devices agency advizes that "a decision to scan should be made at the time by the referring clinician, an MRI radiologist and the patient, based on information about risks versus benefit. Pregnant women should not be exposed above the advised lower levels of restriction, i.e., not to fields above 2.5T."

Safety of Ultrasound

The current data suggest that the use of diagnostic ultrasound is safe. However color Doppler, power, and pulsed Doppler should be used with caution. The main areas of concern are thermal effects and cavitation (13–15). Thermal effects occur due to the loss of energy from the sound wave due to a decrease in wave amplitude at tissue interfaces. Temperature rises of less than 1.5°C are considered safe. Cavitation occurs due to bubble formation at air-water interfaces. As there are no air-water interfaces, cavitation has not been demonstrated in the human fetus. The use of B and M mode ultrasound in clinical practice even in the first trimester is considered safe. These methods do not raise the temperature more than 1.5°C. Doppler techniques however can raise the temperature more than this and the effect on the fetus is unknown. Currently The World Federation of Ultrasound in Medicine and Biology summarize that "a diagnostic exposure that produces a maximum in situ temperature rise of not more than 1.5°C above normal physiological levels may be used without reservation on thermal grounds". "A diagnostic exposure that elevates embryonic and fetal in situ temperature above 41°C for 5 min should be considered potentially hazardous" (16).

Studies that have followed up children exposed in utero to ultrasound and compared them to those not exposed have not demonstrated any detrimental effects. Some of these children were assessed up to 12 years of age for weight, height, general health, visual acuity, hearing ability, cognitive function, behavior, and neurological status (17–21). Two of these studies show an increase in left handedness in males exposed to antenatal ultrasound (22,23), but a meta analysis suggests that this was a chance finding (24).

REFERENCES

1. Whitby E, Paley MN, Davies N, Sprigg A, Griffiths PD. Ultrafast magnetic resonance imaging of central nervous system abnormalities in utero in the second and third trimester of pregnancy: comparison with ultrasound. BJOG 2001; 108:519–526.
2. Whitby E, Paley M, Sprigg A, et al. Outcome of 100 singleton pregnancies with suspected brain abnormalities diagnosed on ultrasound and investigated by in utero MR imaging. Br J Obst Gynaecol 2004. in press.
3. Garel C. 1st ed. MRI of the Fetal Brain. Berlin: Springer, 2004.
4. Kok RD, de Vries MM, Heerschap A, van den Berg PP. Absence of harmful effects of magnetic resonance exposure at 1.5 T in utero during the third trimester of pregnancy: a follow-up study. Magn Reson Imaging 2004; 22:851–854.
5. Myers C, Duncan KR, Gowland PA, Johnson IR, Baker PN. Failure to detect intrauterine growth restriction following in utero exposure to MRI. Br J Radiol 1998; 71:549–551.
6. Clements H, Duncan KR, Fielding K, Gowland PA, Johnson IR, Baker PN. Infants exposed to MRI in utero have a normal paediatric assessment at 9 months of age. Br J Radiol 2000; 73:190–194.
7. Baker PN, Johnson IR, Harvey PR, Gowland PA, Mansfield P. A three-year follow-up of children imaged in utero with echo-planar magnetic resonance. Am J Obstet Gynecol 1994; 170:32–33.
8. Mevissen M, Kietzmann M, Loscher W. In vivo exposure of rats to a weak alternating magnetic field increases ornithine decarboxylase activity in the mammary gland by a similar extent as the carcinogen DMBA. Cancer Lett 1995; 90:207–214.
9. Peeling J, Lewis JS, Samoiloff M, Bock E, Tomchuk E. Biological effects of magnetic fields: chronic exposure of the nematode Panagrellus redivivus. Magn Reson Imaging 1988; 6:655–660.
10. Heinrichs WL, Fong P, Flannery M, et al. Midgestational exposure of pregnant BALB/c mice to magnetic resonance imaging conditions. Magn Reson Imaging 1988; 6:305–313.

11. Carnes KI, Magin RL. Effects of in utero exposure to 4.7 T MR imaging conditions on fetal growth and testicular development in the mouse. Magn Reson Imaging 1996; 14:263–274.

12. Glover P, Hykin J, Gowland P, Wright J, Johnson I, Mansfield P. An assessment of the intrauterine sound intensity level during obstetric echo-planar magnetic resonance imaging. Br J Radiol 1995; 68:1090–1094.

13. Nyborg WL, Steele RB. Temperature elevation in a beam of ultrasound. Ultrasound Med Biol 1983; 9:611–620.

14. Cavicchi TJ, O'Brien WD, Jr. Heat generated by ultrasound in an absorbing medium. J Acoust Soc Am 1984; 76:1244–1245.

15. Flynn HG, Church CC. A mechanism for the generation of cavitation maxima by pulsed ultrasound. J Acoust Soc Am 1984; 76:505–512.

16. Barnett SB, Ter Haar GR, Ziskin MC, Rott HD, Duck FA, Maeda K. International recommendations and guidelines for the safe use of diagnostic ultrasound in medicine. Ultrasound Med Biol 2000; 26:355–366.

17. Kieler H, Ahlsten G, Haglund B, Salvesen K, Axelsson O. Routine ultrasound screening in pregnancy and the children's subsequent neurologic development. Obstet Gynecol 1998; 91:750–756.

18. Salvesen KA, Eik-Nes SH. Ultrasound during pregnancy and birthweight, childhood malignancies and neurological development. Ultrasound Med Biol 1999; 25:1025–1031.

19. Lyons EA, Dyke C, Toms M, Cheang M. In utero exposure to diagnostic ultrasound: a 6-year follow-up. Radiology 1988; 166:687–690.

20. Moore RM, Jr., Diamond EL, Cavalieri RL. The relationship of birth weight and intrauterine diagnostic ultrasound exposure. Obstet Gynecol 1988; 71:513–517.

21. Stark CR, Orleans M, Haverkamp AD, Murphy J. Short- and long-term risks after exposure to diagnostic ultrasound in utero. Obstet Gynecol 1984; 63:194–200.

22. Kieler H, Axelsson O, Haglund B, Nilsson S, Salvesen KA. Routine ultrasound screening in pregnancy and the children's subsequent handedness. Early Hum Dev 1998; 50:233–245.

23. Salvesen KA, Vatten LJ, Eik-Nes SH, Hugdahl K, Bakketeig LS. Routine ultrasonography in utero and subsequent handedness and neurological development. Bmj 1993; 307:159–164.

24. Salvesen KA, Eik-Nes SH. Ultrasound during pregnancy and subsequent childhood non-right handedness: a meta-analysis. Ultrasound Obstet Gynecol 1999; 13:241–246.

2.6

In Utero Magnetic Resonance Imaging of Developmental Abnormalities of the Fetal Cerebellum

Ashley J. Robinson and Susan I. Blaser
The Hospital for Sick Children, Toronto, Ontario, Canada

The preceding chapter summarized the capability of magnetic resonance imaging (MRI) to assess normal and abnormal anatomy with the fetal central nervous system in utero. One of the most difficult structures to assess on ante-natal ultrasonography is the developing cerebellum. Therefore, this chapter concentrates on the normal and abnormal development of that structure. It is important to understand some of the detailed sequential development of the structures in the posterior fossa, particularly the cerebellar vermis. We therefore commence with a description of earlier MRI studies of fetal specimens. This allows us to review the anatomical features that will be important when we perform in utero studies described in the second part of the chapter.

DEVELOPMENT OF THE CEREBELLUM SHOWN BY MRI OF FETAL SPECIMENS

The cerebellar vermis starts development as a thickening of the alar plate of the rhombencephalon during the 5th week of gestation (1). This thickening forms the rhombic lip which is continuous across the midline (Fig. 1). The cerebellar hemispheres grow on both sides, and the vermis forms along their line of fusion in the midline, starting in the 9th week of gestation.

This development can be seen on MRI of fetal specimens in vitro (3), although the gestational age at which the respective features are seen is approximately 5 weeks later than those that seen by histology (4,5). By 6 or 7 weeks the early cerebellum can be seen as a thickening across the superior aspect of the 4th ventricle. By 9 weeks the midline fusion can be seen beginning rostrally and extending extra-ventricularly. By 10 to 11 weeks, the vermis has enlarged rostrally and the hemispheres enlarge laterally, and by 12 to 13 weeks the lobules and folia of the cerebellum proliferate and the mid-part of the vermis swells (Fig. 2A).

At around 13 to 14 weeks the cerebellum and early vermis can be seen rostrally. The fastigial crease can be seen developing along the ventral surface of the cerebellar plate (Fig. 2B), and the roof of the 4th ventricle is just able to be resolved (5,6). The hemispheres enlarge first dorso-laterally and then later caudo-laterally. By 14 to 16 weeks the primary fissure of the vermis is visible (4,5). By 16 weeks, the roof of the 4th ventricle is visible throughout, and the vermis enlarges caudally and "folds" along the fastigial crease, beginning to cover the roof of the 4th ventricle (Fig. 2C). This is commonly referred to as "closure" of the 4th ventricle. By 15 to 17 weeks the secondary, pre-pyramidal, pre-culmenate, and pre-central vermian fissures are visible (4,5).

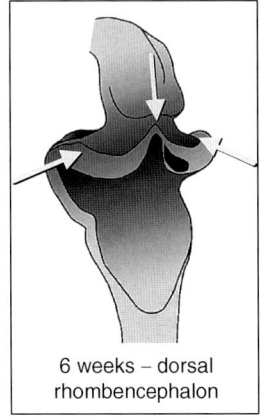

6 weeks – dorsal
rhombencephalon

Figure 1. Diagram of the posterior aspect of the rhombencephalon in a 6-week fetus. The arrows indicate the developing rhombic lips that will form the cerebellum. *Source*: From Ref. 2.

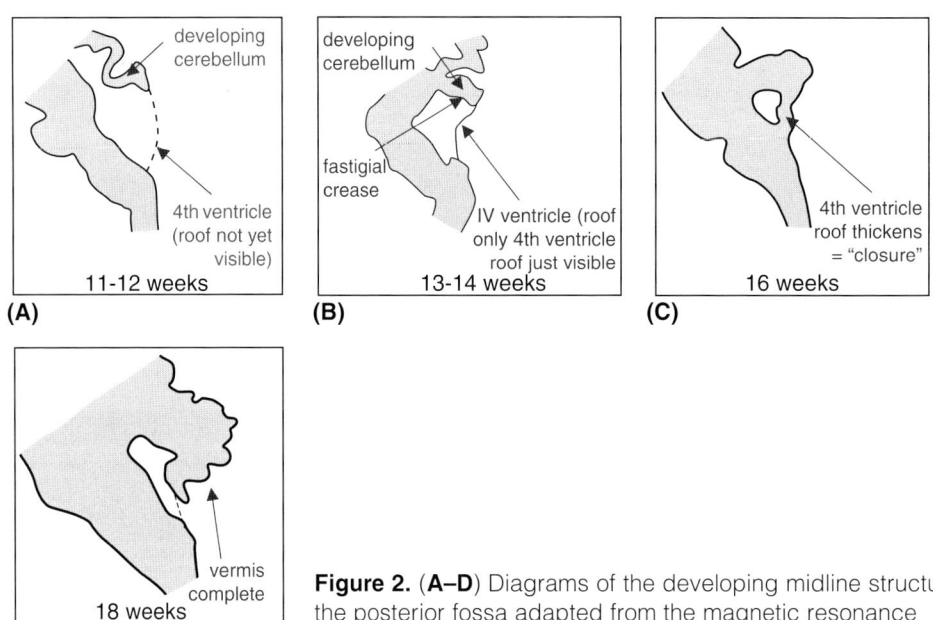

(A)   (B)   (C)

(D)

Figure 2. (**A–D**) Diagrams of the developing midline structures of the posterior fossa adapted from the magnetic resonance appearances of fetal specimens. *Source*: From Refs. 3, 5, 6.

By 18 to 19 weeks the cranio-caudal length of the vermis is equal to that of the cerebellar hemispheres, and the 4th ventricle is almost completely covered (6), as shown in Figure 2D. Although often complete by this gestation (7), coverage of the 4th ventricle as in the normal newborn mature relationship should always occur by 22 to 24 weeks (4,5), a feature also seen by fetal ultrasonography (8,9). Figure 3 shows the complicated lobular structure of the mature cerebellar vermis.

It should be borne in mind that in some fetal specimen studies (4,3) the fetal age is defined as the age from conception, and this is on average approximately 2 weeks less than the menstrual age (i.e., time from last menstrual period) used in clinical studies (5,6).

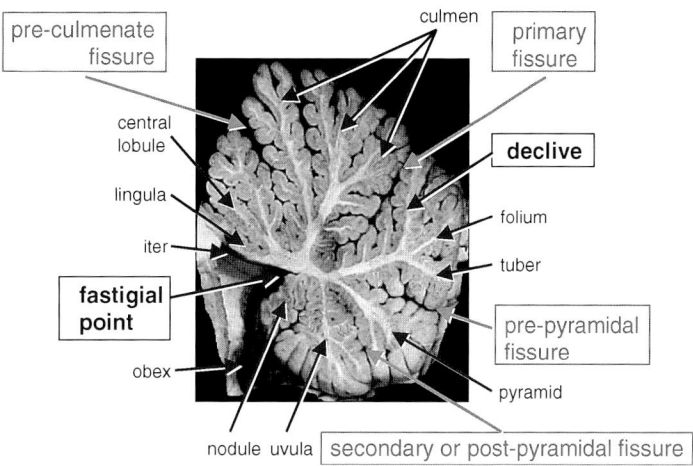

Figure 3. Normal anatomy of the mature cerebellar vermis. *Source*: From Ref. 10.

EARLY DEVELOPMENT OF THE CEREBELLUM SHOWN BY MRI IN UTERO

Development follows the same pattern as in fetal specimen studies; therefore, by 14 to 16 weeks, there should always be a fastigial point and by 22 to 24 weeks, a "closed" 4th ventricle, although there is some physiological variation in timing. However, due to the drop in resolution incurred by imaging in utero (fetal motion, larger field of view, lower signal-to-noise ratio) there is a delay between identification of the vermian fissures in vitro compared to in vivo. In the 17.5-week fetus shown in Figure 4, the fastigial point is visible, the 4th ventricle is covered, and the declive and primary fissures are visible.

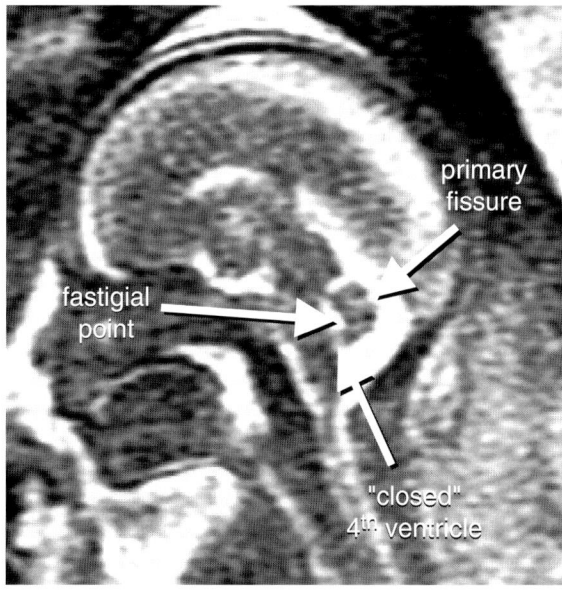

Figure 4. 17.5-Week fetus.

By 21 weeks the pre-pyramidal fissure can be seen, as shown in Figure 5 and soon after the pre-culmenate fissure can be seen (Fig. 6). By 24 weeks (Fig. 7) the secondary fissure can be seen and other lobules are becoming visible; by 27 weeks (Fig. 8), all lobules are visible (11).

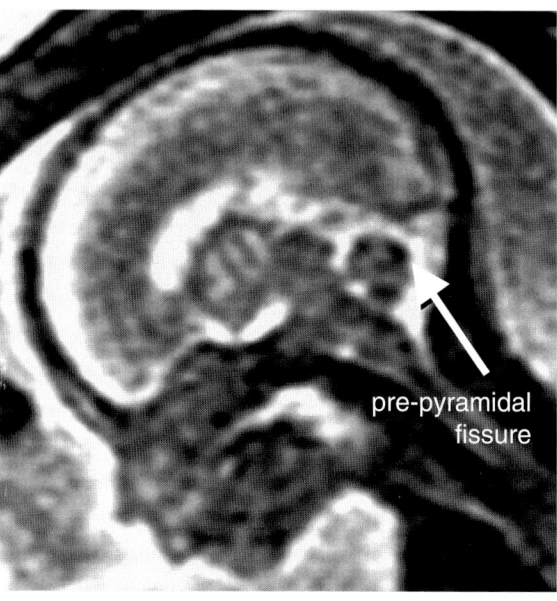

Figure 5. 21-Week fetus.

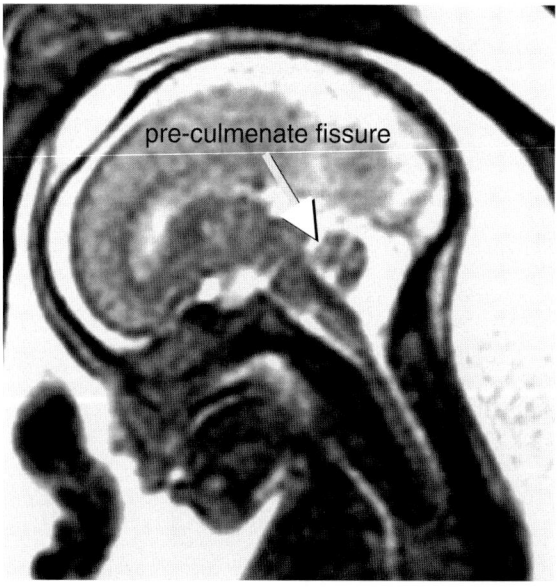

Figure 6. 21- to 22-Week fetus.

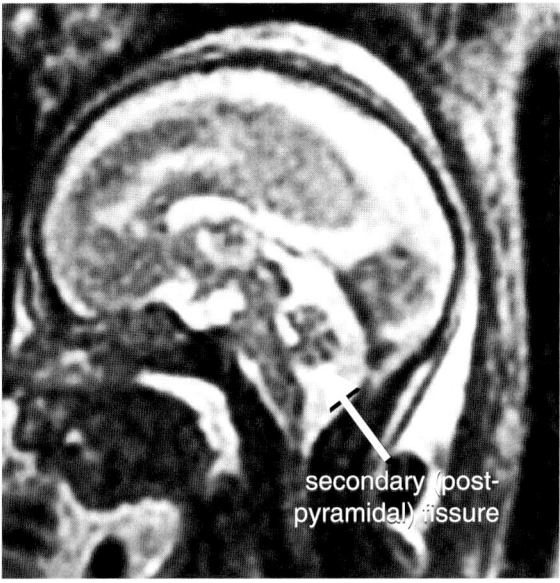

Figure 7. 24-Week fetus.

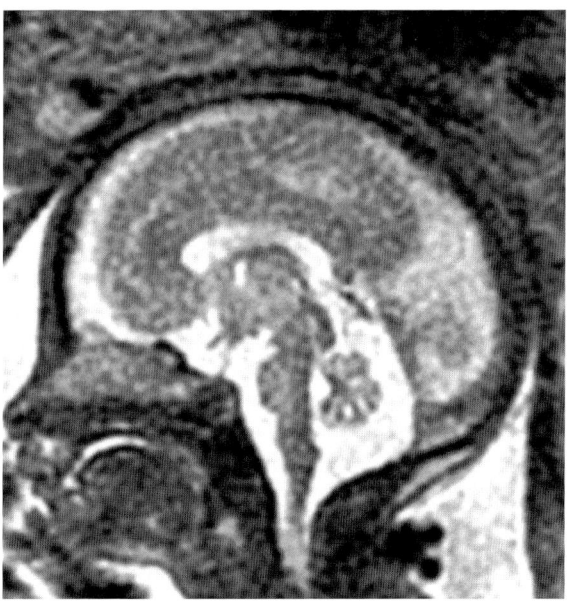

Figure 8. 27-Week fetus.

SYSTEMATIC APPROACH TO ANALYSIS OF VERMIAN DEVELOPMENT

It is important to develop a systematic approach assessing the cerebellum and in particular the cerebellar vermis. This assessment should include asking the following questions:

■ Is the vermis present and are the normal landmarks present; i.e., a fastigial point or crease? Vermian fissures?
■ Is the vermis mature with respect to the chronological dates of the fetus?

IS THE VERMIS PRESENT?

By 18 weeks, one should be able to clearly identify the vermis; the following three cases show the range of abnormalities that may affect the normal development of the vermis. In the fetus at 20 weeks gestation shown in Figure 9, we see a small amount of tissue in the midline between the cerebellar hemispheres, which at first sight could be vermian tissue. On the sagittal view (Fig. 9A) some of what looks to be midline vermis is actually partial volume averaging of adjacent cerebellar hemisphere. There is no fastigial point and the roof of the 4th ventricle has a squared-off shape rather than being triangular and there is no primary fissure. On the axial view (Fig. 9B) there is a "molar tooth" configuration of the brainstem, and the 4th ventricle has an abnormal "batwing" shape. This is an example of Joubert syndrome, the prototype for congenital vermian hypoplasia. The vermis is either aplastic, hypoplastic, or cleft, and the superior medullary velum is absent.

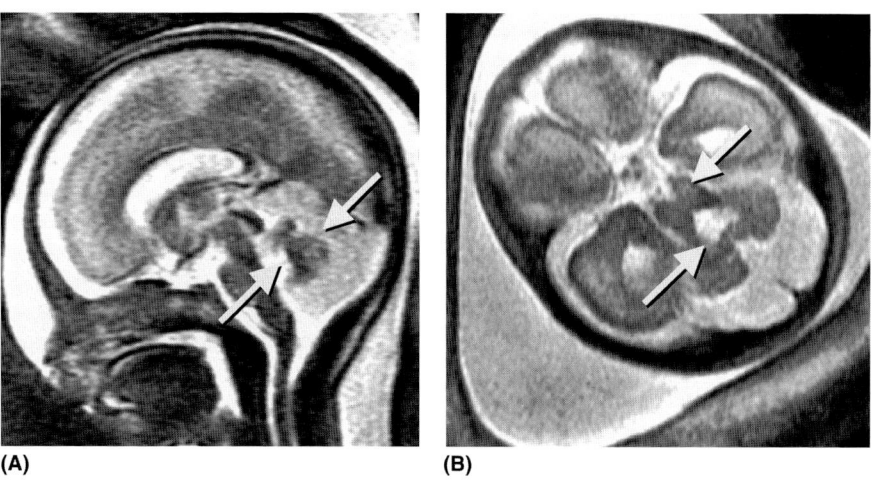

(A) **(B)**

Figure 9. 20-Week fetus showing vermian aplasia and the characteristic features of Joubert's syndome.

Figure 10 shows a 26-week gestation fetus in which the fastigial point is rounded off rather than triangular. There is no primary fissure shown in the sagittal plane (Fig. 10A). On the axial view (Fig. 10B), the cerebellar folia are continuous across the midline. Additionally the cranio–caudal diameter of the "vermis" is too big because it is the cerebellar hemispheres that are being measured rather than the vermis (see below for vermian cranio-caudal diameter measurement). The fetus has rhombencephalosynapsis, which is a fusion anomaly where the vermis does not form and the cerebellar hemispheres are fused across the midline.

Figure 11 is an example of a 20-week fetus with congenital muscular dystrophy. The vermis is incomplete, and there is no fastigial point or primary fissure. The 4th ventricle is uncovered and there are shell-like cerebellar hemispheres. The hindbrain has a configuration similar to a 13 to 14 week fetus (see above). The brainstem has maintained its primitive Z-shaped configuration with a dorsal kink at the ponto-mesencephalic junction. In addition to the vermian hypogenesis, there was thin cortex and callosal agenesis.

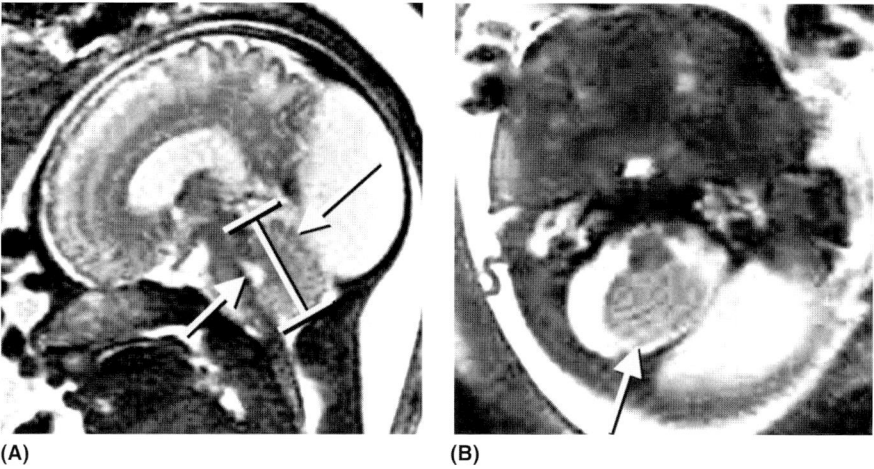

Figure 10. 26-Week fetus with rhombencephalosynapsis. *Source*: From Ref. 12.

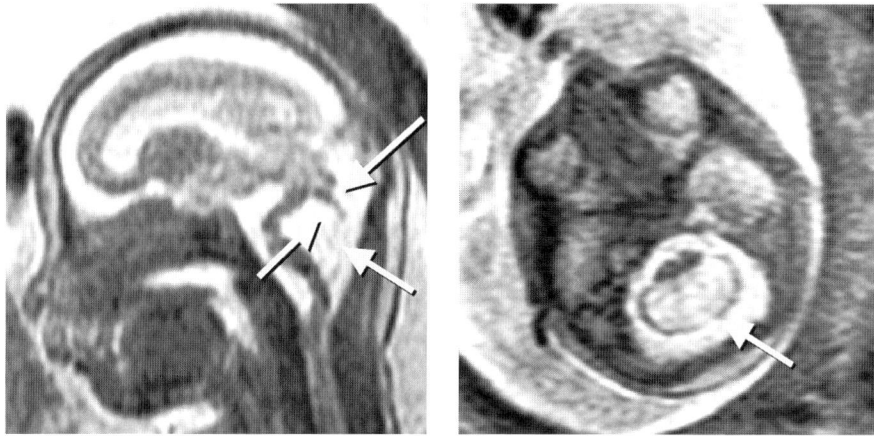

Figure 11. Vermian hypoplasia and complicated brainstem deformity in a 20-week fetus with congenital muscular dystrophy.

IS THE VERMIS MATURE?

The next step is to assess the maturity of the vermian development. In addition to the fastigial point and the vermian fissures, we can assess the following:

■ Tegmento–vermian angle ("closure" of 4th ventricle)
■ Cranio–caudal diameter of the vermis
■ Ratio of vermian tissue above and below the fastigial point

The tegmento–vermian angle is measured by drawing a line along the dorsal surface of the brainstem parallel to the tegmentum. This line usually transects the nucleus gracilis at the obex. A second line is draw along the anterior surface of the vermis as shown in Figure 12.

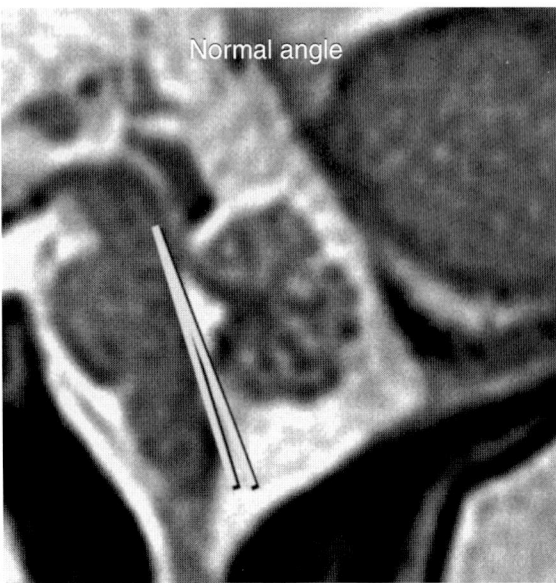

Figure 12. Construction lines used to assess the tegmento–vermian angle.

Tegmento–Vermian Angle

The tegmento–vermian angle is usually close to 0° in normal fetuses. An elevated tegmento–vermian angle is virtually always pathological (Fig. 13) and may represent one of two processes: (1) either arrest of vermian development with failure of "closure" of the 4th ventricle, or (2) a failure of fenestration of the 4th ventricle outflow, leading to secondary elevation of the vermis. Often these two processes are seen together. When an increased tegmento–vermian angle is seen with normal growth and morphology of the vermis and without other abnormalities elsewhere in the fetus, this may represent elevation of the vermis due to a persistent Blake's pouch cyst, and does not indicate an adverse outcome (13).

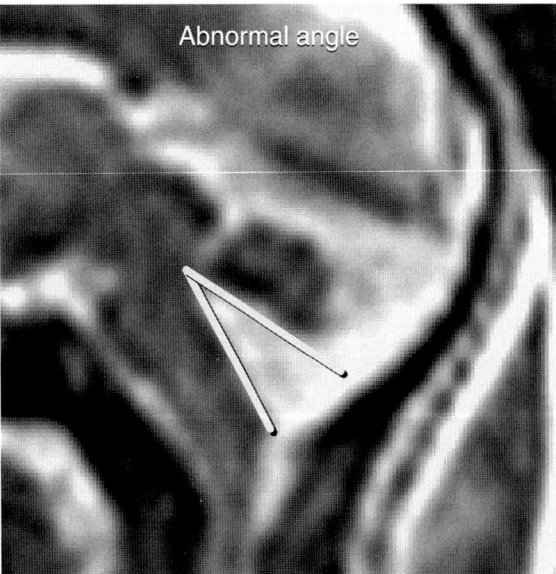

Figure 13. An example of abnormally increased tegmento–vermian angle.

The fetus shown in Figure 14 is of 22-weeks gestational age. The tegmento–vermian angle is increased with the 4th ventricle uncovered. The vermis is very small; there is no primary fissure or fastigial point. The cerebellar hemispheres are small. The overall configuration is similar to that of an 11- to 12-week fetus. This fetus would fall into the classification of Dandy–Walker continuum; however it is more severe than a classic Dandy–Walker malformation because of the additional hypoplasia of the brainstem and absence of the pons. A poor outcome would be expected. The 22-week fetus shown in Figure 15 demonstrates more typical findings of Dandy–Walker malformation. The tegmento–vermian angle is increased with the 4th ventricle uncovered. The vermis is small, but not as small as the previous case. There is no primary fissure and the fastigial point is visible but relatively flattened compared to what is expected at this gestationage. The cerebellar hemispheres are hypoplastic, but are larger than in the previous case. Once again the configuration is similar to that of an 11- to 12- week fetus.

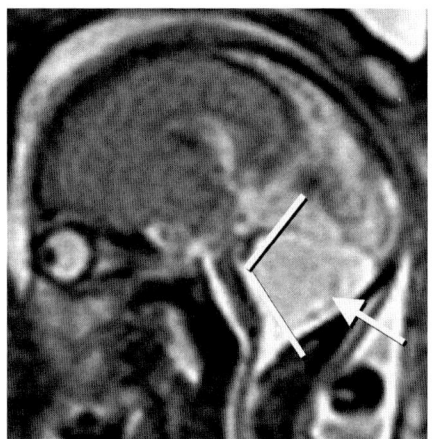 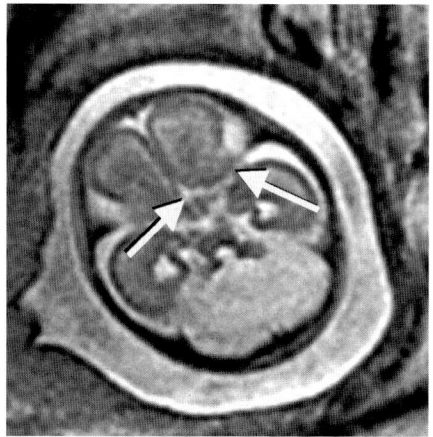

Figure 14. Marked increase of the tegmento–vermian angle in an extreme case of Dandy–Walker malformation.

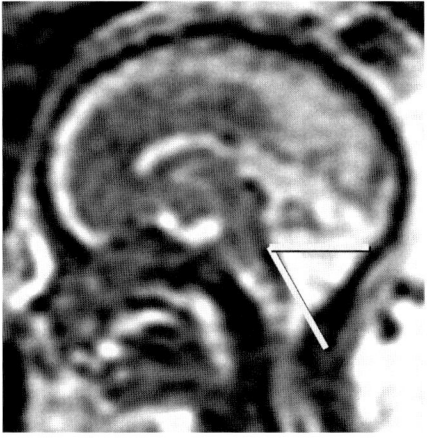 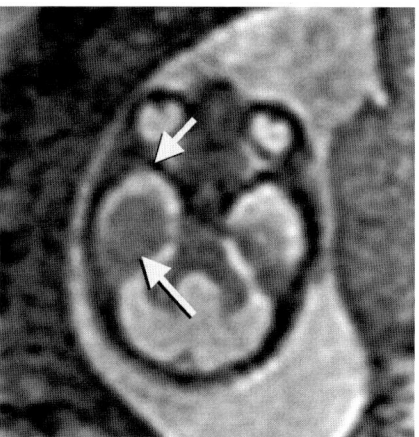

Figure 15. Increase of the tegmento–vermian angle in a more typical case of Dandy–Walker malformation.

In the example shown in Figure 16, a fetus at 34 weeks shows elevation of the tegmento–vermian angle, with the 4th ventricle uncovered. The vermis is hypoplastic but the primary fissure is seen. The fastigial point is less flattened, and the cerebellar hemispheres quite well-formed. This fetus again falls into the Dandy–Walker continuum, however the degree of severity is less than in the previous cases. Postnatally, the child was deaf but had otherwise normal neurological development. Post-natal MR imaging (Fig. 16C) confirms the in utero brain findings while high resolution CT of the temporal bones (Fig. 16D) demonstrated bilateral cochlear dysplasia consisting of modiolar deficiencies.

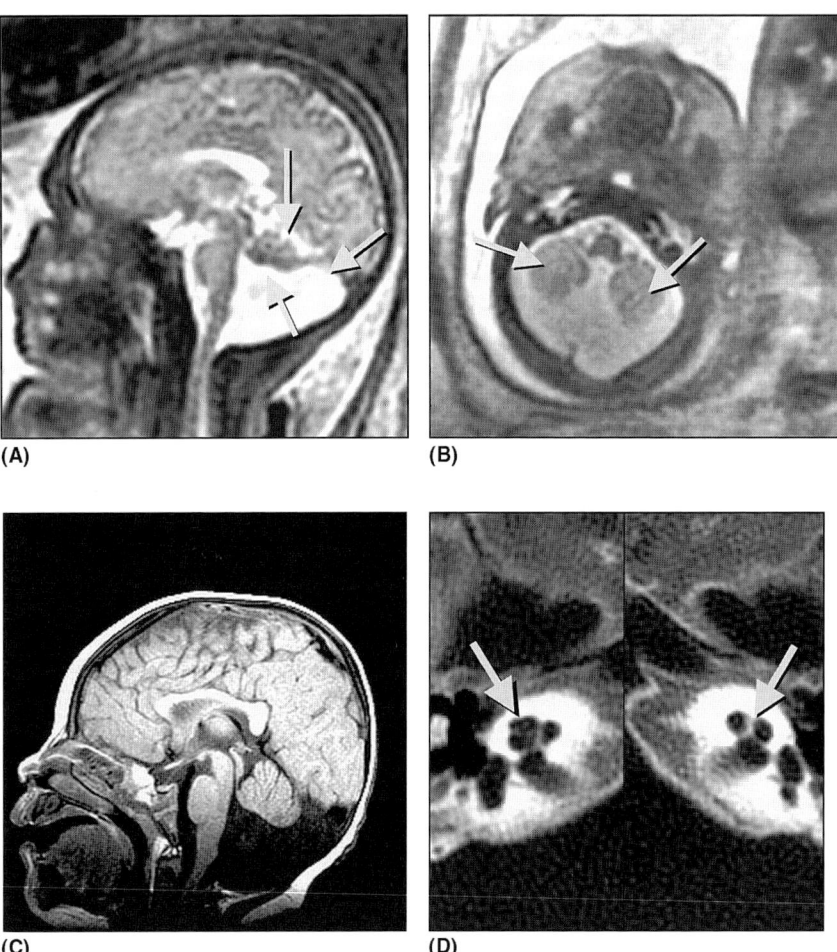

(A)

(B)

(C)

(D)

Figure 16. Dandy–Walker continuum diagnosed in utero (**A**,**B**) and confirmed post-natally (**C**). Post-natal CT of the temporal bones shows cochlear dysplasia (**D**).

Cerebellar and labyrinthine anomalies often co-exist because the rhombic lip forms the cerebellum and the cochlear nucleus, and the rhombencephalon induces the otocyst to form.

In this next case of a 21-week fetus, the tegmento–vermian angle is increased, with the 4th ventricle uncovered inferiorly (Fig. 17). The fastigial point is visible and vermian lobulation is seen. Again this would fall into the Dandy–Walker continuum and this fetus had other facial, visceral, and skeletal anomalies. The autopsy diagnosis was

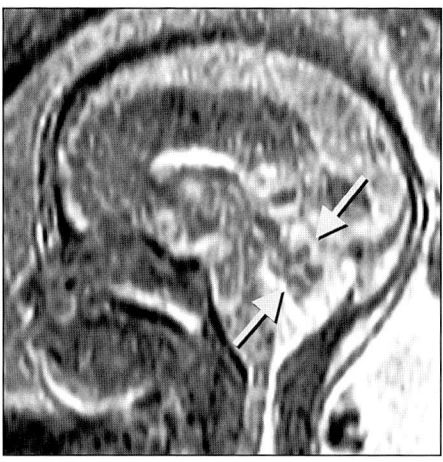

Figure 17. Relatively mild variety of Dandy–Walker continuum in fetus subsequently shown to have Wolf–Hirschhorn syndrome.

Wolf–Hirschhorn syndrome, characterized by multiple congenital anomalies including midline fusion defects, associated with a chromosomal deletion of the short arm of chromosome 4 (14).

These cases demonstrate an important aspect of the Dandy–Walker continuum. The infants can have a wide range of clinical outcomes, although syndromic cases usually have poor outcomes. The different outcomes are based on the degree of vermian dysplasia plus any associated abnormalities, which can be anatomic, genetic, or chromosomal. This makes counseling extremely difficult.

Cranio–Caudal Diameter of the Vermis

The fastigial point and the primary fissure should always be visible in normal fetuses. The declive is seen as a low intensity area immediately below the primary fissure. A line can therefore be drawn through the fastigial point and declive in normal fetuses (the fastigium–declive line), and often also in fetuses where the tegmento–vermian angle is increased. The cranio–caudal diameter of the vermis is measured perpendicular to this line (Fig. 18).

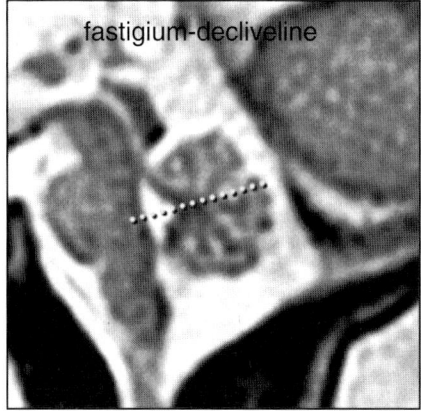
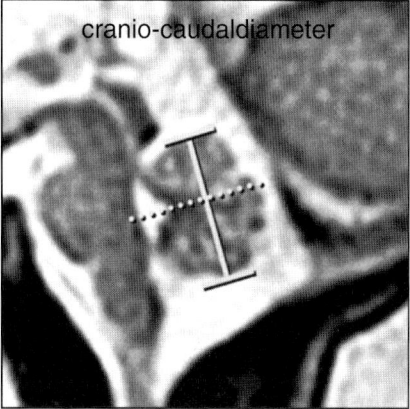

Figure 18. Construction lines for measuring the cranio–caudal diameter of the vermis.

Table 1. Predicted Cranio–Caudal Diameter of the Vermis Between Gestational Ages 14 to 40 Weeks

Gestational Age (wk)	Cranio-Caudal Dimension (mm)	Gestational Age (wk)	Cranio-Caudal Dimension (mm)
14	4.6	28	14.8
15	5.3	29	15.6
16	6.1	30	16.3
17	6.8	31	17.0
18	7.5	32	17.7
19	8.3	33	18.5
20	9.0	34	19.2
21	9.7	35	19.9
22	10.4	36	20.7
23	11.2	37	21.4
24	11.9	38	22.1
25	12.6	39	22.9
26	13.4	40	23.6
27	14.1		

The cranio–caudal diameter of the vermis grows linearly:

Diameter (mm) $= 0.74 \times$ Gestational age (weeks) $- 6.11$

Linear growth of the cerebellar vermis is also confirmed by ultrasonographic studies (15–17). From this we can predict the expected cranio-caudal diameter for any given gestational age, as shown in Table 1.

The case shown in Figure 19 is a 28-week fetus. The vermis is fully formed, the 4th ventricle is "closed," and the fastigial point is present. The expected cranio-caudal diameter of the vermis is 14.8 mm at this maturity (Table 1) but it actually measures 10.9 mm (22 weeks equivalent). Additionally the trans-cerebellar diameter is small in keeping with global cerebellar hypoplasia. Additionally on the sagittal view there is a sloping forehead in keeping with microcephaly, and the CSF spaces are prominent. On autopsy, this fetus had severe microcephaly with dysmorphic features, proptosis, and mild hypotelorism.

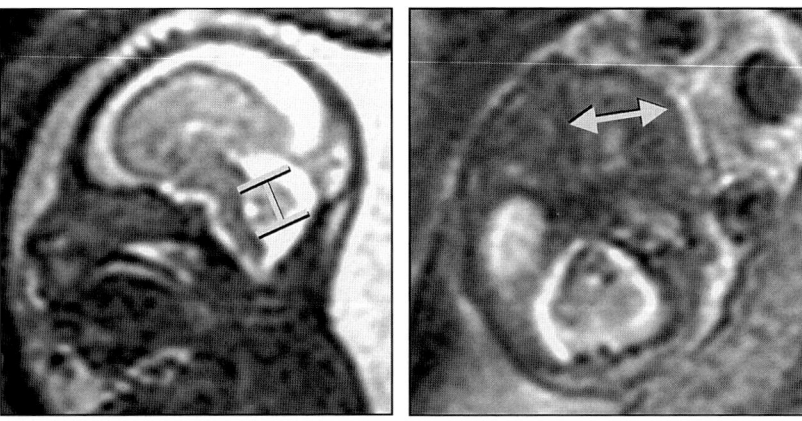

Figure 19. 28-Week fetus with microcephaly with small cerebellum and small cerebral hemispheres.

Ratio of Vermian Tissue Above and Below the Fastigial Point

The second measurement that is useful reflects the relative growth of the superior and inferior portions of the vermis. This is useful in cases of suspected vermian hypoplasia where the inferior vermis is usually affected most severely. The same construct line is used as in assessing the cranio-caudal diameter but the amount of vermis above and below that line is measured (Fig. 20). There should be linear and symmetrical growth of the vermis throughout gestation. The average height above and below the fastigial point should increase linearly, with average percentages above and below of 47.9% and 52.1%, respectively, and no significant change in this ratio with gestational age.

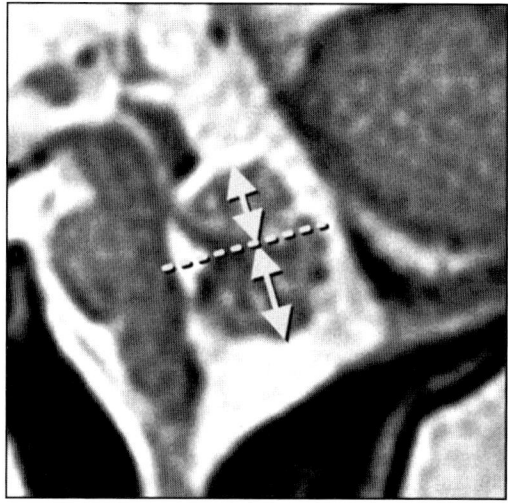

Figure 20. Assessment of the relative growth of the superior and inferior portions of the cerebellar vermis.

The 25-week fetus in Figure 21 has a normal tegmento–vermian angle and normal 4th ventricle (closed), but the vermis is small overall and also relatively small inferiorly. This is an example of inferior vermian hypoplasia. On the postnatal MRI, it can be seen that the inferior vermis is deficient (there is some partial volume artefact from the adjacent cerebellar hemisphere). The 4th ventricle is not distended and its roof can be seen in almost its expected position. There were additional cortical heterotopias.

This case is important because it demonstrates that the cystic dilatation of the 4th ventricle is not necessarily secondary to a deficiency of the vermis (or vice versa); it is probably due to a failure of fenestration of the 4th ventricle outflow foramina. Conversely, there can be cystic dilatation of the 4th ventricle with an elevated tegmento–vermian angle and normal vermian morphology. Therefore, there are two separate processes—namely failure of fenestration and failure of vermian growth—which may be seen separately or together, most likely the latter because of global arrest of development at an early stage.

Other cystic abnormalities in the posterior fossa may easily be confused with Dandy–Walker continuum (as explained in chap. 1.3). The case shown in Figure 22 is a 23-week fetus with an increased tegmento–vermian angle. The fastigial point is present, and there is apparently normal lobulation. At first glance the appearances are suggestive of Dandy–Walker continuum; however the cranio-caudal diameter of the vermis was 10.7 mm (within normal limits for gestational age) and there is as much vermian tissue above the fastigial point as below. There is, therefore, no indication of vermian hypoplasia. There were no other fetal abnormalities, however the mother had

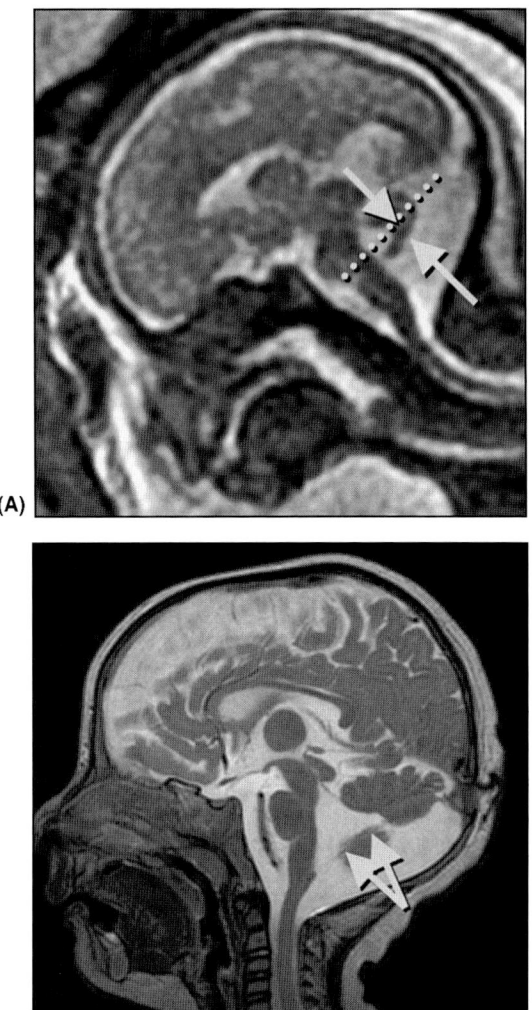

(A)

(B)

Figure 21. Inferior vermian hypoplasia diagnosed antenatally (**A**) and confirmed postnatally (**B**).

sickle-cell anemia and ultimately there was fetal demise in utero due to placental insufficiency. Autopsy demonstrated a normal fetal karyotype and apparently normal cerebellar pathology. This was a case thought to represent a Blake's pouch cyst that had collapsed by the time of autopsy. It is recognized that posterior fossa cysts can easily be missed at autopsy unless the specimen is examined under water (13). The other possibility would be that there was physiological delay in closure of the 4th ventricle. This is unlikely at this gestation age, however it should be borne in mind that abnormalities within the Dandy–Walker continuum cannot be reliably ruled out at earlier gestations (7,9).

In this next example (Fig. 23), a fetus at 36 weeks has a cisterna magna that is too big; however, the vermis is fully formed with a normal tegmento–vermian angle, fastigial point, and lobulation. The child was completely normal on follow-up.

In contrast the fetus in Figure 24 is at 29-weeks gestation; the vermis is the correct size, with a normal tegmento–vermian angle and a fastigial point. Lobulation is not clearly seen and the cerebrospinal fluid space behind the cerebellum is too large. Additionally the cerebellar hemispheres are displaced anteriorly. This was thought to represent a posterior fossa arachnoid cyst, with anterior displacement and compression of the cerebellum and vermis and confirmed on postnatal MRI. The baby had

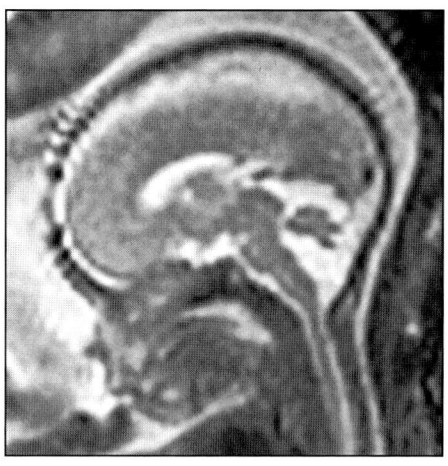

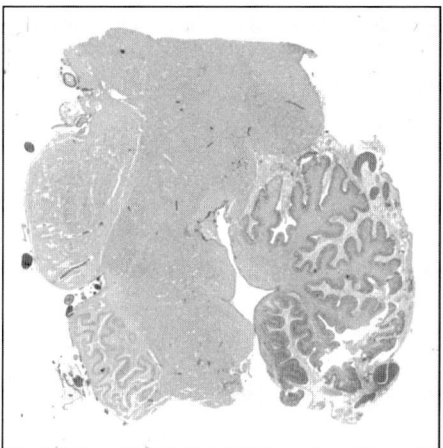

Figure 22. Elevated tegmento–vermian angle but normal vermis (Blake's pouch cyst).

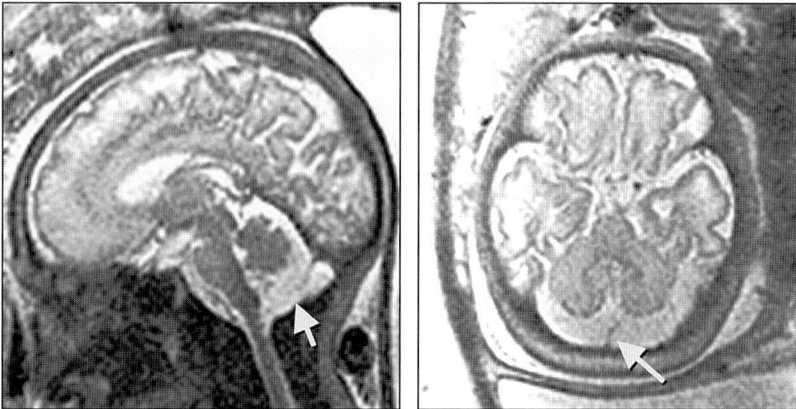

Figure 23. Mega cisterna magna in a 36-week fetus.

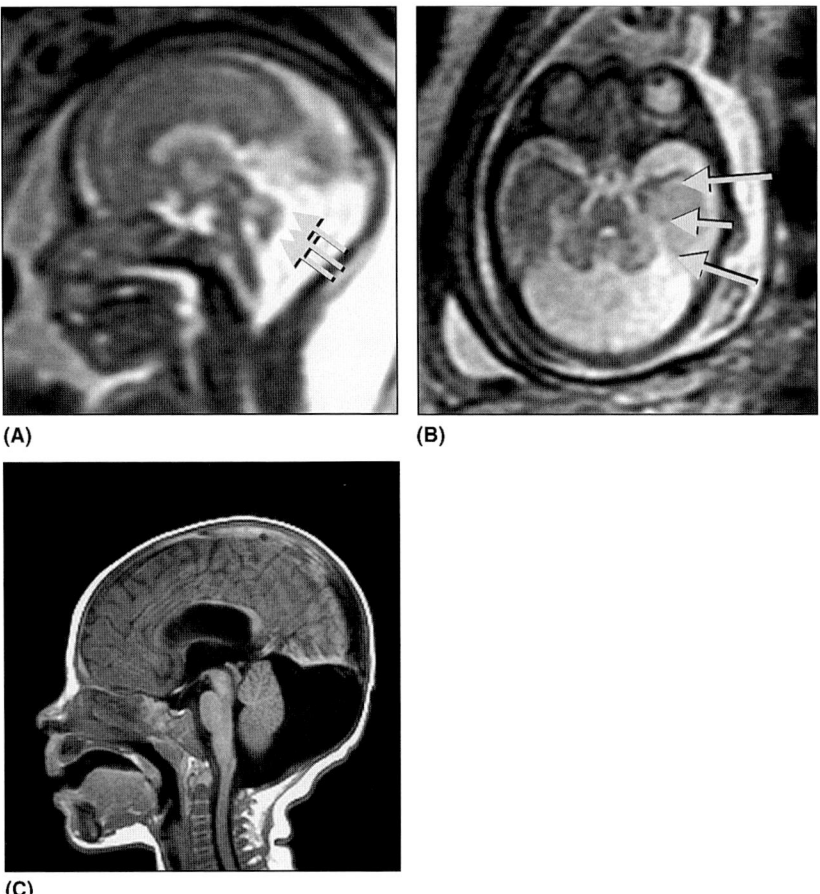

(A) (B)

(C)

Figure 24. Posterior fossa arachnoid cyst diagnosed antenatally (**A,B**) and confirmed postnatally (**C**).

ventriculomegaly as a secondary mechanical phenomenon but neurodevelopmental follow-up was normal.

SUMMARY

We provide several easily identified anatomic criteria for abnormal vermian development including:

- Presence of the vermis and its landmarks: Fastigial point and primary fissure
- Tegmento–vermian angle ("closure" of 4th ventricle)
- Cranio-caudal diameter of the vermis
- Ratio of vermian tissue above and below the fastigial point
- Causes of an apparently enlarged cisterna magna

REFERENCES

1. Pediatric Neuroimaging. Barkovich. 3rd Ed. Lippincott Williams & Wilkins, 2000.
2. Williams, ed. Gray's Anatomy. 37th ed. London, Edinburgh: Churchill Livingstone, 1989.
3. Hansen PE, Ballesteros MC, Soila K, Garcia L, Howard JM. MR imaging of the developing human brain. Part 1. Prenatal development. Radiographics 1993; 13:21–36.

4. Nakayama T, Yamada R. MR imaging of posterior fossa structures of human embryos and fetuses. Radiat Med 1999; 17:105–114.
5. Chong BW, Babcook CJ, Pang D, Ellis WG. A magnetic resonance template for normal cerebellar development in the human fetus. Neurosurgery 1997; 41:924–928 discussion 928–929.
6. Babcook CJ, Chong BW, Salamat MS, Ellis WG, Goldstein RB. Sonographic anatomy of the developing cerebellum: normal embryology can resemble pathology. AJR Am J Roentgenol 1996; 166:427–433.
7. Bromley B, Nadel AS, Pauker S, Estroff JA, Benacerraf BR. Closure of the cerebellar vermis: evaluation with second trimester US. Radiology 1994; 193:761–763.
8. Ben-Amin M, Perlitz Y, Peleg D. Transvaginal sonographic appearance of the cerebellar vermis at 14–16 weeks' gestation. Ultrasound Obstet Gynecol 2002; 19:208–209.
9. Bronshtein M, Zimmer EZ, Blazer S. Isolated large 4th ventricle in early pregnancy—a possible benign transient phenomenon. Prenat Diagn 1998; 18:997–1000.
10. Duvernoy H. The Human Brainstem and Cerebellum. Verlag: Springer, 1995.
11. Stazzone MM, Hubbard AM, Bilaniuk LT, et al. Ultrafast MR imaging of the normal posterior fossa in fetuses. AJR Am J Roentgenol 2000; 175:835–839.
12. Dr. Anne Michelle Fink, The University of Melbourne, Royal Children's, and Royal Women's Hospitals, Melbourne, Australia.
13. Nelson MD, Jr., Maher K, Gilles FH. A different approach to cysts of the posterior fossa. Pediatr Radiol 2004; 34:720–732.
14. Zollino M, Di Stefano C, Zampino G, et al. Genotype-phenotype correlations and clinical diagnostic criteria in Wolf-Hirschhorn syndrome. Am J Med Genet 2000; 94:254–261.
15. Smith PA, Johansson D, Tzannatos C, Campbell S. Prenatal measurement of the fetal cerebellum and cisterna cerebellomedullaris by ultrasound. Prenat Diagn 1986; 6:133–141.
16. Chang CH, Chang FM, Yu CH, Ko HC, Chen HY. Three-dimensional ultrasound in the assessment of fetal cerebellar transverse and antero-posterior diameters. Ultrasound Med Biol 2000; 26:175–182.
17. Malinger G, Ginath S, Lerman-Sagie T, Watemberg N, Lev D, Glezerman M. The fetal cerebellar vermis: normal development as shown by transvaginal ultrasound. Prenat Diagn 2001; 21:687–692.

3.1

Neonatal Cranial Ultrasound

Alan Sprigg
Sheffield NHS Trust, Sheffield, U.K.

The first publications of reasonable quality real time cranial ultrasound scanning (US) were in the early 1980s (1–3). Progressive refinements of computer technology, portability of equipment and probe design provided improved image quality and resolution of normal anatomy and pathological processes (4,5). The addition of pulsed or continuous wave Doppler and color flow imaging has given further research opportunity to assess the pathological processes leading to neonatal neurological damage.

Ultrasound is used in obstetrics to screen for normality of brain structure. The fetal skull vault is thin and allows ultrasonic assessment of fetal brain structure before 20 weeks gestation. Image quality deteriorates in later pregnancy as skull ossification progresses. Postnatally, US can only assess the brain using a patent fontanel as an acoustic window.

Cranial US is non-invasive, easily repeatable, and causes minimal disturbance to the sick neonate. Cranial US was rapidly accepted as a "routine" part of assessment of the neonate requiring special or intensive care. US helps to exclude hemorrhagic or other brain injury and can monitor progress or complications, e.g., porencephaly following neonatal intracerebral hemorrhage, or hydrocephalus following intraventricular hemorrhage (IVH) or meningitis.

Neonates with extreme prematurity, prolonged labor, or following instrumental delivery are at greater risk of brain injury, either due to the effects of hemorrhage or ischemia.

Most fetuses born after 24 weeks are considered viable, but are often clinically unstable and poorly tolerate transportation to a radiology department for computed tomography (CT)/magnetic resonance imaging (MRI). US can be performed at the bed-side and this is the initial imaging modality of choice in the neonatal nursery. Cranial US is available at any time, provided there is a trained operator. As with any other operator dependant imaging modality, it requires a significant amount of operator skill to perform a scan adequately, together with experience in reporting and interpretation.

There is no agreement on how soon after birth the first scan should be performed or the utility or frequency of follow-up examinations. This is usually determined by the clinical course of the baby. Most units have their own protocol for the low-risk baby, dependent on the gestation and birth weight.

LIMITATIONS OF ULTRASOUND

Cranial US is has several limitations especially in the assessment of acute hypoxic ischemic injury and neonatal stroke, but it is primarily because of the ease of access and bed-side assessment that US is the initial imaging modality in most neonatal nurseries. The wider availability of neonatal CT and MRI has further defined the strengths and limitations of US. Fresh intraventricular hemorrhage may not be immediately identified on US until it clots (becomes white) but US is sensitive for intraparenchymal hemorrhage and IVH. US is less sensitive for subarachnoid and surface hemorrhage than CT, especially over the convexities.

As US image quality has progressed, so has the recognition of brain pathology. Initial observations of "bright thalami" were correlated with athetoid cerebral palsy, but now we recognize that increased reflectivity in the thalami is not always associated with neurological damage. Similarly thalamostriate flare (thalamostriate vasculopathy) (Figs. 1–3) was initially associated with infection (syphilis, TORCH, etc.) but is now

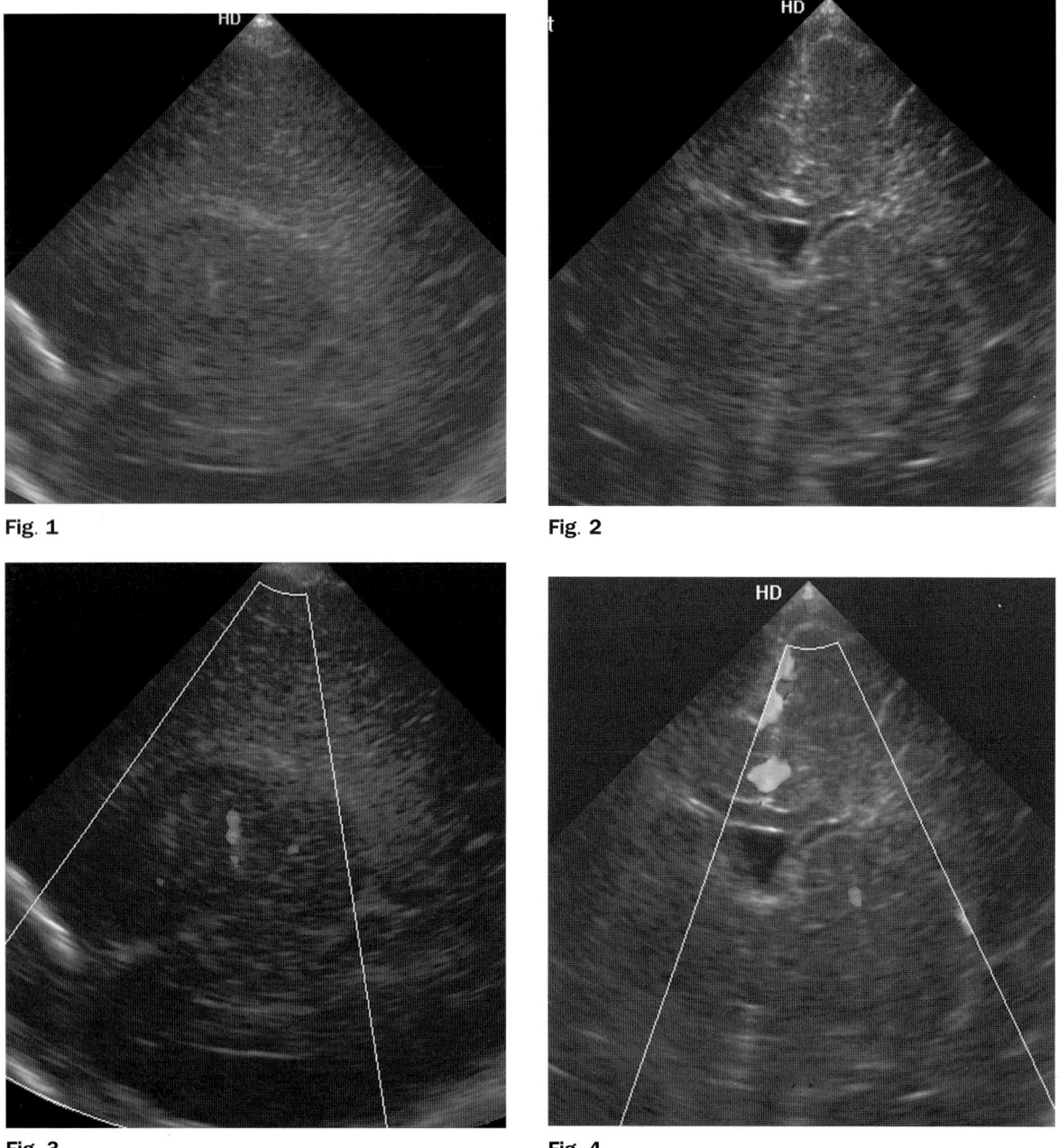

Fig. 1

Fig. 2

Fig. 3

Fig. 4

Figures 1–4. Sagittal and coronal view (Fig. 1); 2-D images (Fig. 2) with color flow imaging. Figs. 3 and 4 show caudothalamic "vasculopathy" (white lines along the course of the caudothalamic arteries). In most neonates, this is a nonspecific finding.

recognized as a non-specific finding in about 1% of neonates scanned on the intensive care unit (6). Subependymal cystic change was initially associated with congenital infection, but we now recognize that this as a coincidental finding. Hence, developments in imaging quality have lead to new findings and clinical correlation of US findings with clinical status over time (Figs. 5–7).

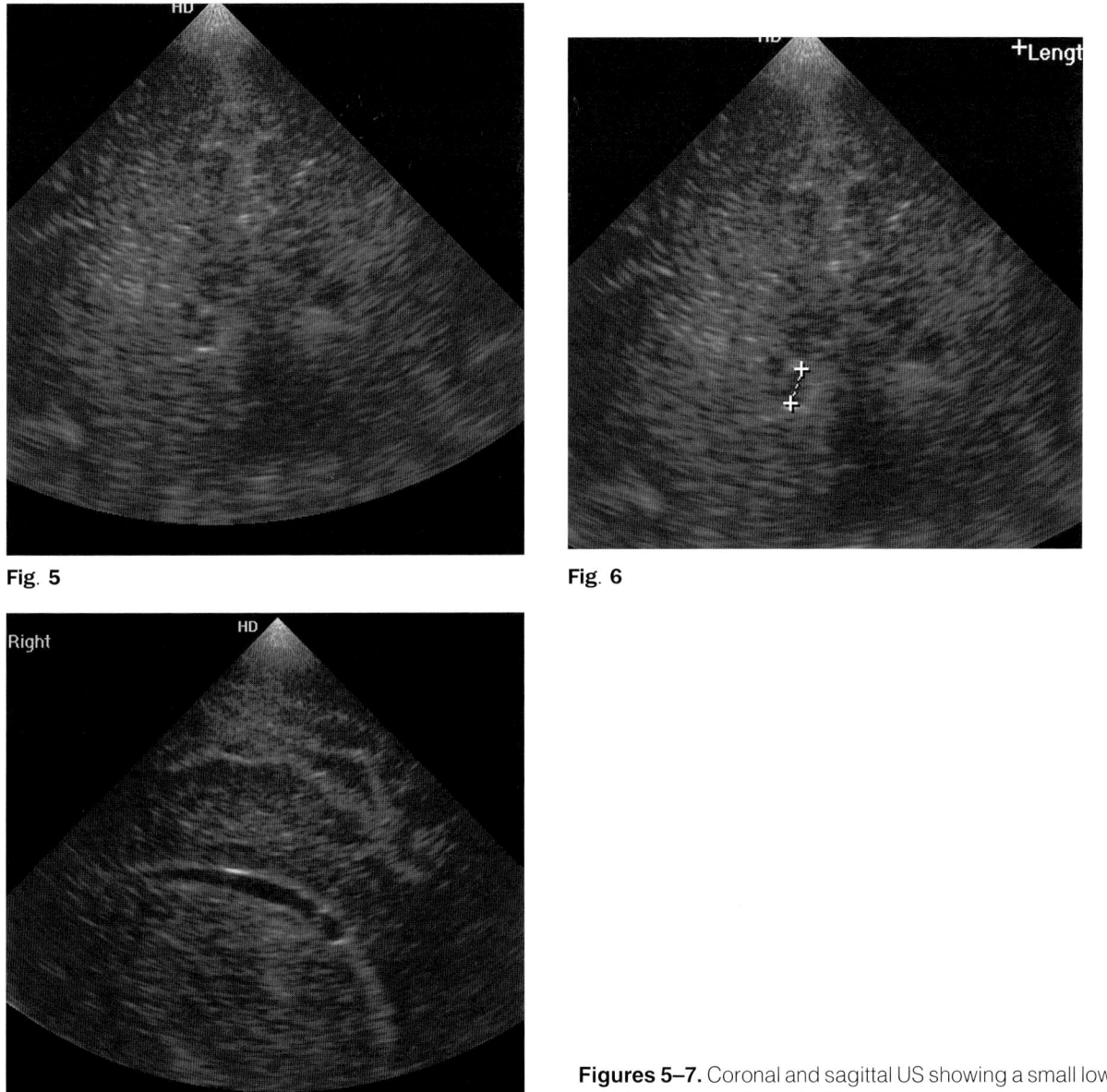

Fig. 5

Fig. 6

Fig. 7

Figures 5–7. Coronal and sagittal US showing a small low echo cyst (between callipers) within the choroid plexus, a coincidental finding on a postnatal scan.

HAZARDS OF NEONATAL ULTRASOUND

There are no known biological hazards from repeated cranial ultrasound in neonates with the intensity or duration of US used in clinical practice. Some neonates are sensitive to pressure on the anterior fontanel—prolonged pressure may cause bradycardia and apnea. This occurs mainly in sick or premature neonates.

WHO SCANS?

Cranial US is performed mainly by general or pediatric radiologists but less commonly by neuroradiologists. In many centers neuroradiologists interpret MRI and CT images, but cranial US is performed and/or interpreted by other radiologists or pediatricians. As ultrasound does not use ionizing radiation, there are no specific restrictions on the personnel performing the scan. Scans on the neonatal unit are performed by various disciplines including radiologists, sonographers, pediatricians or advanced nurse practitioners/midwives. The initial professional background of the person performing the scan does not matter, provided they are well trained and understand the technique and pathologies likely to be seen (7).

ULTRASOUND TECHNIQUE

There are specific machine requirements, which are not normally found on departmental "adult" US machines—many neonatal nurseries have their own dedicated machine. A high frequency (usually 5 MHz to 12 MHz) probe is used to scan the full depth of the neonatal head at different ages—from premature to 6-month old infant. The probe requires a small footprint to fit the small fontanel (i.e., it is usually a specific probe dedicated to neonatal scanning). Specific ultrasound pre-sets are needed to optimize the image for scanning a baby's head compared with other structures. Color flow imaging and power, continuous wave and pulsed Doppler features are advantageous provided they are used with appropriate power settings and for a short duration. A high frequency linear probe is also needed for brain surface scanning (and spinal imaging).

Ultrasound images were correlated with anatomical and pathological findings in many early publications (8,9) and clinical outcomes (10).

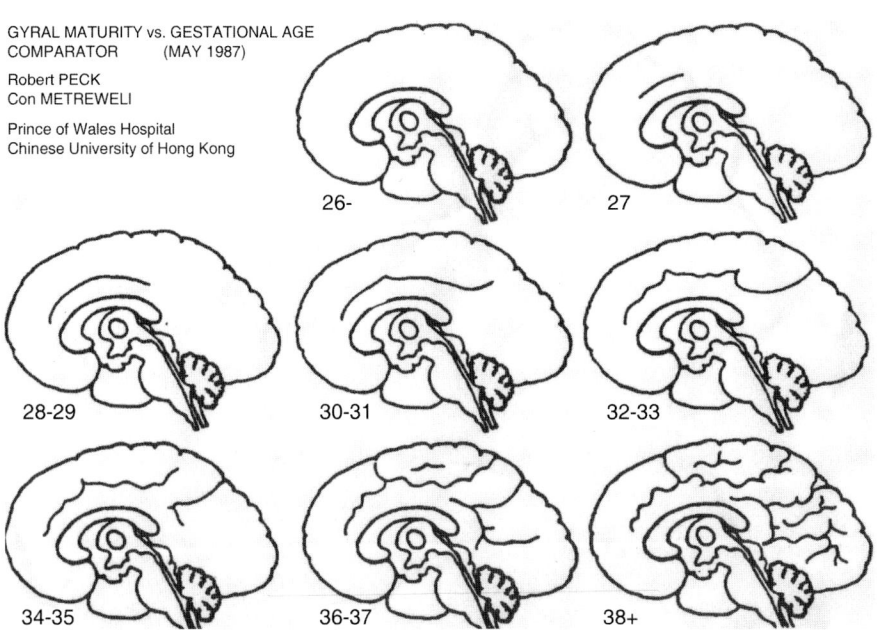

GYRAL MATURITY vs. GESTATIONAL AGE COMPARATOR   (MAY 1987)

Robert PECK
Con METREWELI

Prince of Wales Hospital
Chinese University of Hong Kong

Figure 8. Showing comparative sagittal and coronal sections of gyral pattern in full term, 33-week and 24-week gestation neonates.

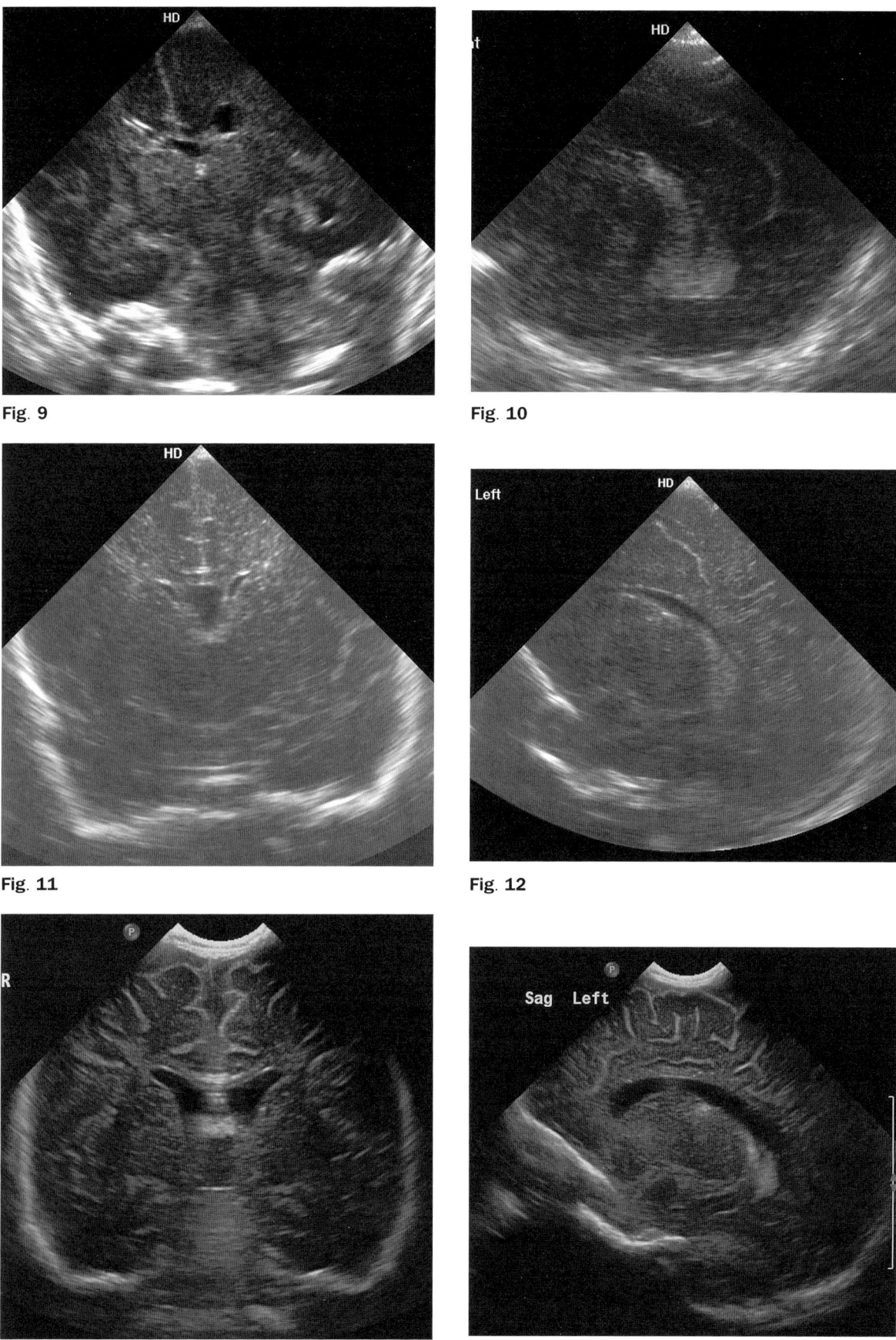

Fig. 9

Fig. 10

Fig. 11

Fig. 12

Fig. 13

Fig. 14

Figures 9–14. Comparative coronal and sagittal scans showing maturation of sulcal-gyral pattern in 24-weeks (Figs. 9 and 10), 33-weeks (Figs. 11 and 12), and term neonates. (Figs. 13 and 14 show term sprigg prem cor vents SCP.)

Cranial US via the anterior cranial fossa allows images to be performed in the coronal, sagittal, and parasagittal planes. As postnatal scanning can only be performed through a patent fontanel (ultrasound will not penetrate bones for any significant distance) the orientation of coronal and parasagittal images are in different planes to CT or MRI images. US images from the anterior fontanel can be supplemented by axial imaging via the mastoid foramen or via the posterior fontanel or cranio-cervical junction. The appearance of the brain surface varies with gestation and progressive sulcation (Figs. 9–14).

There are no internationally recognized standards of how to perform a pediatric cranial ultrasound scan. The British Society of Paediatric Radiologists (www.bspr.org.uk) has produced a technical standard for neonatal cranial US scans to improve reproducibility between operators and standard of performance between different institutions.

Scanning is performed in real time and is best interpreted by the sonographer that performs the scan. Currently there is no requirement to record a standardized set of images in cranial US. On some neonatal units the scan is performed and an opinion written in the notes without any hard (or soft) copy record. Most ultrasound machines are equipped with printers for producing paper images and more recent digital machines will allow electronic recording of images, including video clips for retrospective review, further opinions, and audit. Standardization of technique in US scanning lags behind cranial CT and MR imaging.

STANDARD IMAGING PLANES

The following images demonstrate use of some of the standard scan planes. Standard series of six coronal scans (Figs. 15–21):

1. Anterior
2. At the level of the sylvian fissures
3. At the level of the temporal horns
4. At the level of the hippocampi
5. At the level of the choroid plexi
6. Posterior parietal/occipital horns

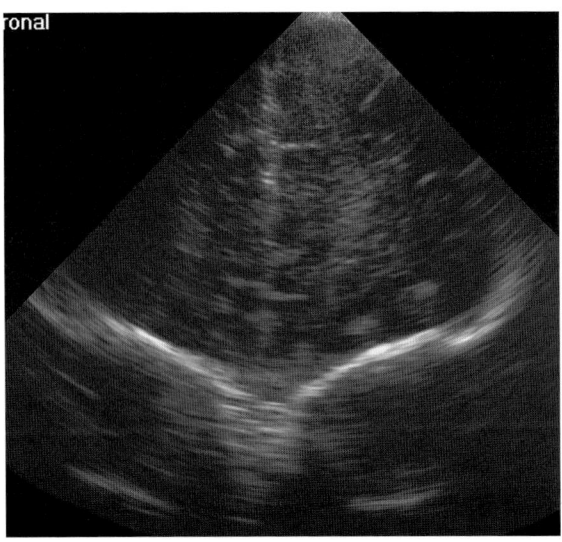

Figures 15. Frontal lobes anterior to the lateral ventricles.

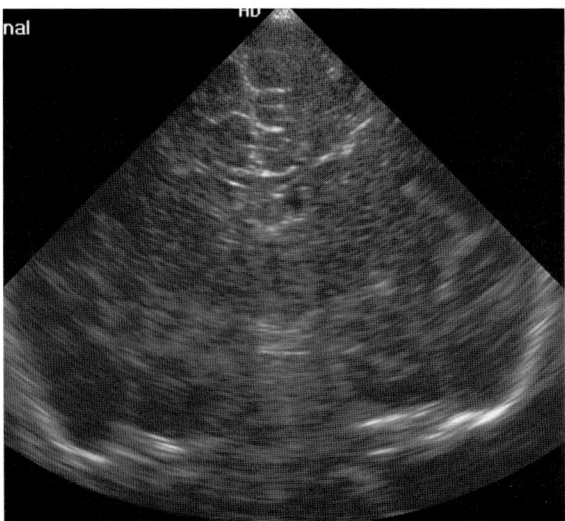

Figure 16. Sylvian fissures and the third ventricle and lateral ventricles (normal small ventricles).

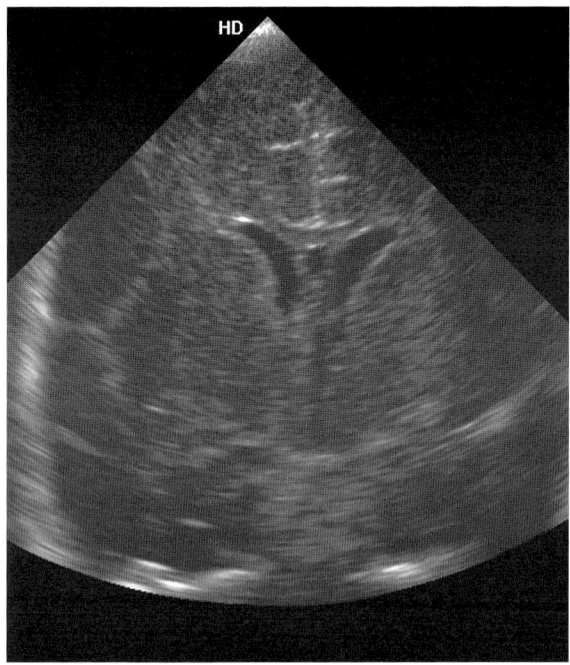

Figure 17. Third ventricle, septum cavum pellucidum thalami and corpus callosum near the level of the foramina of Munro (normal size ventricles).

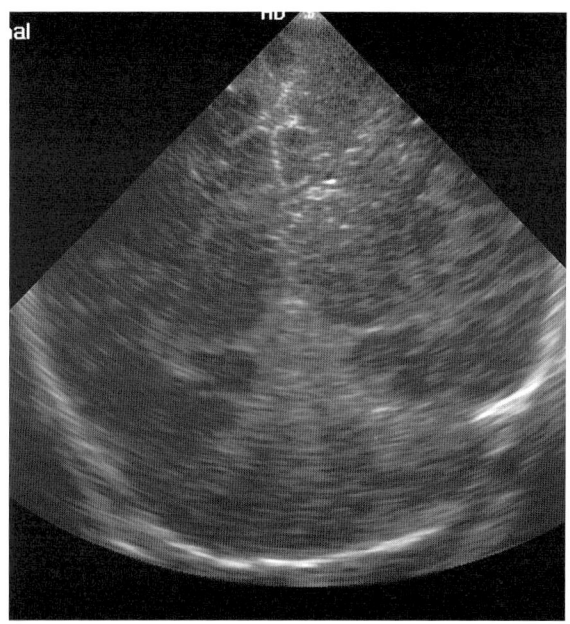

Figure 18. Hippocampi and the tentorium and anterior cerebellum.

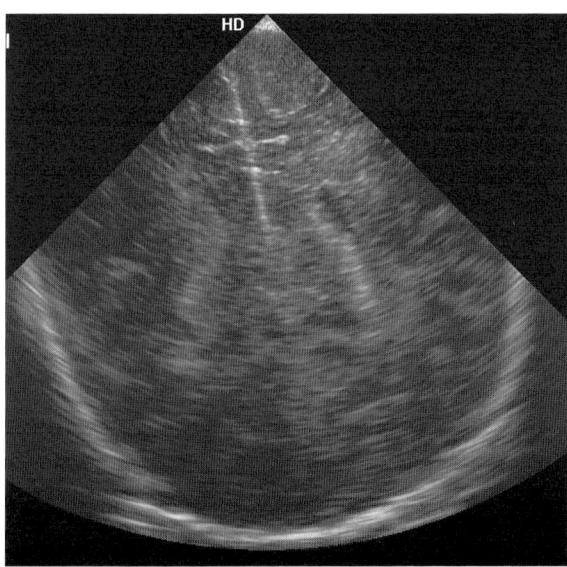

Figure 19. Posterior section showing choroids in the trigone of the lateral ventricles.

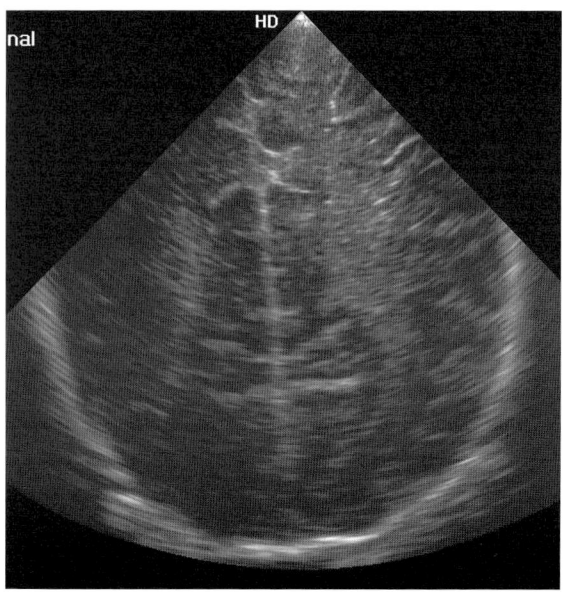

Figure 20. Most posterior section showing periventricular white matter in the parietal lobe.

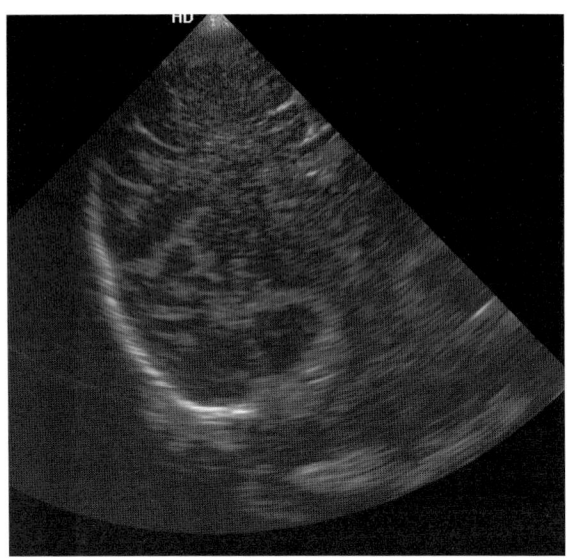

Figure 21. Lateral angulation of the probe shows the periventricular white matter and sulcation pattern—an area that may be omitted from a standard scan due to the limited field of the sector probe, or a small fontanel.

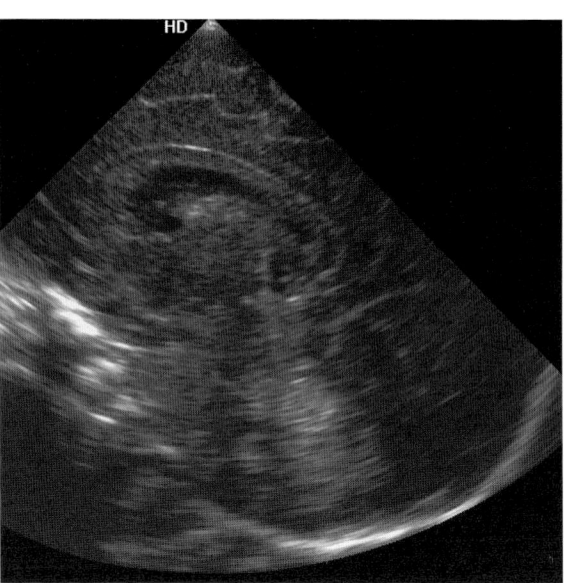

Figure 22. Midline sagittal section showing the corpus callosum and septum cavum pellucidum (SCP) and cerebellum (normal—very bright) with 4th ventricle. The third ventricle is slit-like and below the SCP. The third ventricle is usually difficult to define on sagittal US. It is usually only seen when it is starting to dilate.

Standard series of five (minimum) sagittal views are recorded:

1. Midline sagittal including corpus callosum, septum cavum pellucidum, and cerebellum with 4th ventricle.
2 and 3. Parasagittal scans including the caudothalamic notch, atrium of the lateral ventricle and parietal white matter (left and right).
4 and 5. More lettered parasagittal scan including perventricular white matter (left and right).

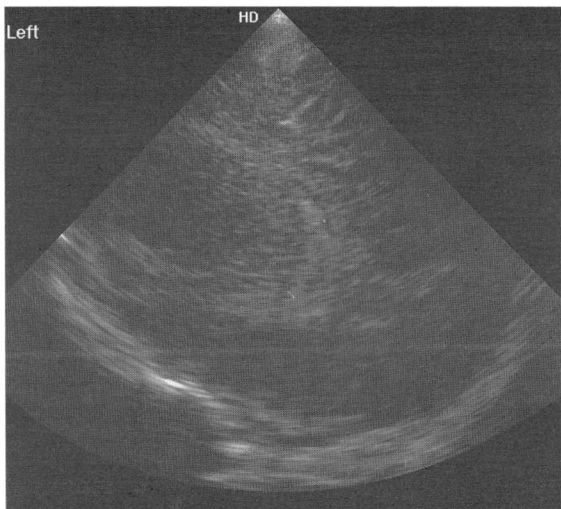

Figure 23. Parasagittal scan of normal term baby with small lateral ventricles. Normal bright choroid at the trigone.

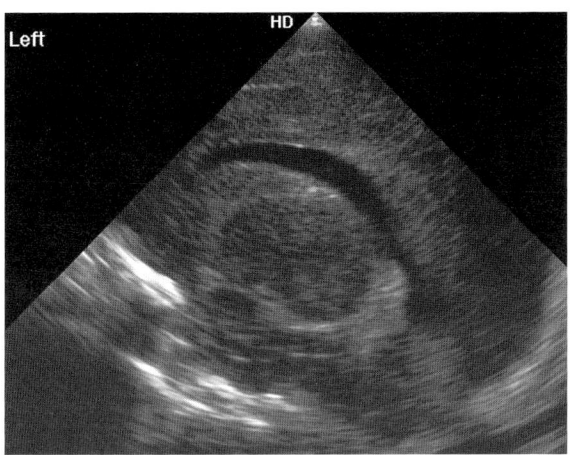

Figure 24. Parasagittal scan in a baby with normal but prominent ventricles. The presence of more CSF in the lateral ventricles helps define the bright choroid, the caudate, and the thalamus.

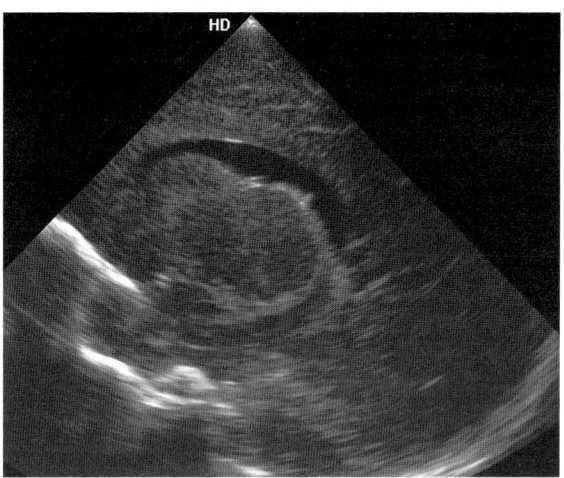

Figure 25. An oblique parasagittal scan with normal ventricles with the head of the caudate and the thalamus. The caudothalamic notch is easily identified as a concavity at the level of the germinal matrix—defining the anterior limit of the choroid (bright).

Alternative scan planes:

1. Axial cerebellum
2. Axial scan showing mild ventricular dilatation
3. Axial cerebral peduncles
4. Limitations of posterior fossa imaging by US
5. Posterior fossa hemorrhage
6. Posterior fossa hemorrhage on CT

The skill of the operator is in adjusting the scan field and gains settings to give an appropriate echo pattern throughout the brain. If the section is recorded with a degree of rotation (due to a wriggling infant) this may simulate pathology. The early work used skull base landmarks to determine optimum position (11) but recent improvements

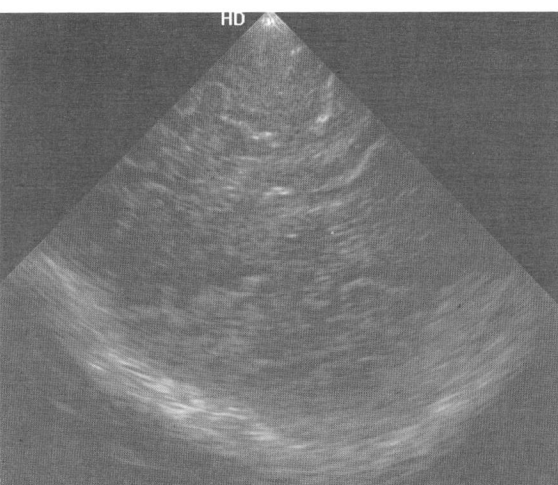

Figure 26. Parasagittal scan with lateral angulation gives better assessment of the periventricular white matter and surface sulcation.

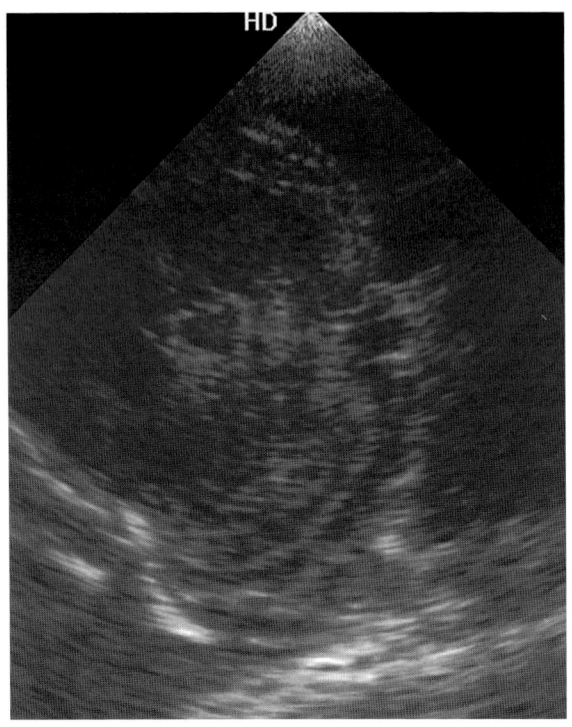

Figure 27. Arial scan via the mastoid foramen shows a normal cerebellum and 4th ventricle in a premature neonate.

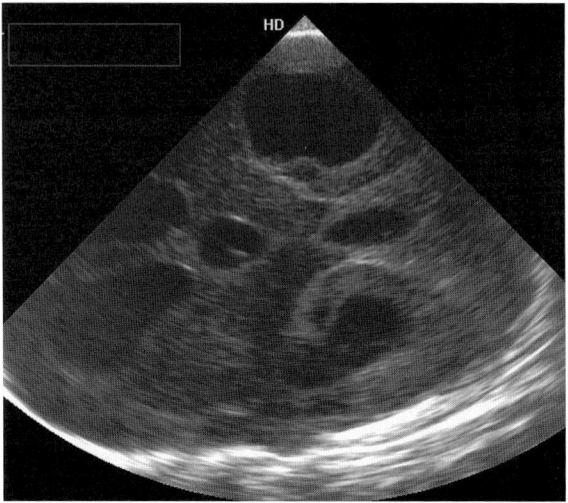

Figure 28. Axial scan with mild ventricular dilatation showing anterior and temporal horns of the lateral ventricles, third ventricle, and the apex of the fourth ventricle.

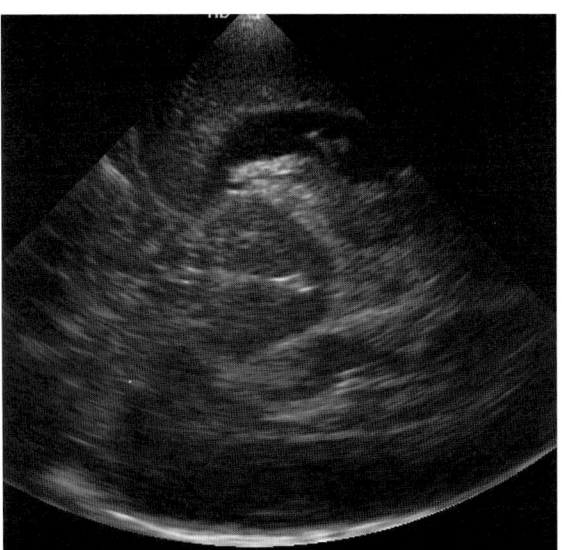

Figure 29. Axial scan showing cerebral peduncles and early dilatation of the temporal horn of the lateral ventricles.

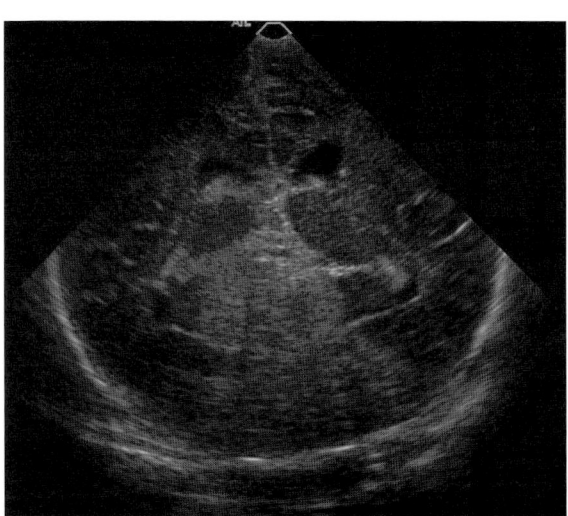

Figure 30. Posterior coronal view with a bright tentorium and loss of the fourth ventricle. The changes are relatively subtle compared to the CT scan—emphazing the difficulties of US imaging in the posterior fossa.

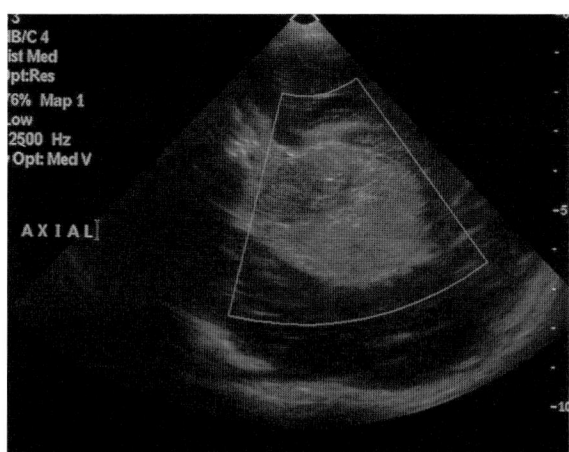

Figure 31. Posterior fossa hemorrhage is evident on axial US.

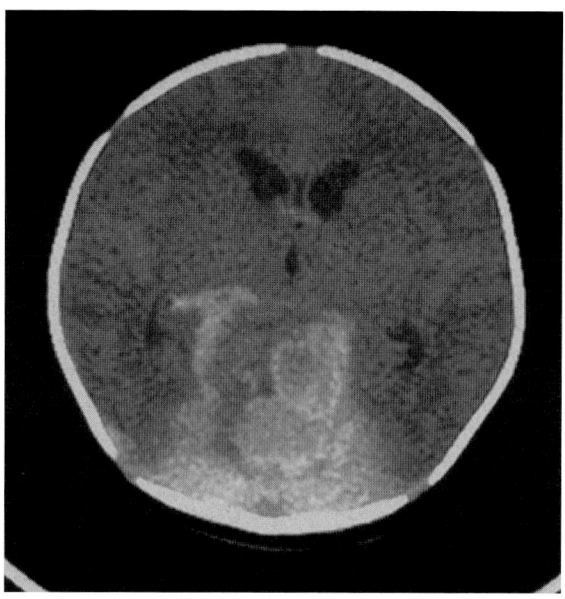

Figure 32. Posterior fossa hemorrhage is evident on CT.

in image quality allow assessment of detailed brain anatomy within imaging planes and sections.

The best quality image is obtained when the US wave from the probe is perpendicular to the structure being imaged. This produces a clear reflected wave signal (e.g., the body of the corpus callosum on a sagittal scan). A structure that lies parallel to the plane of the probe creates a poor quality echo and is poorly visualized (e.g., 3rd ventricle on a coronal scan vs. axial scan) (Figs. 33 and 34) (12). Ventricular size is variable in the neonate.

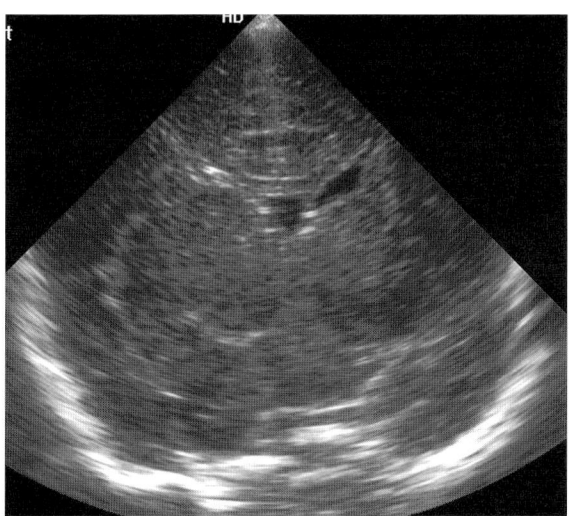

Figure 33. The right lateral ventricle is smaller than the left due to postural changes.

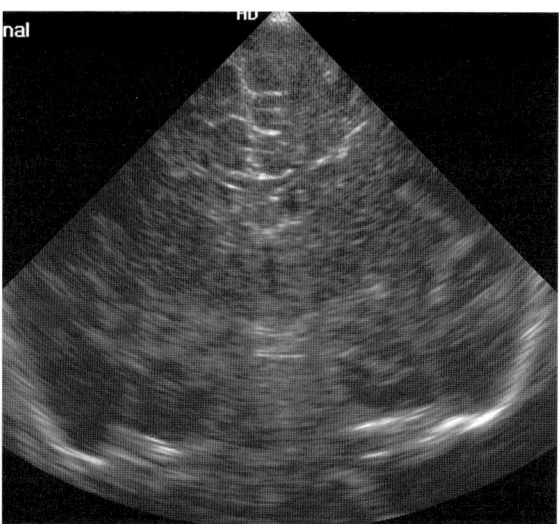

Figure 34. Small lateral ventricles can be normal after vaginal delivery and should not be misdiagnosed as "cerebral edema" in an infant with clinically suspected asphyxia.

PITFALLS AND LIMITATIONS OF ULTRASOUND SCANNING

Cranial US produces a "V" shaped sector image. Further assessment of brain substance needs lateral and posterior angulation of the probe—access to the brain may be limited by the size of the anterior fontanel. Standard images from the anterior fontanel are supplemented by ultrasound images via the mastoid fontanel to produce axial images. The axial plane creates good views of the third ventricle and the cerebral substance of the hemisphere *opposite* to the side of the probe (e.g., the right hemisphere is visualised from the left mastoid foramen and vice-versa). The hemisphere nearer the probe is not well seen due to near-field artifact. Imaging via the midline posterior fontanel or cranio-cervical junction supplements posterior fossa assessment (13,14).

If the initial ultrasound shows displacement of midline structures, then further cranial imaging is indicated using CT or MRI. This should be performed rapidly to determine whether there is a need for neurosurgical intervention (e.g., a significant extra-axial collection or major intra-cerebral or intra-cerebellar hemorrhage).

Cranial US is performed regularly in infants born prematurely as they have a high incidence of cranial complications. Periventricular leukomalacia (PVL) is a common cause of neuro-developmental handicap in prematurity (15). An early sign of PVL on postnatal cranial US is a bright area in the periventricular white matter—a "periventricular flare" (highly reflective area = white). This is a relatively subjective change to the operator and can be confused with the normal corona-radiata on a sagittal scan. This artifact is recognized by sonographers. Abnormal reflectivity from areas of edema/ischemia must be confirmed in both coronal and sagittal planes before diagnosing early PVL. The normal radiating fibers of the corona-radiata are most commonly bright only on the sagittal view but not on the coronal view. If the operator uses high gain settings this may produce artifactual periventricular "flaring."

PVL progresses at a variable rate on US. The bright areas seen initially with PVL are replaced by cystic change within the periventricular white matter. Identifiable cyst formation occurs at a variable time following the insult, with a minimum of seven days but up to several weeks. Hence changes of cystic PVL seen on a scan on the day of birth reflect an antenatal event, not an intra-partum event due to obstetric mismanagement. As healing progresses with gliosis, the amount of periventricular white matter decreases leading to ex-vacuo ventricular dilatation and irregularity of the ventricular margins in the parietal lobes. PVL may develop in infants outside the neonatal period—long term follow-up is needed of infants born prematurely (16).

PVL is often detected postnatally and is related to premature birth. However neurocranial insults may occur antenatally including trauma, ischemia, placental malfunction or twin–twin transfusion (17). Many insults that were once considered due to intrapartum or postnatal events are thought to have their origin in antepartum events. There is significant debate in medical and legal circles regarding intrapartum events causing cerebral palsy (18).

SURFACE (NEAR FIELD) IMAGING

If standard views from the anterior fontanel are not supplemented by near field imaging, surface collections may be missed due to the near field artifact on the standard coronal views. Near field ultrasound can be used to identify the compartment of enlargement of surface spaces, e.g., subarachnoid space enlargement (benign enlargement of the subarachnoid space) (19) from subdural space enlargement (due to effusions, sepsis or hemorrhage). Although US may detect surface collections, contrast enhanced MRI or CT is more sensitive in determining extent and in locating posterior fossa collections and collections over the convexity (especially in neonatal meningitis). The improved sensitivity of CT or MRI over ultrasound has to be balanced against the problems in transporting a sick neonate from the neonatal nursery to the main imaging department (in most hospitals) (Figs. 35–38).

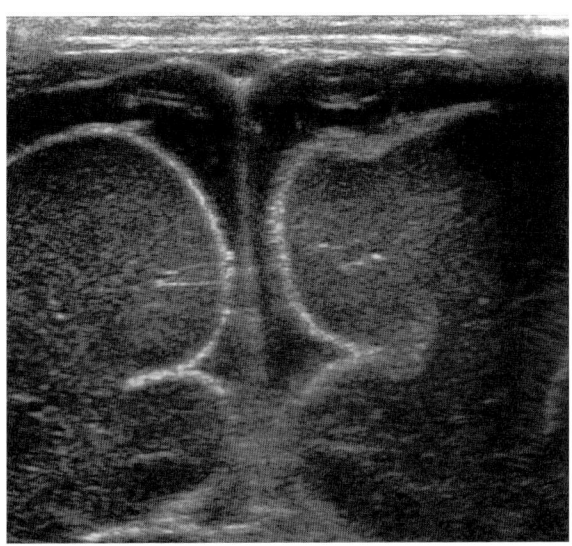

Figure 35. Normal surface subarachnoid space.

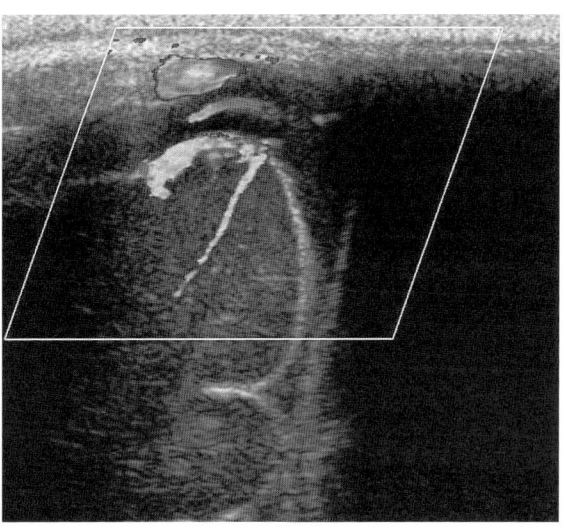

Figure 36. Normal surface subarachnoid color Doppler showing arterial system limited to the subarachnoid space.

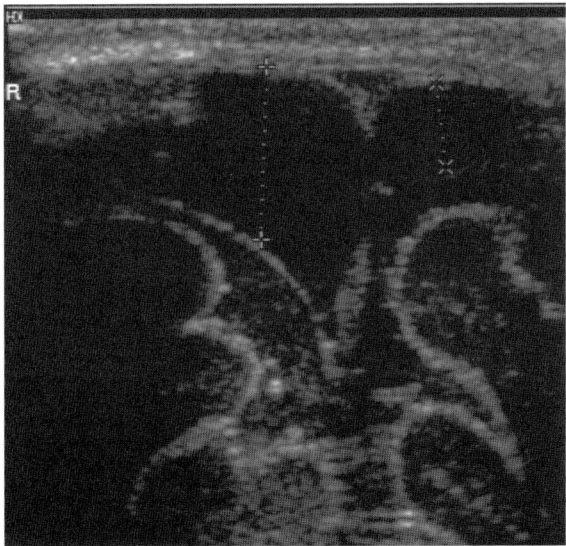

Figure 37. Normal surface subarachnoid and abnormal subdural spaces (calliper).

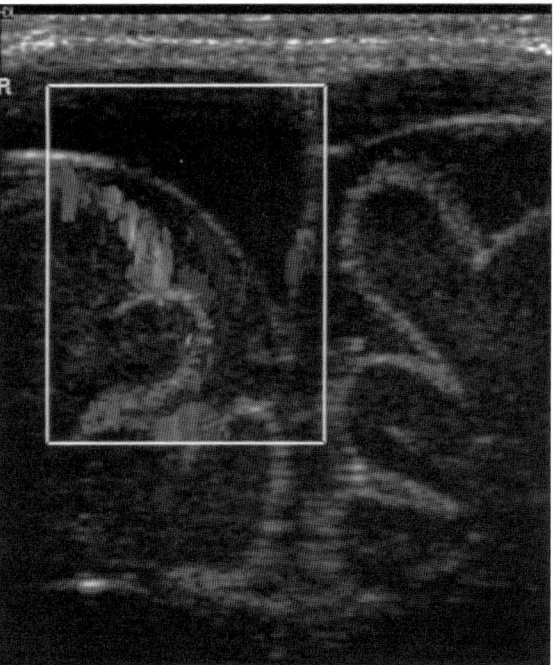

Figure 38. Normal surface subarachnoid and abnormal subdural spaces. Color Doppler showing arterial system limited by the arachnoid membrane and not crossing into the subdural space. If scanning is limited to sector probes then the surface anatomy is lost in the near field. Surface imaging is best performed with a high frequency linear probe.

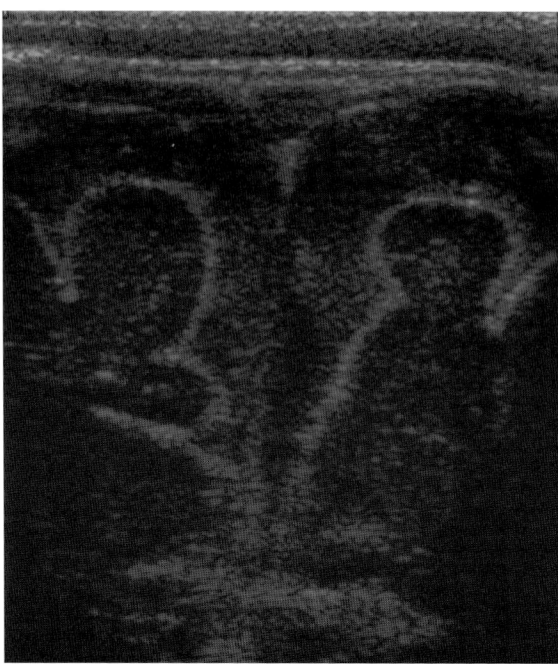

Figure 39. Surface imaging shows increased echo pattern in the subarachnoid space in a baby with meningitis.

Surface collections may complicate meningitis, coagulation disturbance, or metabolic disorders (Fig. 39). They are also frequently seen in association with non-accidental injury (Figs. 35–38). US may also detect shearing lesions at the grey and white matter interface due to acceleration/deceleration injury interface due to shaking in the older infant (20). These will be missed if the operator fails to scan using a near field probe (high frequency linear).

DOPPLER AND OTHER ULTRASOUND SCANNING DEVELOPMENTS

Pulse wave, continuous wave, and color flow Doppler imaging can be used to demonstrate normal intracranial anatomy and occasionally may be used to demonstrate vascular malformations (e.g., vein of Galen varix) (21). Pulsed and continuous wave Doppler US are used to assess cranial blood flow in many pathological states including hypoxic ischemic change and congenital abnormalities and to assess the need for shunt placement in hydrocephalus (Figs. 40–49).

The dynamics of cerebral flow control are complex and further research is needed on the validity of use of Doppler flow signal in various arteries relating to findings on other imaging modalities. In cerebral dysregulation (e.g., hypoxic ischemic change) there is loss of the normal vascular resistive pattern on color flow imaging with a high diastolic trough. A resistive index of less than 0.5 is associated with significant hypoxic ischemic damage. This is due to preservation of the normal systolic peak velocity but a rise of diastolic velocities due to loss of auto-regulation of cerebral blood flow.

The Doppler signal obtained depends on intra-cerebral and extra-cranial factors. Cardiac output fluctuates in an unstable neonate, altering carotid artery perfusion. In a compromised hypoxic ischemic baby, cardiomyopathy may co-exist with cerebral dysregulation. Hypoxic cerebral change is also common in babies with cyanotic congenital heart disease. In many premature babies the ductus arteriosus opens and closes intermittently which further affects the waveform on Doppler imaging of the intra-cranial arteries due to extra-cerebral diastolic "run-off" change.

Color Doppler imaging is useful in defining the limit of the arterial system within the subarachnoid space. This helps differentiate fluid in the subdural space from adhesions

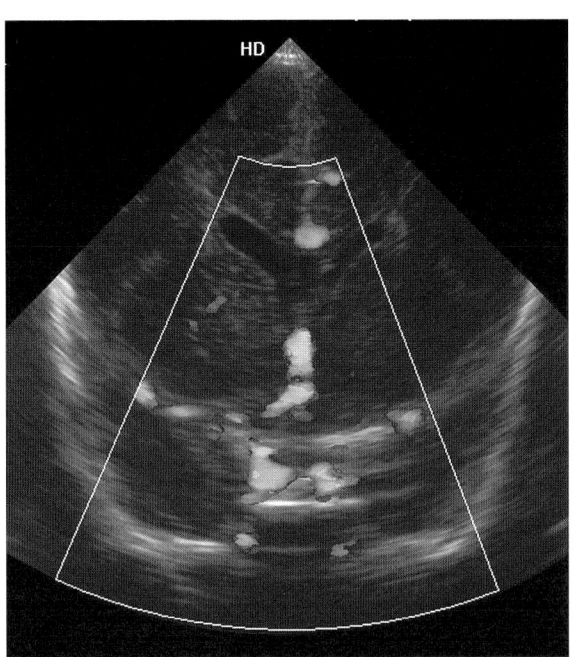

Figure 40. Coronal color scan shows circle of Willis and middle cerebral arteries.

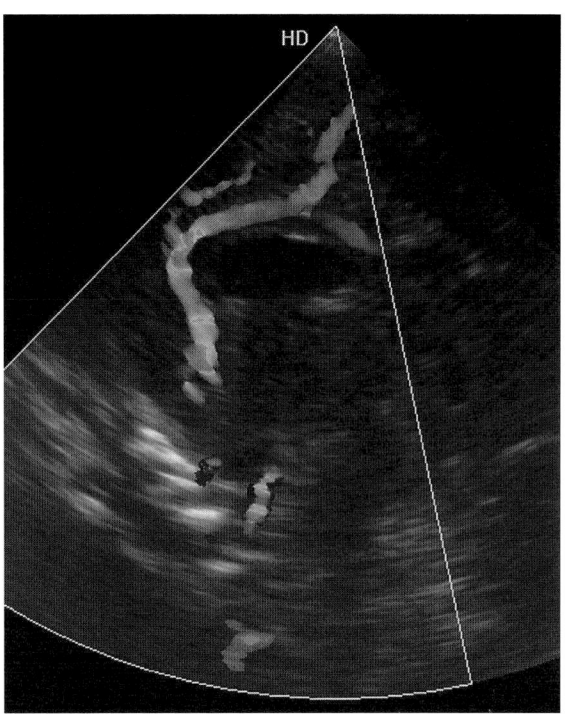

Figure 41. Sagittal midline color scan shows the basilar artery, anterior cerebral artery and pericallosal artery.

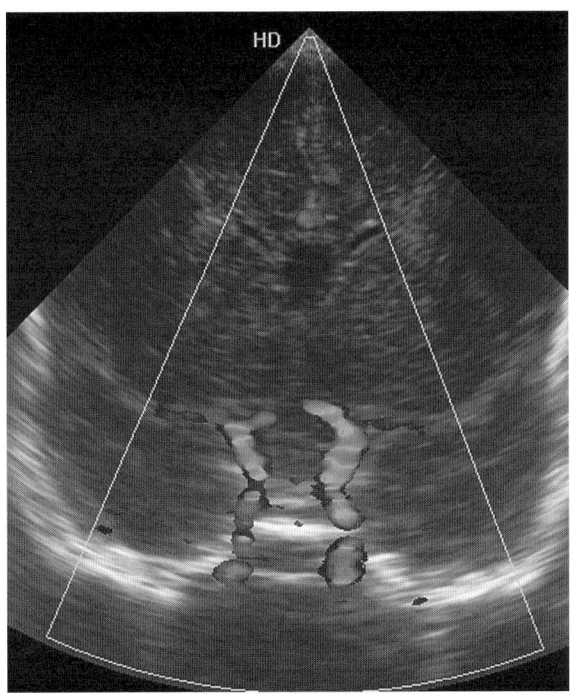

Figure 42. Coronal color scan shows the carotid bifurcation and pericallosal artery.

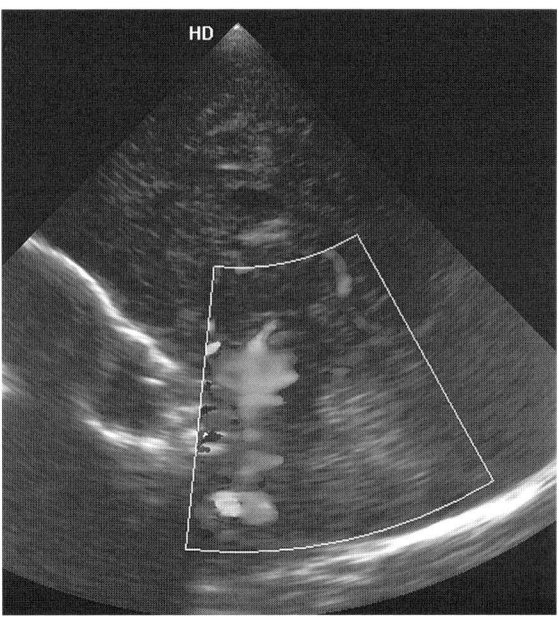

Figure 43. Midline sagittal color scan shows the basilar artery and midline veins.

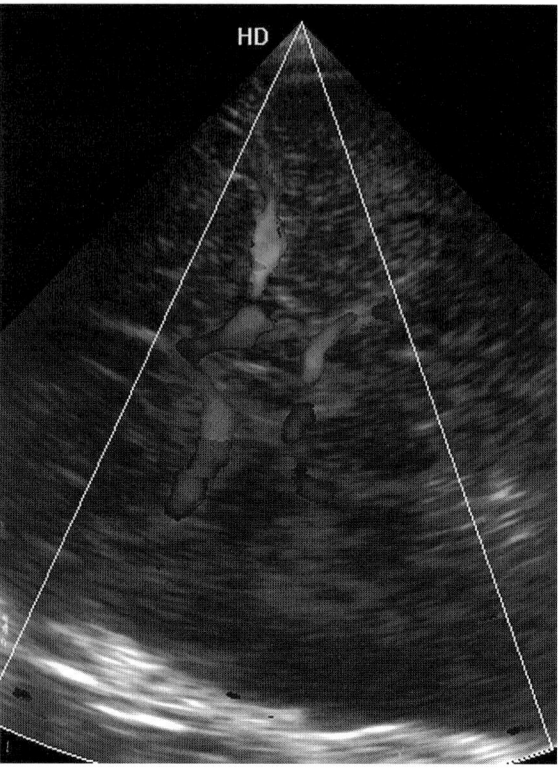

Figure 44. Axial scan with color flow imaging showing a normal circle of Willis.

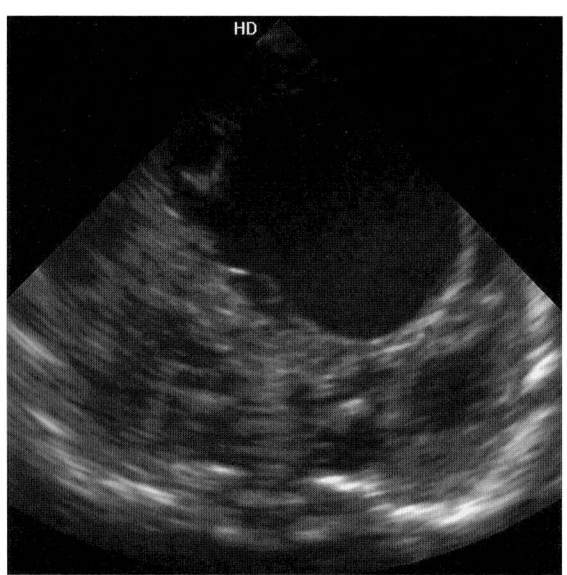

Figure 45. Premature neonate with a cystic area in the left hemisphere. In real time "swirling" was seen within the cyst suggesting vascular malformation.

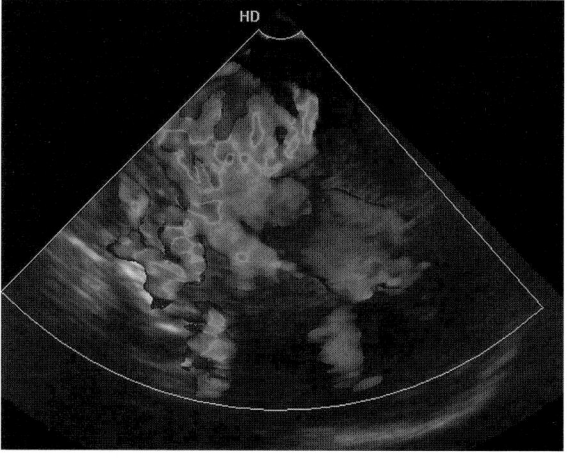

Figure 46. Sagittal color Doppler shows vascular flow within multiple areas (same patient as Fig. 45).

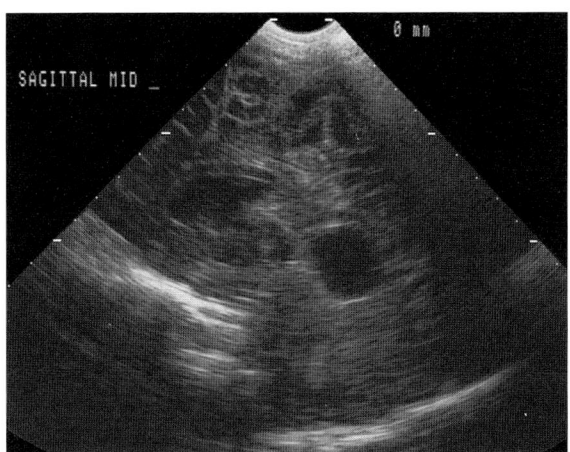

Fig. 47

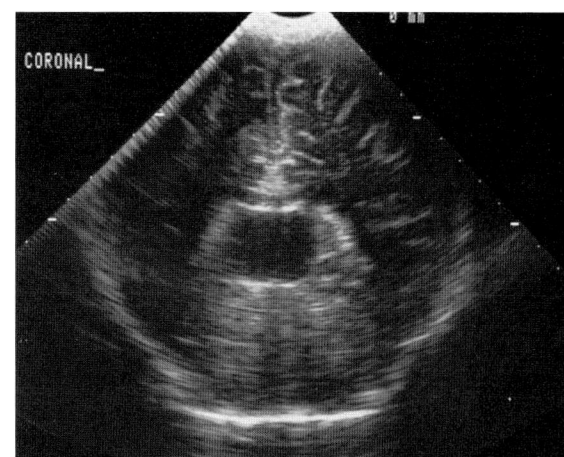

Fig. 48

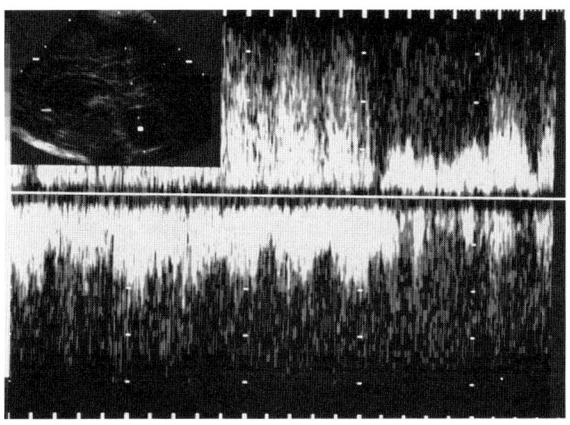

Fig. 49

Figures 47–49. Sagittal (Fig. 47) and coronal (Fig. 48) US show a midline posterior cystic structure in the supratentorial compartment. Pulsed Doppler confirms turbulent flow within the "cyst" (Fig. 49).

within the arachnoid space, as the arterial system is confined to the subarachnoid space (19). Power Doppler has also been used to assess hypoxic ischemic injury (22).

Coronal and midline sagittal Doppler US is used to assess the patency of the superior sagittal venous sinus. This is only accessible in the region beneath the patent anterior fontanel—US assessment of the torcular region is difficult.

More recently 3D US has become available. Its utility in the neonatal nursery needs further assessment, but it may be useful in assessing ventricular volumes and producing more meaningful images for the pediatricians to show to parents to demonstrate major cerebral damage, if there is an issue of withdrawing intensive care (23).

ASSESSMENT OF VENTRICULAR DILATATION

US is sensitive to ventricular dilatation and minor degrees of ventricular asymmetry due to posture. Neonates are often nursed in different positions during the day. If a neonate is nursed on its side, the dependent ventricle will be slightly compressed compared to the uppermost lateral ventricle, hence mild ventricular asymmetry is acceptable (Figs. 33 and 34).

In the clinically normal term infant the ventricles are often small (slit-like) for the few days after vaginal delivery. This may be misinterpreted as a sign of cerebral edema by operators unfamiliar with the normal range of postnatal ventricular size (24,25).

True cerebral edema, which is usually related to hypoxic ischemic damage, requires a change in cerebral architecture—a "bright brain" (with normal gain settings) with loss of definition of surface sulcal pattern in a term infant. These signs within the cerebral substance may take several days to become evident.

Levine (12) described normal ranges of ventricular size at differing gestation with defined centiles. This is regarded as a "standard table" for assessment of ventricular dilatation. Ventricular dilatation on cranial US does not always equate with raised intra-cranial pressure needing shunting—hydrocephalus is a dynamic process between production and re-absorption of cerebrospinal fluid. Following IVH, ventricular dilatation is frequently demonstrated on US but this may arrest, or even revert to normal ventricular size as IVH resolves with time (26). It may be complicated by progressive hydrocephalus, which may need shunting. Serial assessment of ventricular size by US using a standardized technique has a high reliability with a low inter- and intra-operator variability. It is easily performed at the bed-side and repeated assessments can be made over time.

"Ventricular dilatation" may also, associated with failure of brain growth due to a global insult (ex vacuo effect), hence clinical assessment (rate of rise of occipito-frontal circumference (OFC)) and clinical assessment of increased tension in the anterior fontanel by palpation is needed prior to considering shunt insertion for "hydrocephalus." Some neonatal units manage post-hemorrhagic hydrocephalus with serial ventricular (or lumbar) taps via the anterior fontanelle (with US guidance) as a temporizing measure before requesting shunt placement. A ventricular tap also allows pressure measurement. As the sutures have not fused in a neonate, the hydrodynamics of raised pressure hydrocephalus are complex and cannot be assessed purely by measurement of a "ventricular index" on US (Figs. 50–53).

Ultrasound is also used in the neonatal nursery to monitor changes in ventricular dilatation following shunt placement. It may also determine the position of the shunt tip relative to the ventricle to confirm that it is within the ventricular space rather than with

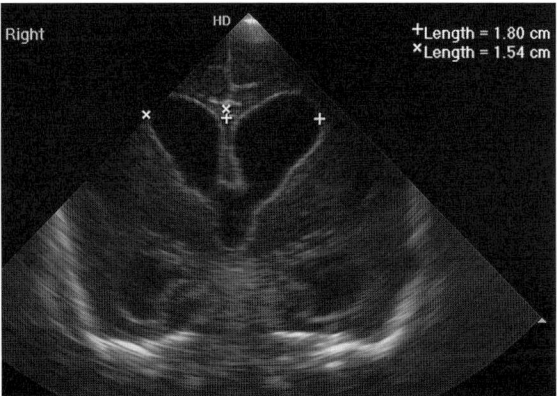

Figure 50. The ventricular index (coronal) is measured from midline to the outermost part of the lateral ventricle at the level of the foramina of Munro.

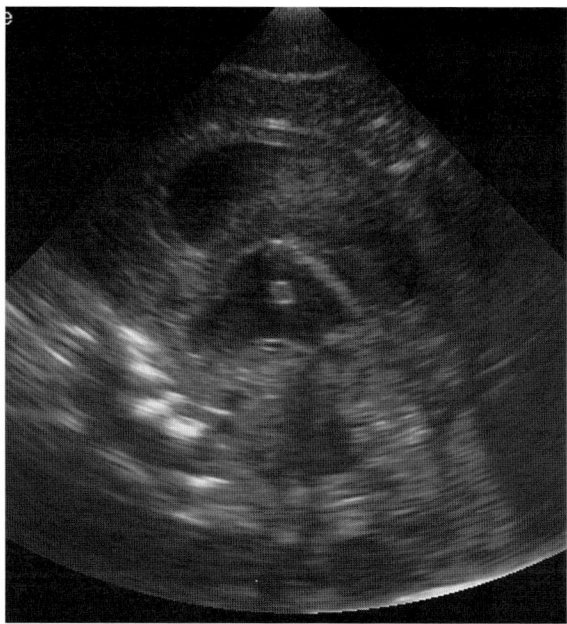

Figure 51. Hydrocephalus—midline sagittal section. The interthalamic connection in the third ventricle is easily identified when there is hydrocephalus.

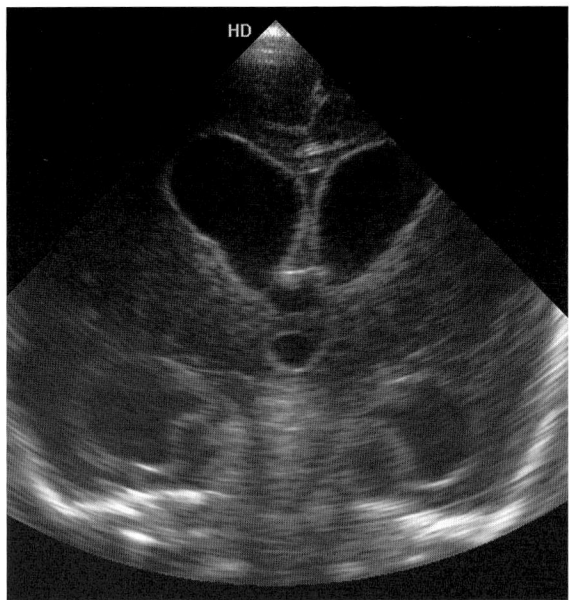

Figure 52. Hydrocephalus—coronal section. The temporal horns of the lateral ventricles are dilated and the inter-thalamic connection is seen in the third ventricle. The bright ventricular lining is due to post hemorrhagic "ventriculitis."

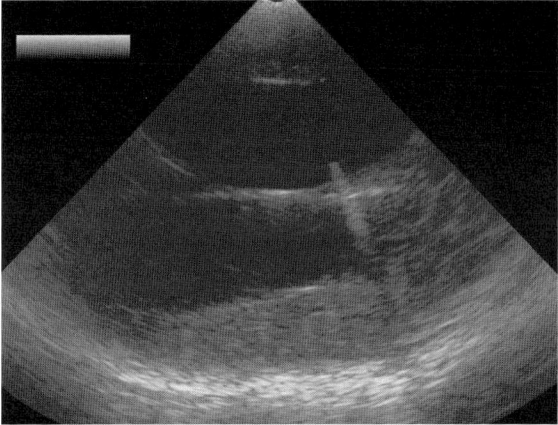

Figure 53. Axial scan shows a shunt placed from the left side crossing the midline with its tip in the posterior part of the right lateral ventricle surrounded by CSF.

the tip being in cerebral substance (i.e., non-functioning). US can also demonstrate loculated fluid collections around the lower end of VP shunts as a cause of shunt malfunction. This is most often seen after VP shunt placement for hydrocephalus in babies with NEC (necrotizing enterocolitis—an ischemic gut disorder of premature neonates).

CONGENITAL ABNORMALITIES

Often congenital abnormalities suspected on obstetric ultrasound are imaged with antenatal MR cranio-spinal imaging. Postnatal US is useful in assessing ventricular dilatation and monitoring progress, but US is not sensitive in detecting migrational or white matter abnormalities. Hydrocephalus is a dynamic process and may develop during the last trimester of pregnancy, despite a normal anomaly scan at 20 weeks. Many cortical structural abnormalities are not formed or detectable at the time of routine fetal anomaly scanning (18–20 weeks gestation). In the newborn period cranial US can be used as the initial modality to exclude a major structural malformation or ventricular dilatation that might need neurosurgical intervention. US is also useful as an initial "screen" with a family history of hydrocephalus or major structural malformation. Detailed assessment of neurocranial anatomy by MRI or CT may be performed electively if the initial cranial US is normal.

USE OF CRANIAL ULTRASOUND OUTSIDE THE NEONATAL PERIOD

Ultrasound is most commonly used in the neonatal intensive care unit, but it is also used for non-invasive imaging up until the fontanel closes, prior to 12 months of age. Before requesting US imaging the pediatrician should assess the adequacy of the fontanel!

Pediatricians may request cranial ultrasound rather than CT or MRI as a rapid screen in an infant with a disproportionately large head (OFC) to exclude hydrocephalus or surface space enlargement or "benign macrocephaly." US is frequently requested in the infant presenting with apnea, fits, faints or vacant episodes as it will rapidly exclude displacement of midline structures and significant hydrocephalus.

Pediatricians favor US as an initial screen modality in a baby with a patent fontanel as it does not use ionizing radiation and does not have the same sedation/anesthesia and monitoring problems as with CT and MRI. US is more rapidly available than CT in most imaging departments, which in turn is more rapidly accessible than MRI in an infant with a low clinical probability of intracranial anomaly. While US may detect parenchymal abnormalities it is much less sensitive than CT and MRI—hence the pediatrician still needs to consider further elective imaging by CT/MRI, if the initial US is "normal"—especially if there are persistent clinical features or focal neurology.

ULTRASOUND AND SPINAL IMAGING

Ultrasound does not penetrate through bone but in the neonate the posterior spinal arches are poorly mineralized, allowing US assessment of the cord and dural sac from the foramen magnum down to the sacral hiatus. This is performed in sagittal and axial orientation. As the infant matures and the posterior bony arch ossifies, access for spinal imaging is increasingly limited and MRI is needed (Figs. 54–59).

There is a high incidence of spinal abnormalities in babies who have other congenital syndromes, e.g., ano-rectal malformation, cloacal exstrophy, caudal regression and spinal segmentation abnormalities—the VATER/VACTEROL anomaly. Spinal US is used as an initial screening tool in the neonate unless there is rapid access to spinal MRI.

COMPARISON WITH OTHER IMAGING MODALITIES

Basic Physics

US: Uses high frequency sound waves. Images are produced due to differences in reflectivity of the ultrasound beam.

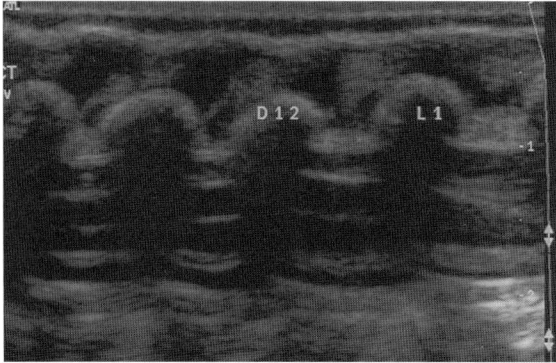

Figure 54. Midline sagittal section. The normal expansion of the lower cord is shown, and the bright central canal and terminus. The spinous processes are counted from the lowest rib. Normal conus at L1/2 level. The baby is lying prone and the conus moves to the dependent part of the dural sac.

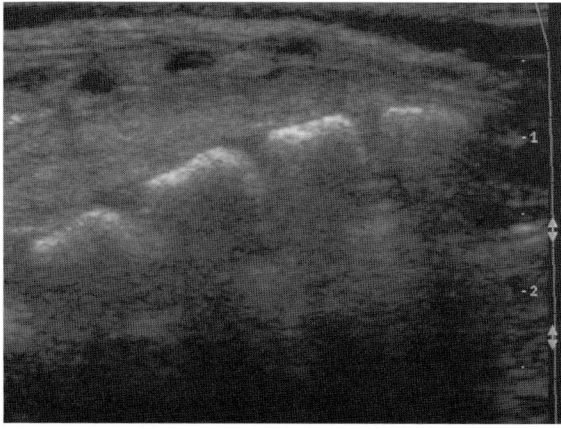

Figure 55. Sagittal view of the cauda equina in the sacral hiatus anterior to the sacral spine vertebral bodies.

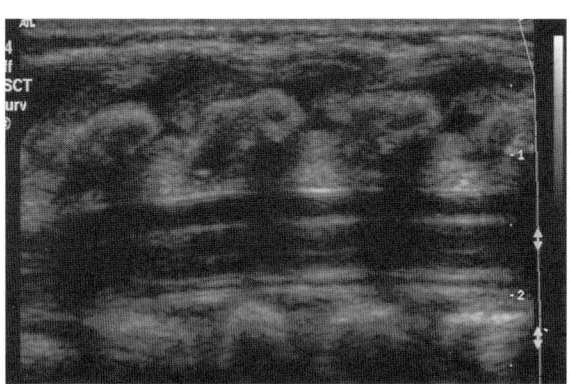

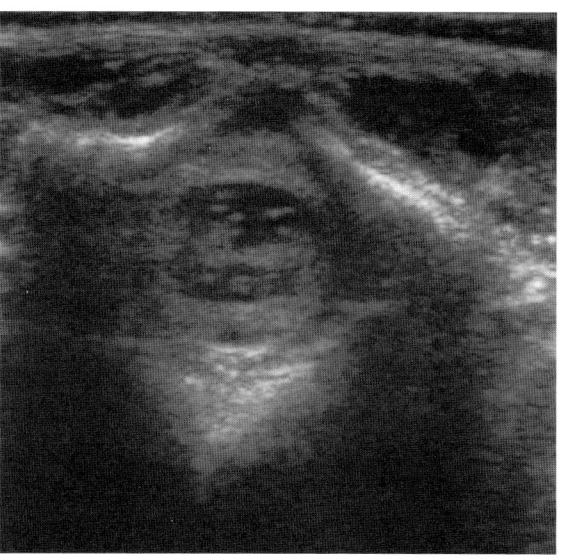

Figure 56. Sagittal view of cord in the mid thoracic region. Normal—low echo cord with narrow bright central canal.

Figure 57. Axial section of canal below the conus shows nerve roots moving in the dural sac. The separate dorsal and ventral roots are identifiable.

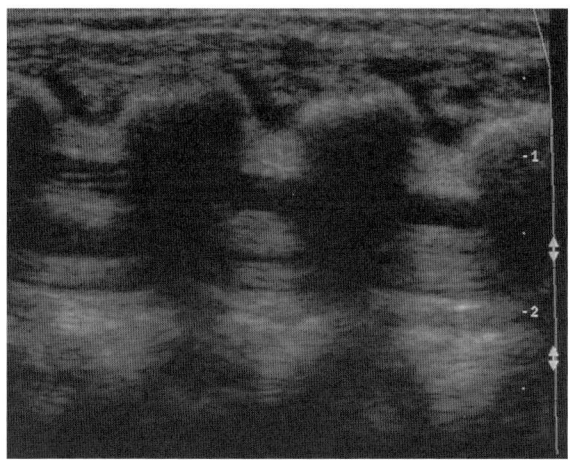

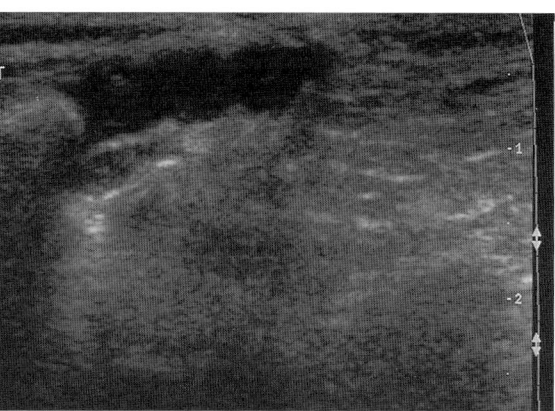

Figure 58. Sagittal section shows the conus (dark) with the mobile nerve roots of the cauda equina in the dural sac.

Figure 59. The low echo unossified coccyx is seen below the ossified S5 segment.

CT: Uses ionizing radiation. Images depend on differences in X-ray attenuation of different brain structures and skull.

MRI: Uses high field magnetic fields and radio-frequency signals. Signal intensity depends on varying distribution of protons (H) in the normal brain and pathological areas. The imaged signal depends on the sequence used.

Ultrasound Advantages

- Easily portable to the bed-side
- Does not use ionizing radiation
- Good tolerance of patient movement

- Minimal disturbance to a sick neonate
- Easily repeated
- Sensitive to major intra-cranial hemorrhage and ventricular dilatation

Ultrasound Disadvantages

- Imaging planes coronal and sagittal supplemented by posterior fossa and axial imaging
- Needs a patent fontanel (restricted to infants)
- Operator dependent
- Reporting variability
- Limited sensitivity to hypoxic ischemic change
- Limited views of the convexity over both cerebral hemispheres
- Limited views of the posterior fossa
- Limited assessment of acute extra-axial hemorrhage

CT Advantages

- Sensitive to acute hemorrhage
- Reproducible
- Gives some imaging of bone
- Some assessment of arterial and venous system with intravenous contrast

CT Disadvantages

- Uses ionizing radiation
- Limited tolerance of movement
- The neonate has to be transported to the machine (usually in imaging department)
- Reporting variability (in neonatal CT)—especially in myelination pattern
- Mainly limited to the axial plane
- May not show acute ischemic change
- May not show white matter disorder

MRI Advantages

- Multiplanar capability
- Sensitive to white matter change/edema/hypoxic ischemic change
- Good at posterior fossa imaging
- Reproducible, but depends on multiplicity of sequences
- Sensitive to heterotopia and congenital cortical abnormalities
- Assesses myelination
- Diffusion weighted imaging (DWI and/or ADC)
- MR Angiography/MR Venography capability

MRI Disadvantages

- May miss acute hemorrhage
- The neonate requires transporting to the department (most high field MRI machines are in imaging departments)
- Radio-frequency signals determine specific ventilator/monitoring requirements

■ Pattern of neonatal imaging is different from adult anatomy due to variation in maturity of patient and progressive myelination

■ Very limited tolerance of neonatal movement i.e., may require several attempts at MRI: feed and wrap, sedation or general anesthesia

REFERENCES

1. Grant E, Schellinger D, Borts F, et al. Real time sonography of the neonatal and infant head. Am J Neuroradiol 1980; 1:487–492.
2. Dewbury KC, Aluwihare APR. The anterior fontanelle as a window for study of the brain: a preliminary report. Br J Radiol 1980; 53:81–84.
3. Dewbury KC, Bates RI. The value of transfontanellar ultrasound in infants. Br J Radiol 1981; 54:1044–1052.
4. Babcock DS, Han BK. The accuracy of high resolution real time ultrasonography of the head in infancy. Radiology 1981; 139:665–676.
5. Babcock DS. Sonography of the brain: role in evaluating neurologic abnormalities. AJR 1995; 165:417–423.
6. Makhoul IR, Eisenstein I, Sujov P, et al. Neonatal lenticulostriate vasculopathy: further characterization. Arch Dis Child Neonatal Ed 2003; 88:F275–F279.
7. Royal college of radiologists: Ultrasound training recommendations for medical and surgical specialities. Royal College of radiologists, London, 2005.
8. Shuman WP, Rogers JV, Mack LA, Alvord EC, Christie DP. Real time sonographic sector scanning of the neonatal cranium: technique and normal anatomy. AJR 1981; 137:821–828.
9. Pigadas A, Thompson JR, Grube GL. Normal infant brain anatomy: real time sonograms and brain specimens. AJR 1981; 137:815–820.
10. Stewart AL, Thorburn RJ, Hope PL, Goldsmith M, Lipscomb AP, Reynolds EO. Ultrasound appearance of the brain in very preterm infants and neurodevelopmental outcome at 18 months of age. Arch Dis Child 1983; 58:598–604.
11. Cremin BJ. Anatomical landmarks in anterior fontanelle ultrasonography. Br J Radiol 1983; 56:517–526.
12. Levine MI. Measurement of the growth of the lateral ventricles in pre-term infants with real time ultrasound. Arch Dis Child 1981; 56:900–904.
13. Buckley KM, Taylor GA, Estroff JA, Barnewolt CE, Share JC, Palteil HJ. Use of the mastoid fontanelle for improved sonographic vizualilization of the neonatal midbrain and posterior fossa. AJR 1997; 168:1021–1025.
14. Yousefzadeh DK, Naidich TP. US anatomy of the posterior fossa in children: correlation with brain sections. Radiology 1985; 156:353–361.
15. Decillion T, N'Guyen SN, Muet A, Quere MP, Mousally F, Roze JC. Limitations of ultrasonography for diagnosing white matter damage in preterm infants. Arch Dis Child Neonatal Ed 2003; 88:F410–F414.
16. Townsend SF, Rumack CM, Thilo EH, Merenstein GB, Rosenberg AA. Late neurosongraphic screening is important to the diagnosis of periventricular leukomalaicia and ventricular enlargement in preterm infants. Pediatr Radiol 1999; 29:347–352.
17. Weeks AD, Davies NP, Sprigg A, Fairlie FM. Sequential in-utero death of hetrokaryotypic monozygotic twins. A case report and literature review. Prenat Diagn 1996; 16:657–663.
18. MacLennan A. A template for defining a causal relation between acute intrapartum events and cerebral palsy: international consensus statement. Br Med J 1999; 319:1054–1059.
19. Libicher M, Troger J. US measurement of the subarachnoid space in infants: normal values. Radiology 1992; 184:749–751.
20. Jaspan T, Narborough G, Punt JAG, Lowe J. Cerebral contusional tears as a marker of child abuse—detection by cranial sonography. Pediatr Radiol 1992; 22:237–245.
21. Soto G, Daneman A, Hellman J. Doppler evaluation of cerebral arteries in a galenic malformation. J Ultrasound Med 1985; 4:673–675.
22. Steventon DM, John PR. Power doppler ultrasound appearances of neonatal ischaemic brain injury. Pediatr Radiol 1997; 27:147–149.
23. Riccabona M, Nelson TR, Weitzer C, Resch B, Pretorius DP. Potential of three-dimensional ultrasound in neonatal and paediatric neurosonography. Eur J Radiol 2003; 13:2082–2093.

24. Mercuri E, Dubowitz L, Paterson-Brown S, Cowan F. Incidence of cranial ultrasound abnormalities in apparently well neonates on a postnatal ward: correlation with antenatal and perinatal factors and neurological status. Arch Dis Child Fetal Neonatal Ed 1998; 79:F185–F189.

25. Nelson MD, Jr., Tavare CJ, Petrus L, Kim P, Gilles FH. Changes in the lateral ventricles in the normal-term newborn following vaginal delivery. Pediatr Radiol 2003; 831:835.

26. London DA, Carroll BA, Enzmann DR. Sonography of ventricular size and germinal matrix hemorrhage in premature infants. AJR 1980; 135:559–564.

FURTHER READING

1. Rennie JM. Neonatal Cerebral Ultrasound. Cambridge: Cambridge University Press, 1997.

2. Govaert P, de Vries LS. An atlas of brain sonography. Clinics in Developmental Medicine. London: Cambridge University Press, 1997 pp. 141–142.

3. Rennie JM, Roberton NRC. Textbook of Neonatology. 3rd ed. Edinburgh: Churchill Livingstone, 1999.

4. Sarnat HB, Sarnat MS. Neonatal encephalopathy following fetal distress. Arch Neurol 1976; 33:696–705.

5. US adaptation of Papile classification Levene MI, De Crespigny L. Classification of intraventricular haemorrhage. Lancet 1983; 1:643.

6. Papile L-A, Burstein J, Burstein R, Koffler H. Incidence and evolution of subependymal and intraventricular haemorrhage: a study of infants with birth weight less than 1500 gram. J Pediat 1978; 92:529–534.

7. De Vries LS, Eken P, Dubowitz LMS. The spectrum of leukomalacia using cranial ultrasound. Behav Brain Res 1992; 49:1–6.

3.2

Magnetic Resonance Imaging of the Neonatal Brain

Elspeth H. Whitby and Martyn N. J. Paley
Academic Unit of Radiology, University of Sheffield, Sheffield, U.K.

MAGNETIC RESONANCE IMAGING (MRI) OF THE NEONATAL BRAIN

With the increasing developments in neonatal and reproductive medicine there are greater numbers of premature neonates surviving. These babies are at a higher risk of diseases and trauma that result in long-term neurodevelopmental and behavioral problems than those born at term.

Traditionally ultrasound imaging has been the reference standard for neonates on the neonatal intensive care unit (NICU), as it is easy to perform by trained personnel, causes minimal disruption to the neonate, and is transportable. However the technique is operator dependent, unable to differentiate gray and white matter, and is poor at delineating posterior fossa and peripheral anomalies, although new anatomical views are helping in that regard (1).

Computed tomography (CT) is of value but the gray/white matter differentiation is poor, the equipment is static, and the neonate needs to be removed from the stable environment of the NICU and transported to the imaging department. CT uses ionizing radiation, which should be avoided if at all possible.

MRI has been available for over 20 years, but again has been limited to fixed locations as the capital and running costs have meant that only large centers have had access to such equipment. The size of the machines and costs are decreasing and there is correspondingly increasing experience in imaging the neonate by MRI, however difficulties still remain. Most units only have access to MRI scanners in the imaging department, which involves transfer of the neonate. MRI-compatible life support equipment has made this easier, but it still places the neonate under additional stress. Ideally imaging should take place on the NICU in a clinical environment designed to support the neonate (2). Several units now have a dedicated MRI scanner situated on the NICUs which provide an ideal location for scanning the neonate; not having the clinical demands of the large departments gives the greater flexibility to work around the neonate (3).

In our institution we have developed a small 0.2T magnet (Innervision MRI Ltd., London, U.K.) for such work (4), which is situated on the NICU (Fig. 1). The fringe field is within the outer Faraday cage and a standard resuscitator can be used to mechanically ventilate the neonate if required. Waveguides allow all medication to be continued throughout the duration of the scan and if necessary a member of staff can sit in the unit and have continual access to the child throughout the scan time. The magnet is virtually noiseless, allowing us to image the neonate after a feed without the need for sedation or anesthesia. We have shown that this magnet can detect over 50% more pathology than ultrasound, or detect changes earlier than ultrasound, allowing earlier treatment (4). We have also shown that the majority of pathologies are detected at 0.2T, allowing diagnosis

159

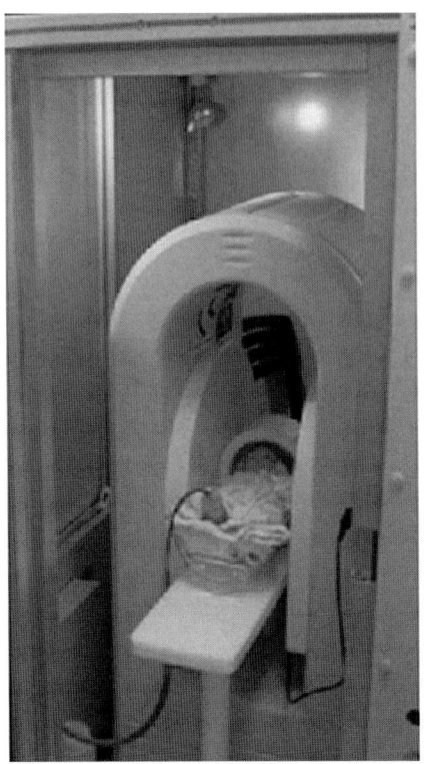

Figure 1. 0.2T MRI scanner.

on the NICU without the need for transfer to the imaging department. Our work has shown that the multiplanar capability of MRI is a distinct advantage when imaging structural abnormalities, especially complex ones that cannot be easily recognized as a distinct pathology. The ability of MRI to demonstrate lesions adjacent to the skull is essential when defining hydranencephaly rather than gross hydrocephalus as this area is difficult with ultrasound. It is similar for lesions in the posterior fossa when bony structures affect the quality of the ultrasound. Certain pathologies can be detected earlier with MRI than ultrasound, e.g., hypoxic damage, and this will allow earlier treatment if available.

An additional advantage of low field over high field MRI is the cost. It is a permanent magnet that does not require cryogens. The capital outlay is a lot less than the larger magnets and the running costs are minimal, resulting in a piece of equipment that is competitive with best available ultrasound machines. In addition conventional resuscitation and ventilation equipment can be used in the magnet room and extension tubes can be added to allow ventilation of the neonate with conventional equipment 'negating' the need to purchase MRI compatible equipment.

The low field scanner has a low specific absorption ratio and low acoustic noise. Vital signs have not been affected in any of the neonates that we have imaged. The open that access design allows rapid removal of the neonate if required.

Currently we image all neonates at 0.2T and a minority of them at 1.5T after the initial 0.2T scan. In most cases this is to obtain good quality DWI not yet possible at 0.2T.

The alternative approach is to use an MRI-compatible incubator for transport and imaging of the neonate at 1.5T. Currently only one such incubator is commercially available and has been used in a research capacity in the U.K. (5) and U.S.A. (6); another is under development. We have tried the incubator on a 1.5T system (5). The incubator allows fast imaging in a safe environment, reducing the risk of adverse events occurring during the transport and imaging of the neonate.

The neonatal incubator would allow sites without a dedicated MRI scanner to image neonates safely. Further developments will overcome the main problems with the incubator, which are poor visibility of the neonate from the control room (it is safer to have a member of staff in the room throughout the scan), and the need for additional monitoring for electrocardiography and oxygen saturation. This is discussed further in the following chapter.

MRI can provide both structural and functional information. The structural MR imaging uses standard T1 and T2 weighted techniques or fast imaging techniques and not only provides a means of differentiating gray and white matter but also can differentiate unmyelinated and myelinated white matter.

Developmental changes can be shown on structural imaging and are related to changes in hydration and myelination. The MRI intensities of the neonatal brain are the opposite of those of the adult brain. Immature white matter is of lower signal intensity than gray matter on T1 weighted images and higher on T2 weighted images. As the white matter matures, the changes in composition result in the signal intensity increasing and becoming higher than that of gray matter. Knowledge of the myelination process is important for accurate interpretation of the images. Myelination occurs in a rostral to caudal direction. During the second trimester, the spinal roots and cord start to myelinate and in the third trimester the brainstem becomes myelinated. At term the superior and inferior cerebella peduncles, the posterior limb of the internal capsule, and the corona radiata are myelinated. It has been shown as early as 25 weeks that the inferior cerebellar peduncles are myelinated, followed by inferior colliculi, posterior brain stem, and ventro-lateral nucleus of the thalamus (7,8). Little seems to myelinate in the period between 28 and 35 weeks. Diffusion weighted imaging (DWI) and diffusion tensor imaging (DTI) are adding to our understanding of myelination (9,10).

Structural malformations in the newborn depend on the gestational age at which the insult occurred. Imaging the neonate allows accurate delineation of the anatomy and the use of fast techniques has reduced the need for general anesthesia (GA) and/or sedation. Without fast imaging techniques, movement artifact makes the image obtained non diagnostic. Ultrafast imaging techniques that allow rapid acquisition of 20 interleaved slices over 20 seconds result in high quality images in short times. Standard T1 and T2 weighted techniques used on sedated neonates or ultrafast T2 weighted techniques provide accurate anatomical information and are ideal for structural abnormalities and damage. The low field strength magnet in our institution enables us to do standard T1 (Fig. 2) and T2 weighted scans without sedation or anesthesia in both pre-term and term neonates and provides information not available by ultrasound (4). Further developments will allow rapid imaging techniques and DWI.

As with the in utero imaging, the appearance depends on the gestational age at the time of birth and the events prior to, during, and post delivery. In all cases it is essential that clinical information is available at the time of imaging and reporting. Knowledge of the normal appearance at each gestational age is increasing from the post-mortem and in utero work and also from various groups involved in imaging of the premature neonate. Knowledge of brain development is essential to ensure optimization of the imaging parameters. It has been shown that T2 measurements gradually decrease from 24 weeks to term but this does not significantly affect the imaging appearances. However, changes are more dramatic in the first year of life as myelination progresses rapidly (11). Several groups (7,12) have documented the developmental stages in terms of sulci and gyri seen in premature neonates on MRI.

Other MRI techniques are used for different conditions affecting the neonate. Both hypoxic and ischemic insults are comparatively common in the term newborn and several different methods of intervention have been described to help reduce the severity of the deficit caused; however, these are interventions that need accurate assessment and if used inappropriately may cause more harm than good (13). MRI is an ideal tool to follow changes in the neonatal brain in response to treatment. Standard T1 (Figs. 2–4) and T2 weighted images will provide diagnostic information (4,14).

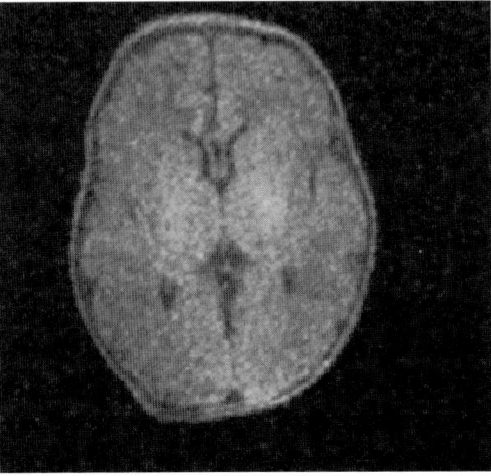

Figure 2. T1 weighted image obtained at 0.2T from a 38-week-gestation neonate at 2 days of age.

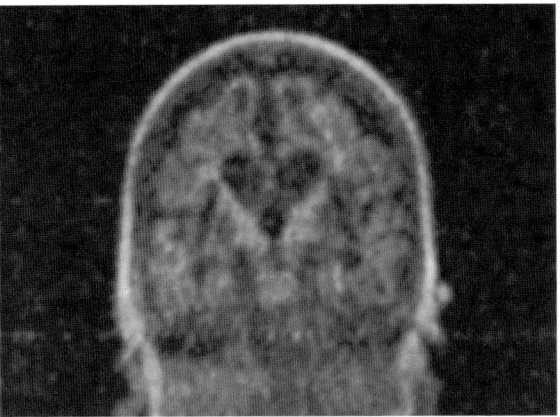

Figure 3. Late hypoxic ischemic damage in a neonate born at term and now 14 days old.

In acute asphyxia in the term infant the basal ganglia, thalami, and corticospinal tracts show high signal on T1 weighted scans. DWI is particularly useful to image ischemic insults (14). DWI measures movement of water molecules, which is completely random but influenced by axonal pathways that restrict diffusion in certain directions. Hence the importance of understanding the pattern of myelination as this will affect the DWI pattern. The technique allows us to obtain DWI maps of the section of the brain imaged. The information obtained depends on the direction in which the orientation of the gradient is applied and it requires information to be obtained in three

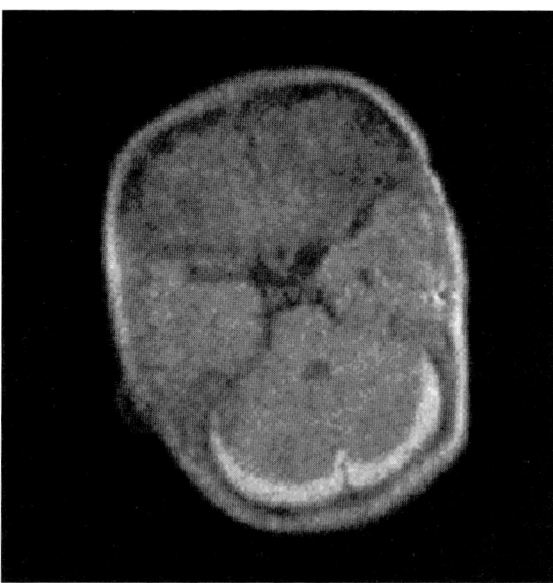

Figure 4. Acute posterior fossa subdural hemorrhage in a term infant age 12 hours.

or more planes. This provides useful information in the early alteration of water movement secondary to an insult, especially an ischemic insult where DWI is abnormal very early in the process when other techniques appear normal, e.g., cell swelling post ischemic injury following a stroke results in further restriction of movement of the water molecules. Recent research shows that diffusion imaging can also be used to evaluate the effects of white matter injury on subsequent microstructural brain development. This has shown that there is not only tissue destruction but also disruption of subsequent brain development (9); again, accurate understanding of development at different gestational ages is essential for interpretation of the data obtained. Despite several reports on the use of DWI for accurate imaging of ischemic injury, a recent publication suggests that conventional MRI methods may be more accurate at detecting ischemic injury, in the deep gray matter than DWI (14). The differences in the groups' results may depend not only on the site of the injury but also on the age of the injury, the technical parameters used for imaging, and the subjects involved as the technique is very sensitive to movement. Reports with conflicting results highlight the nature of imaging neonates where multiple factors are involved in the data collection and its interpretation.

Inborn errors of metabolism may have imaging abnormalities; although these are non-specific, they may aid in the differential diagnosis. For example gray matter is primarily involved in Tay-Sachs and Menke's kinky hair syndrome, whereas white matter is primarily involved in metochromatic leukodystrophy and Krabbes disease. Others involve both, e.g., Leigh disease (subacute neotizing encephalomyelopathy). In these diseases research has shown that MR spectroscopy techniques may be able to identify metabolites that further delineate the diagnosis (15). Normal MR spectroscopy changes as proliferation, organization, and myelination occur in the neonatal brain. The spectrum obtained not only depends on the age of the neonate but also on the area within the brain that is imaged and any insults that have occurred, e.g., asphyxia increases the lactate level and this can remain high for several weeks or months depending on the severity of the injury (16). MR spectroscopy is used to study nuclei with a non-zero magnetic moment. In practical terms this usually includes ^{1}H, ^{23}Na, and ^{31}P. The signal obtained is proportional to the number of nuclei present and hence is a measure of concentration, although this is complicated by relaxation effects necessitating long TRs and short TEs. MR spectroscopy requires high field strengths, tends to sample mix of cell types, e.g., glial cells, cerebrospinal fluid, and white and gray matter, and take several minutes to acquire the data. These factors limit the use of spectroscopy in the neonate, but further developments may speed up the technique, refine the area sampled and allow further research in this group of patients.

With current neonatal care it is increasingly important to know what the impact of any insult to the neonatal brain is likely to have on neurological outcome. With new techniques developing all the time and outcome measures taking years to collect the data, we will not be able to evaluate long-term outcome of new methods for several years.

SUMMARY

Neonatal MRI is a rapidly expanding field. The studies are important but should be interpreted with caution. The changes occurring at this stage of development are immense and rapid. We are only just beginning to understand the "normal" developmental pattern in terms of MRI appearance and the normal age range over which this occurs. The histological basis for the MRI appearance is not fully evaluated for normal or pathological and multiple factors are involved in all cases. Further evaluation is required "with" long-term follow up on large numbers of neonates before we can evaluate the use of new imaging methods for diagnosis or for evaluating the efficacy of new treatment regimes.

REFERENCES

1. Di Salvo DN. A new view of the neonatal brain: clinical utility of supplemental neurologic US imaging windows. Radiographics 2001; 21:943–955.
2. Blickman JG, Jaramillo D, Cleveland RH. Neonatal cranial ultrasonography. Curr Probl Diagn Radiol 1991; 20:91–119.
3. Bradley WBG. 1st ed. Advanced MR imaging techniques. London: martin Dunitz, 1997.
4. Whitby EH, Paley MN, Smith MF, Sprigg A, Woodhouse N, Griffiths PD. Low field strength magnetic resonance imaging of the neonatal brain. Arch Dis Child Fetal Neonatal Ed 2003; 88:F203–F208.
5. Whitby EH, Griffiths PD, Lonneker-Lammers T, et al. Ultrafast magnetic resonance imaging of the neonate in a magnetic resonance-compatible incubator with a built-in coil. Pediatrics 2004; 113:e150–e152.
6. Erberich SG, Friedlich P, Seri I, Nelson MD, Jr., Bluml S. Functional MRI in neonates using neonatal head coil and MRI compatible incubator. Neuroimage 2003; 20:683–692.
7. van der Knaap MS, van Wezel-Meijler G, Barth PG, Barkhof F, Ader HJ, Valk J. Normal gyration and sulcation in preterm and term neonates: appearance on MR images. Radiology 1996; 200:389–396.
8. Huppi PS, Warfield S, Kikinis R, et al. Quantitative magnetic resonance imaging of brain development in premature and mature newborns. Ann Neurol 1998; 43:224–235.
9. Huppi PS, Murphy B, Maier SE. Microstructural brain development after perinatal cerebral white matter injury assessed by diffusion tensor magnetic resonance imaging. Pediatrics 2001; 107:455–460.
10. Cowan FM, Pennock JM, Hanrahan JD, Manji KP, Edwards AD. Early detection of cerebral infarction and hypoxic ischemic encephalopathy in neonates using diffusion-weighted magnetic resonance imaging. Neuropediatrics 1994; 25:172–175.
11. Johnson MA, Pennock JM, Bydder GM, et al. Clinical NMR imaging of the brain in children: normal and neurologic disease. Am J Roentgenol 1983; 141:1005–1018.
12. Ruoss K, Lovblad K, Schroth G, Moessinger AC, Fusch C. Brain development (sulci and gyri) as assessed by early postnatal MR imaging in preterm and term newborn infants. Neuropediatrics 2001; 32:69–74.
13. Gunn AJ, Gluckman PD, Gunn TR. Selective head cooling in newborn infants after perinatal asphyxia: a safety study. Pediatrics 1998; 102:885–892.

14. Forbes KP, Pipe JG, Bird R. Neonatal hypoxic-ischemic encephalopathy: detection with diffusion-weighted MR imaging. Am J Neuroradiol 2000; 21:1490–1496.

15. Chabrol B, Salvan AM, Confort-Gouny S, Vion-Dury J, Cozzone PJ. Localized proton magnetic resonance spectroscopy of the brain differentiates the inborn metabolic encephalopathies in children. C R Acad Sci III 1995; 318:985–992.

16. Hanrahan JD, Cox IJ, Edwards AD, et al. Persistent increases in cerebral lactate concentration after birth asphyxia. Pediatr Res 1998; 44:304–311.

3.3

Neonatal Hypoxic Ischemic Brain Injury

Elysa Widjaja
Academic Unit of Radiology, University of Sheffield, Sheffield, U.K.

Alan Sprigg
Sheffield NHS Trust, Sheffield, U.K.

HYPOXIC ISCHEMIC BRAIN INJURY

Hypoxic ischemic brain injury (HIBI) may result in permanent neurologic injury that manifests as cerebral palsy. There is still a belief among the lay public that HIBI is a major cause of cerebral palsy, hence the high incidence of parties raising medico-legal issues in children with cerebral palsy. In this chapter, we will discuss the major features and potential causes of cerebral palsy, followed by the pathophysiology of HIBI and imaging features of HIBI.

CEREBRAL PALSY

Cerebral palsy is used to describe a group of disorders of the central nervous system manifested by aberrant control of movement or posture, present early in life, and that are not the result of a recognized progressive disease. It is caused by a broad range of developmental, genetic, metabolic, ischemic, infectious, and other acquired etiologies that produce a common group of neurologic phenotypes (1). Though the brain disorder is static, the clinical effects are usually dynamic as the brain matures and the child develops. Cerebral palsy is also commonly associated with a spectrum of developmental disabilities: epilepsy, and visual, hearing, speech, cognitive, and behavioral abnormalities.

Cerebral palsy syndromes are classified according to the type of motor disorder or the topographic distribution of the condition (2,3). The motor disorders included spastic, hypotonic, dystonic, athetoid or mixed varieties of motor problems. Spasticity was the commonest motor impairment, reported to be present in 85% in one series (4), occurring in approximately 1:500 children. Dyskinetic cerebral palsy was found in 8.5% (about 1:5000) and simple ataxia in 6.5% (about 1:6500) children. Topographic taxonomy describes the extremities involved. Hemiplegia describes cerebral palsy affecting one half of the body, predominantly the upper limb more than the lower limb, normally sparing the bulbar muscles. Quadriplegia, or tetraplegia affects all four limbs, the upper limbs more than the lower limbs, and is usually associated with a bulbar palsy. When there is predominant involvement of the lower limbs, this is described as diplegia. If there is predominant involvement of the bulbar muscles, this is described as congenital suprabulbar paresis or Worster–Drought syndrome (5). Cerebral palsy syndromes differ according to the pattern of neurologic involvement, neuropathology, and etiology (Table 1).

Cerebral palsy is the most common disabling and costly form of chronic neurologic disorder affecting approximately 2 in 1000 children (6,7). There is a greater

Table 1. Classification of Cerebral Palsy and Major Causes

Motor Syndrome	Neuropathology	Major Causes
Spastic diplegia	Periventricular Leukomalacia (PVL)	Prematurity Ischemia Infection Endocrine/metabolic (e.g., thyroid)
Spastic quadriplegia	PVL Multicystic encephalomalacia Malformations	Ischemia Infection Endocrine/metabolic Genetic/developmental
Hemiplegia	Stroke: in utero or neonatal	Thrombophilic disorders Infection Genetic/developmental Periventricular hemorrhagic infarction
Extrapyramidal (athetoid, dyskinetic)	Basal ganglia Pathology: putamen, globus pallidus, thalamus	Asphyxia Kernicterus Mitochondrial Genetic/metabolic

number of premature infants who survive, and some of these infants develop cerebral palsy. There is a shift in the number of those with cerebral palsy due to traumatic delivery of term infants to the higher proportion of very low birth weight survivors who would have died in the past. Hence, the overall prevalence of cerebral palsy remains little changed. In 1862, the orthopedic surgeon Little ascribed cerebral palsy to perinatal causes (8). The widespread lay belief that cerebral palsy is likely to be the consequence of asphyxia at birth has led to extensive litigation.

Studies now suggest that the perinatal asphyxial origin of cerebral palsy is much less common than previously thought (9–11). Antepartum events account for a significant portion of cerebral palsy in the term infants (9,10). In more than 75% of cases of cerebral palsy, a single identifiable cause cannot be elucidated (12). Fewer than 10% of children with cerebral palsy had evidence of intrapartum asphyxia (10,12). Many of the factors and conditions associated with cerebral palsy have been extensively reviewed by Nelson et al. (9,13,14), Freeman et al. (15), and Torfs et al. (11). These factors include maternal conditions, congenital anomalies, prematurity or low birth weight, multifetal gestations and placental abnormalities.

Maternal factors associated with cerebral palsy include mental retardation, hyperthyroidism, proteinuria, and long menstrual cycles (9,11). A substantial number of children had congenital anomalies external to the central nervous system. Nelson et al. (13) reported a relative risk of 3.8 for cerebral palsy when major congenital malformations (excluding the central nervous system) were present in the newborn. Torf et al. (11) reported that three-fourths of those children with cerebral palsy in their cohort had either severe (41%) or minor (32%) birth defects. These defects were heterogenous. Intrauterine exposure to maternal infection (e.g., chorioamnionitis, inflammation of placental membranes, umbilical cord inflammation, foul-smelling amniotic fluid, maternal sepsis, temperature greater than 38°C during labor, and urinary tract infection) is associated with a significant increase in the risk of cerebral palsy in normal birthweight infants. The greater number of premature infants who survive with cerebral palsy reflects a greater survival of such infants, most of whom survive in a healthy condition (16), rather than an increased risk of cerebral palsy for such children. Cerebral palsy in the preterm infants is primarily due to hemorrhage and periventricular leukomalacia (PVL). Although the incidence of intracerebral haemorrhage has declined significantly, PVL remains a major problem.

HYPOXIC ISCHEMIC BRAIN INJURY

Hypoxia/ischemia is a significant cause of neurologic damage arising in the pre-and perinatal periods. Sixty percent of premature infants with HIBI die, 13% survive with significant neurologic deficit and 27% develop normally (17). Term infants with HIBI have a better prognosis, with death in 11%, neurological deficit in 25% and normal development in 64% (17). The 25% that survive with neurological deficits often need prolonged care, which affects the life of parents and siblings and is expensive. For this reason they frequently enter the medico-legal environment. However, only a small number of neonates with birth asphyxia have cerebral palsy and similarly only a small proportion of cerebral palsy is due to birth asphyxia. However, establishing the causative link between cerebral palsy and hypoxia/ischemia is fraught with problems. Criteria to define an acute intrapartum hypoxic event as sufficient to cause cerebral palsy was first proposed by the American College of Obstetricians and Gynecologists (ACOG) (18). These criteria were refined by the International Cerebral Palsy Task Force Consensus Statement (19). This was subsequently updated by the ACOG and American Academy of Pediatrics Task Force on Neonatal Encephalopathy and Cerebral Palsy (20). The use of these criteria will help to evaluate the probability that the pathology causing the cerebral palsy occurred during labor and hence might have been avoided by intervention.

The four essential criteria to define an acute intrapartum event sufficient to cause cerebral palsy are as follows (21):

1. Evidence of a metabolic acidosis in fetal umbilical cord arterial blood obtained at delivery (pH less than 7 and base deficit of at least 12 mmol/L).
2. Early onset of severe or moderate neonatal encephalopathy in infants born at 34 or more weeks of gestation. The examination is characterized by abnormalities in (i) cortical function (lethargy, stupor, coma with or without seizures), (ii) brainstem function (i.e., papillary and cranial nerve abnormalities), (iii) tone (hypotonia), and (iv) reflexes (absent, hyporeflexia). The outcome is related to the severity of the encephalopathy (17).
3. Cerebral palsy of the spastic quadriplegic or dyskinetic type.
4. Exclusion of other identifiable etiologies. A large proportion of cerebral palsy cases are associated with maternal and antenatal factors, such as preterm birth, fetal growth restriction, intrauterine infection, maternal or fetal coagulation disorders, multiple pregnancy, antepartum hemorrhage, breech presentation, and chromosomal or congenital abnormalities (9,10,22,23).

The criteria that collectively suggest an intrapartum timing (within close proximity to labor and delivery—for example, 0-48 hours) but that are non-specific for an asphyxial insult are as follows:

1. A hypoxic event occurring immediately before or during labor. These include uterine rupture, placental abruption, umbilical cord prolapse, amniotic fluid embolus, maternal cardiopulmonary arrest, and fetal exsanguination from either vasaprevia or massive fetomaternal hemorrhage.
2. A sudden and sustained fetal bradycardia or the absence of fetal heart rate variability in the presence of persistent late or persistent variable deceleration, usually after a hypoxic event when the pattern was previously normal.
3. Apgar scores of 0-3 beyond 5 minutes. The 1 or 5 minutes Apgar score is a poor predictor of long-term neurological outcome in the individual patient (24). However,

there is good correlation between an extremely low Apgar score at 15 and 20 minutes and subsequent neurological dysfunction (24).

4. Onset of multisystem involvement within 72 hours of birth. This includes acute bowel injury, renal failure, hepatic injury, cardiac damage, respiratory complications and hematologic abnormalities (25).

5. Early imaging studies showing evidence of acute non-focal cerebral abnormality.

The pattern of brain damage depends on (i) the maturity of the brain at the time of the insult, (ii) the severity of the insult and (iii) the duration of the damaging event. Selective vulnerability occurs in different parts of the brain depending on the gestational age (26,27). Early in pregnancy (mainly before 20 weeks of gestation), HIBI may cause a wide range of brain malformations. Periventricular white matter damage resulting in PVL is the typical sequelae of HIBI between 24 and 34 gestational weeks, with relative sparing of the subcortical white matter and cerebral cortex. Insults to the brain between 34 to 42 gestational weeks usually result in one of two patterns of damage depending on the severity or duration of hypoxia. Short periods of severe hypoxia result in damage to the basal ganglia, thalami, and perirolandic gyri, while milder but more prolonged hypoxia/ischemia affects the parasagittal watershed regions. This chapter will focus mainly on the imaging appearance of HIBI in the preterm and term infants.

HIBI IN THE PRETERM INFANTS

HIBI affecting premature infants results in injury to the periventricular white matter with relative sparing of the subcortical white matter and cerebral cortex, producing PVL. The predilection of the periventricular white matter to injury was previously thought to be due to the poorly developed ventriculofugal blood vessels in the brain (28–30). However, this explanation is not widely accepted (31,32). The limited vasodilatory capability of the cerebral vessels in premature infants plays a role in exacerbating the hypoxic damage. Periventricular white matter in a premature infant is a site of oligodendrocyte proliferation in preparation for myelination (33) and hence very active metabolically. During episodes of ischemia, the periventricular white matter responds by undergoing anaerobic glycolysis that results in depletion of high-energy phosphates and acidosis that contributes to tissue injury (34). There is an intrinsic developmental susceptibility of the oligodendrocyte, particularly of the immature oligodendrocyte (pro-OL), to the consequences of ischemia and subsequent reperfusion, mediated via free radical attack and to a lesser degree, glutamate toxicity (17,35,36). In a rat model, hypoxia/ischemia damages the stem/progenitor cells in the subventricular zone (SVZ), resulting in a permanent depletion of oligodendrocytes, increase in astrocytes, and dysmyelination of the subcortical white matter (37).

Perinatal infections and inflammatory conditions have also been implicated in the pathogenesis of PVL (38–42). The risk of antenatal white matter damage was ninefold greater in preterm neonates with purulent amniotic fluid (43). Experimental studies showed that injection of infectious agents caused fetal or neonatal brain white matter lesions similar to those seen in PVL (44,45). Proinflammatory cytokines (tumor necrosis factor α and interleukin 1β and interleukin 6) are increased in neonatal blood or in amniotic fluid during ischemia, which can result in PVL (41,42,45–47). Cytokines were detected in both infected and noninfected neonates with PVL, but the levels have been found to be higher in the infected neonates (48). These cytokines are produced by hematogenous and neural cells that can produce expression of adhesion molecules such as intercellular adhesion molecule (ICAM)-1 and vascular cell adhesion molecule (VCAM)-1 in CNS parenchymal and vascular endothelial cells, and can promote microglial activation and demyelination (49). The hypothesis that infectious or inflammatory factors play an important role in the pathophysiology of PVL is further supported by the findings that prenatal glucocorticoid administration, which is a potent inhibitor of proinflammatory cytokine synthesis, is associated with a decreased risk of PVL (40,47).

Cerebral palsy in premature infants is commonly due to periventricular white matter damage (1). The children often develop spastic diplegia due to involvement of the more medial fibers that supply the lower extremity. Visual impairment is also common in prematurely born children with spastic diplegia, and has been reported in up to 70% of patients (50–53). Visual impairment is often due to damage to the optic radiations that passes close to the ventricles. Visual impairment is manifest as loss of visual acuity, reduced visual field, abnormal ocular motility, and blindness (54,55).

IMAGING OF PERIVENTRICULAR LEUKOMALACIA

In the neonatal period, ultrasound is the only imaging modality that can be readily performed in the intensive care unit in most centers. It is portable and can be performed at the bedside, but is operator dependent. As the changes in the periventricular region and the size of the ventricles are well evaluated with sonography, ultrasound is well suited to monitoring the intracranial abnormalities. Moreover, ultrasound will exclude major intracranial hemorrhage as a cause of cerebral symptoms. In the first 24 to 48 hours, PVL is seen as areas of increased echogenicity in the periventricular areas. The periventricular areas of increased reflectivity need to be visualized in two planes and persist for more than seven days. These echogenic areas may gradually cavitate and form cysts over a two-to four-week period (56). These cysts may shrink over time. The appearance of PVL on ultrasound may be classified according to the extent and severity of the cysts (Table 2) (57). As cystic changes require a period of time to develop, it

Table 2. Classification of PVL Based on Ultrasound

Grade I	Areas of increased echogenicity, usually seen within 24–48 hr after an insult and persisting beyond day seven, but not evolving into cysts
Grade II	Periventricular increased echogenicity evolving into small cysts, often located in the fronto-parietal periventricular white matter
Grade III	Periventricular increased echogenicity evolving into extensive cysts, particularly prominent in the parieto-occipital periventricular white matter. The cysts do not usually communicate with the lateral ventricles. They collapse after several weeks and are no longer visible on cranial ultrasound in two to three months. After several months, atrophy of the periventricular white matter leads to ventricular dilatation with irregular walls
Grade IV	Periventricular increased echogenicity evolve into extensive cysts which extend into the deep white matter

follows that periventricular cysts seen on ultrasound immediately after birth is due to an antenatal event rather than intra-partum or immediate post-partum events. Although ultrasound is useful in the acute hypoxic/ischemic injury and in detecting cystic white matter injury (58,59), it is less sensitive for non-cystic periventricular white matter injury than MRI, an injury which is probably more common than cystic white matter injury (Figs. 1–4) (60).

Due to the difficulty in transferring and monitoring sick premature neonates, MRI scans are not frequently performed in the early stages of PVL. In the few centers where this has been done, MRI in the first 2–3 days of PVL shows punctate short T1 and long T2 areas in the periventricular white matter. T2 shortening appears around the first 6 to 7 days. Gradually, the periventricular tissue undergoes necrosis, resulting in the

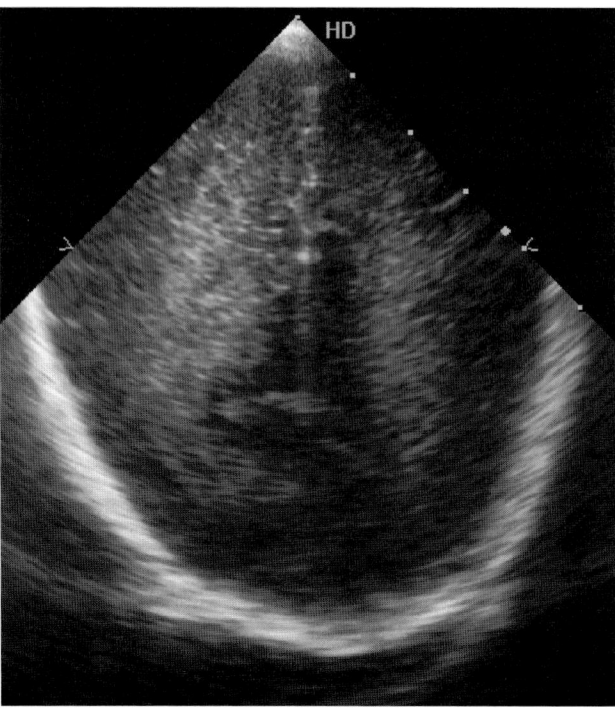

Figure 1. Posterior coronal ultrasound shows bilateral flare (high reflectivity) right more than left—the "bright/flare" phase of PVL. This was present in both coronal and sagittal scans using low gain settings to exclude artifact.

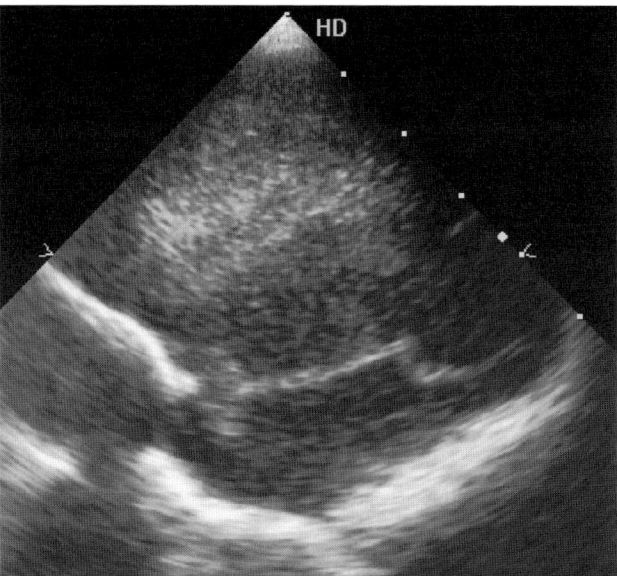

Figure 2. Sagittal ultrasound shows a bright area in the frontal white matter confirmed in the coronal plane, indicative of the "flare" phase of PVL.

development of cysts in the white matter that become smaller and incorporate into the ventricular wall. Diffusion weighted imaging showed marked abnormalities of water diffusion in the cerebral white matter, which can be detected prior to any changes visible on the conventional MRI or cranial ultrasound (61). MR spectroscopy performed in preterm infants in the subacute phase showed high lactate and myo-inositol and reduced N-acetyl group in the region of periventricular white matter (62).

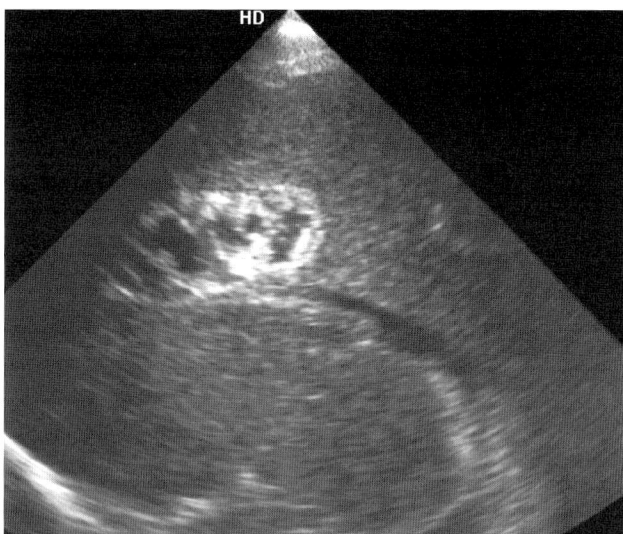

Figure 3. Sagittal ultrasound several weeks later the frontal lobe flare has progressed into fluid-filled cyst—cystic PVL.

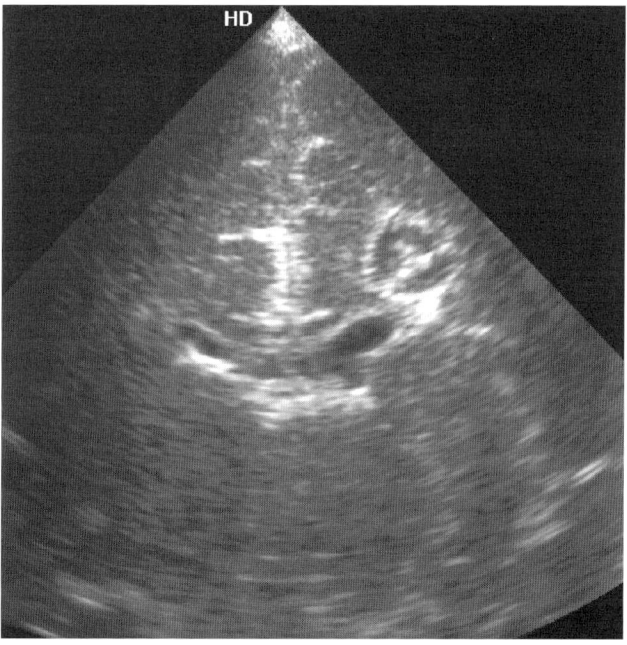

Figure 4. Coronal section showing cystic PVL in the left frontal lobe.

MRI scans are often used to document the final extent of PVL. Hypoxia/ischemia occurring before 26 gestational weeks results in localized ventricular enlargement with irregular ventricular margins, particularly of the body and trigone of the lateral ventricles (Fig. 5). At that gestational age, there is minimal prolongation of T2 relaxation time in the surrounding white matter, suggesting absent or minimal gliosis. As the gestational age at the time of HIBI increases, a rim of prolonged T2 relaxation around the ventricular atria develops and grows thicker (26). Delayed myelination is another feature seen on MRI (63,64), which is more severe with earlier asphyxia (65). Thinning of the corpus callosum may be seen, particularly the posterior body and splenium, which results from degeneration of the transcallosal fibers (66). Abnormalities of the optic radiation were seen in 50% of MRI and in 17% of cases, the visual cortex was also affected (54).

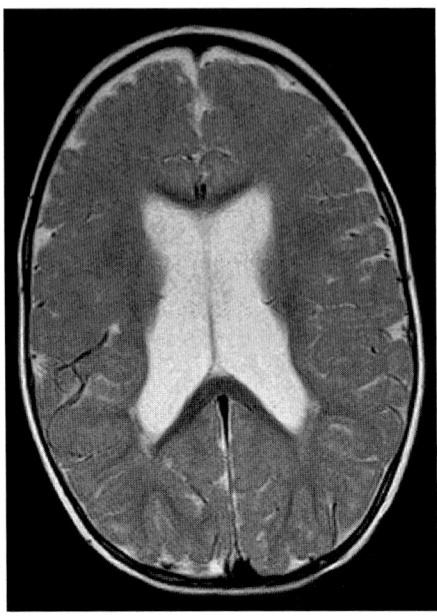

Figure 5. MRI of long standing periventricular leukomalacia. Axial T2-weighted image demonstrates ventriculomegaly with irregular ventricular margins, as well as a rim of hyperintensity in the periventricular white matter.

The severity of MRI abnormalities correlates well with the severity of motor and cognitive sequelae (1,67,68). Normal terminal or delayed myelination dorsal and superior to the trigones of the lateral ventricles should not be mistaken for PVL. The normal regions of unmyelinated white matter are separated from the ventricular wall by a thin band of myelinated white matter and the ventricular contour is smooth. In contrast PVL directly abuts the ventricular wall, has irregular ventricular contour, and is associated with reduced white matter volume.

HIBI IN TERM INFANTS

Despite improvements in perinatal care in the developed world, birth hypoxia/ischemia occurring at or close to term remains a major cause of mortality, resulting in up to 25% of perinatal mortality and morbidity. Studies have shown that perinatal hypoxia/ischemia account-for 8–15% of cerebral palsy (9,1). Intrauterine or perinatal hypoxia/ischemia in neonates greater than 37 gestational weeks often demonstrate, abnormal cardiotocography recordings (late decelerations), low Apgar scores (Apgar score <5 at 5 minutes or <6 at 10 minutes), bradycardia (heart rate <100/min), and reduced scalp or umbilical pH (pH <7.2). Most hypoxic injuries in fetuses and infants reflect combinations of hypoxia and ischemia rather than hypoxia alone (69). It is unlikely that acute hypoxemia will damage the fetal or neonatal brain unless there is superimposed ischemia (70). This reflects the greater resistance of the immature brain to hypoxia compared with the adult and the robustness of its protective mechanisms.

The pattern of injury depends on the type and severity of the insult. Severe but short-term hypoxia/ischemia is frequently associated with damage to the basal ganglia, thalami, brain stem, hippocampi, and perirolandic region (71–74), also known as central cortical-subcortical injury. The clinical sequalae of profound hypoxia/ischemia include choreoathetosis, quadriparesis, seizures, and mental retardation (75–77). Choreoathetosis may not manifest until after the first year of life, the majority presenting between one and four years of age (78,79).

The increased vulnerability of the basal ganglia and thalami is thought to be due to the increased metabolic rate of this region that is actively myelinating at term (80). An alternative explanation is the excitotoxic selective neuronal necrosis. In the term infant, cerebral cortical neurons of certain regions, including the CA1 sector of the hippocampus, are prone to injury due to the accumulation of excitotoxic amino acids such as glutamate. The increased glutamate is due to increased release from nerve endings and failure of glutamate reuptake systems after oxygen deprivation (73). The areas most vulnerable are the areas with highest density of excitatory amino acids, including the hippocampus and the basal ganglia (81–83). There is relative sparing of the cortex except for the perirolandic region.

Mitochondria appear to play a central role to determine the fate of cells subjected to hypoxia/ischemia (84–86). Mitochondria handle multiple oxidation reactions, which may produce toxic oxygen free radicals under conditions of oxidative stress. Neurodegeneration from hypoxia/ischemia can take the form of either necrosis or apoptosis, depending on the severity of mitochondrial dysfunction (84). The more severe insult produced rapid loss of mitochondrial membrane potential, loss of ATP production, and disruption of nuclear and cytoplasmic membranes, consistent with necrosis. On the other hand, neurons subjected to less intense excitotoxic insult have initial losses but later recover the mitochondrial membrane potentials, and will eventually develop nuclear fragmentation of chromatin and shrinkage of nuclear and cytoplasmic contents typical of apoptosis. It has been suggested that damaged mitochondria may signal the apoptotic process by release of cytochrome c or other intramitochondrial proteins, in turn activating cysteine protease enzymes or caspases that fragment DNA and execute apoptotic programs (84,85,87,88). Control of apoptosis and the apoptosis/necrosis continuum may provide potential approaches to modifying the outcome of hypoxia/ischemic brain injury (87,89,90). Moreover, the cascade of biochemical and histopathologic events triggered by hypoxic ischemic events can extend for days to weeks after the insult is triggered, creating the potential for therapeutic interventions (91). Several protein growth factors that have been reported to protect against hypoxic/ischemic brain injury in immature animal models may act by inhibiting apoptosis (92–95). Hypothermia may slow or reduce the excitotoxic cascade by altering processes favoring apoptosis (96–98) or through other mechanisms such as reducing glutamate release.

Chronic low grade or repetitive insults are more likely to involve the cortex and white matter, particularly in the parasagittal distribution involving the arterial border zones (33,99). The injury is frequently bilateral and affects the posterior cerebrum more commonly than the anterior cerebrum (99). The parasagittal zones are particularly vulnerable to a fall in cerebral blood flow, which is likely to occur with systemic hypotension during perinatal asphyxia (100). Cerebral vascular autoregulation is lost, resulating in pressure passive flow (99). As a result of hypoperfusion in the watershed regions, toxic metabolites accumulate and tissue damage occurs (99). Parasagittal injury manifests clinically as spastic tetraplegia with the proximal limbs affected more than the distal limbs and the upper extremities more severely affected than the lower extremities (101).

IMAGING OF HIBI IN TERM INFANTS

Cranial ultrasound is widely available and portable, therefore is used frequently to assess clinically suspected HIBI. Cranial ultrasound is useful in neonates in identifying cerebral edema, intraparenchymal, and intraventricular hemorrhage. The findings may be minimal on ultrasound compared with the clinical state of the baby showing signs of HIBI. On ultrasound, the first sign of cerebral edema is ventricular compression and effacement of cerebral sulci. However the ventricular size in a normal newborn baby may be small and slit-like and therefore is not a specific finding for cerebral edema. This is followed by loss of definition of the sulcal and gyral pattern that can be subtle. Such changes may not be evident for several days after birth. Parenchymal infarcts or basal ganglia changes are seen as areas of increased echogenicity but may take several days to develop. The thalami may show hyperechogenicity, which is predictive of poor neurologic outcome (102).

Doppler ultrasound has been used to demonstrate changes in intracerebral circulation in those with HIBI. Doppler may show slow flow in the superior sagittal sinus due to cerebral edema. Altered flow may also be seen in the anterior and middle cerebral arteries, with loss of pulsatility attributed to loss of cerebral autoregulation (Figs. 6 and 7). The resistive index is reduced, with increased diastolic velocities indicating luxury perfusion or low peak systolic velocities indicating decreased cerebral perfusion (103). However, the waveform may be affected by extracranial factors including co-existent myocardial ischemia causing poor cerebral perfusion or altered run off due to persistent patent ductus arteriosus. Moreover, the resistive index is not predictive of outcome (104). Cranial ultrasound has a role in screening and monitoring patients but is less sensitive than MRI in assessing the extent of the lesion. Moreover, cranial ultrasound is only useful during the first year of life when the fontanel are still open and provide an acoustic window.

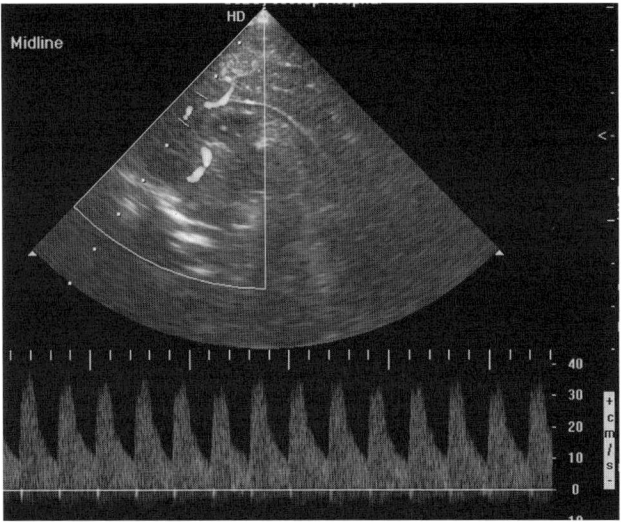

Figure 6. Midline sagittal color pulsed Doppler of normal anterior cerebral artery.

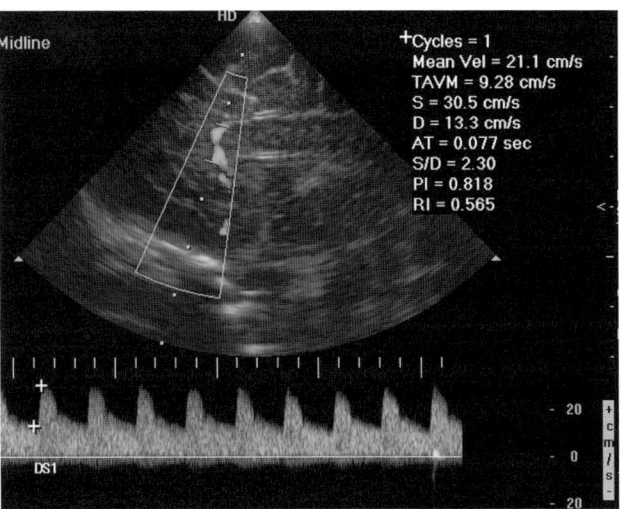

Figure 7. Sagittal color Doppler of anterior cerebral artery shows raised diastolic flow due to loss of cerebral autoregulation (RI=0.56—borderline) in clinical FTA.

CT is less sensitive than MRI in detecting the changes secondary to hypoxia/ischemia and incurs radiation burden on the child. Although MRI is less widely available, the multiplanar capability of MRI, the lack of radiation and the superb definition of the brain compared to ultrasound and CT, makes it the investigation of choice where available. Moreover, MRI has an important role to play in the assessment of the underlying cause of cerebral palsy. However, the interpretation of MRI in neonates and children requires considerable expertise. The MRI sequences that we use in our institution in imaging children with suspected birth hypoxia/ischemia depends on the age of the child and the time interval between the insult and MR imaging. In the acute to subacute phase, rapid sequences which do not require sedation or general anesthetic could be used (Table 3). In the long-standing cases, spin echo and fast spin echo sequences supplemented by FLAIR are used (Table 4). Gradient echo imaging is added to the protocol to detect subtle calcification that may occur in congenital infection, a cause of cerebral palsy.

Table 3. MRI Sequences for Suspected Acute Birth Hypoxia/Ischemia

Axial and coronal ultrafast T2	TR/TE 25000/75, FOV 25.0 cm Flip angle: 90° Slice thickness: 7 mm Resolution: 240 by 256
Axial and sagittal RF-Fast T1	TR/TE 238/3.3 FOV 25.0 cm Flip angle: 70° Slice thickness: 4 mm Resolution: 192 by 256
Diffusion weighted SE EPI imaging with fat saturation	TR/TE 7787/100, Turbo factor 152 Flip angle 90° FOV 24.0 cm Slice thickness: 5 mm Resolution: 152 by 152

Table 4. MRI Sequences for Suspected Long-Standing Birth Hypoxia/Ischemia

Coronal and axial FSE T2	TR/TE 3667/100, turbo factor 8 FOV 24.0 cm Slice thickness 4 mm Resolution 352 by 512
Axial FLAIR	TR/TE/TI 10000/109/2200 FOV 23.0 cm Slice thickness 4.5 mm Resolution 192 by 256
Axial T1	TR/TE 384/16 FOV 24.0 cm Slice thickness 4 mm Resolution 256 by 256
Axial gradient echo T2	TR/TE 999/30 Flip angle 15° FOV 23.0 cm Slice thickness 4 mm Resolution 256 by 256

MRI FINDINGS OF CENTRAL CORTICAL-SUBCORTICAL INJURY

MRI can be performed in the first two weeks of acute severe perinatal hypoxia/ischemia to provide prognostic information (105). In the first two or three days of injury, the posterior putamen, ventrolateral thalami, and perirolandic region show high signal on the T1 and T2 weighted images (Fig. 8). More severe cases may have involvement of the posterior limb of the internal capsule, caudate nuclei, and midbrain, as well as more extensive involvement of the whole basal ganglia and thalami. By 7 to 10 days, heterogenous high and low signal is seen in the basal ganglia and thalami. Abnormalities may also be seen in the hippocampi, which are usually seen as high signal on T1 and do not manifest until two weeks after birth (106). Over time, the affected areas undergo atrophy and show T2 prolongation, which may not become evident in the white matter until myelination has developed (Fig. 9). In the early phase of hypoxia/ischemia, cerebellar white matter hyperintensity has been described (107). In the late phase, vermian and cerebellar hemispheric volume loss have been described (106). Involvement of the anterior lobe of cerebellar vermis has also been reported in those with profound asphyxia (108).

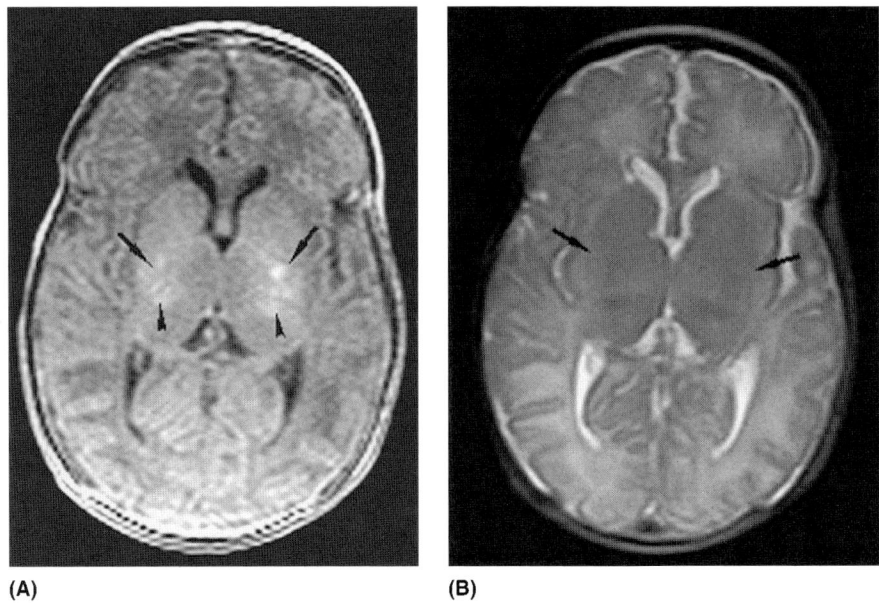

(A)   **(B)**

Figure 8. MRI of profound acute hypoxic ischemic brain injury in term infant. Axial T1 (**A**) and axial T2 (**B**) weighted image demonstrating high signal in the posterior putamen (arrow) and ventrolateral thalami (arrowhead).

Diffusion weighted imaging has been shown to demonstrate abnormalities in the thalami and internal capsule in the first day of HIBI, when conventional MR imaging is normal (109). Diffusion weighted imaging, however, underestimated the extent of the long term injury (109,110). Delayed neuronal and oligodendroglial cell death due to apoptosis in areas with lower metabolic demand may explain the reason that diffusion weighted imaging underestimates the extent of injury (110). Diffusion weighted images obtained between the second and fourth day of life reflects the extent of injury more reliably. By the seventh day, diffusion MRI is less sensitive to perinatal brain injury compared to conventional MRI because of transient pseudonormalization of diffusion images (111).

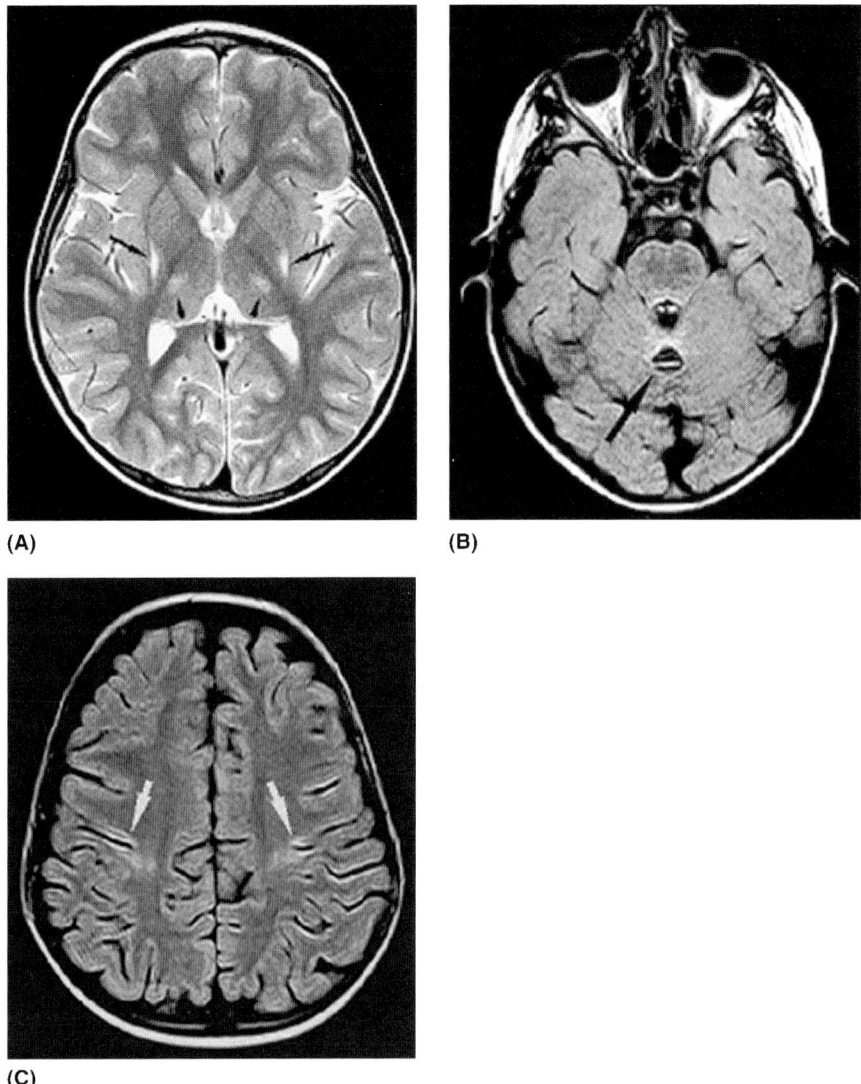

(A)   (B)

(C)

Figure 9. MRI of long standing profound hypoxic ischemic brain injury in term infant. Axial T2 (**A**) and FLAIR (**B**) show high signal and volume loss in the posterior putamen (small black arrow) and ventrolateral thalami (black arrow) as well as in the superior vermis (black arrow). High signal is also seen in the perirolandic region on the axial FLAIR (**C**) (white arrow).

MR spectroscopy has been used to evaluate brain injury in asphyxiated term infants (Figs. 10 and 11) (112–114). The N-acetyl level is reduced and the lactate level is elevated. The lactate level was shown to rise within the first 24 hours of injury and remained elevated after 24 hours (112,114). The elevated lactate levels in the basal ganglia and thalami were shown to predict clinical outcomes (115–117).

MRI FINDINGS OF PARASAGITTAL INJURY

In the early stage of injury, the affected cortex is hyperintense compared with adjacent normal cortex on the T1 weighted images, termed cortical highlighting. The corresponding area is of low signal on T2 weighted images. There is greater vulnerability of the cortex at the depths of the sulci relative to the apex of the gyri due to the greater perfusion at the apices of the gyri (29). Adjacent white matter edema is seen as low

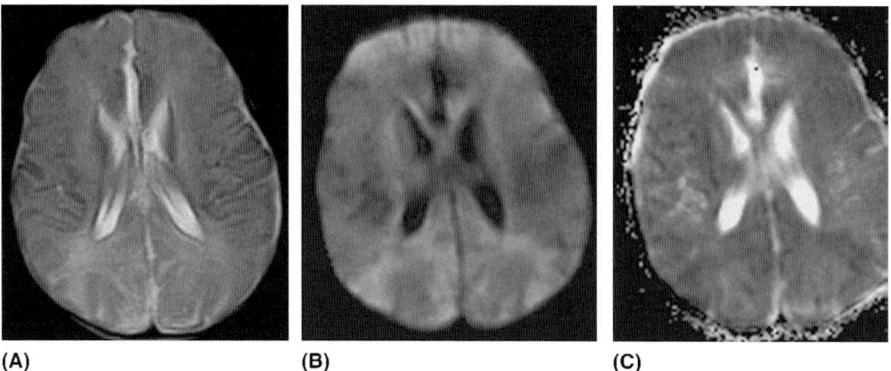

(A)   (B)   (C)

Figure 10. MRI of acute hypoxia/ischemia with involvement of parasagittal area in term infant. (**A**) Axial T2 shows subtle high signal in the watershed region, slightly more prominent in the posterior watershed area. (**B**) On the diffusion-weighted image, the high signal is more pronounced. (**C**) The corresponding ADC map demonstrates restricted diffusion in the watershed region.

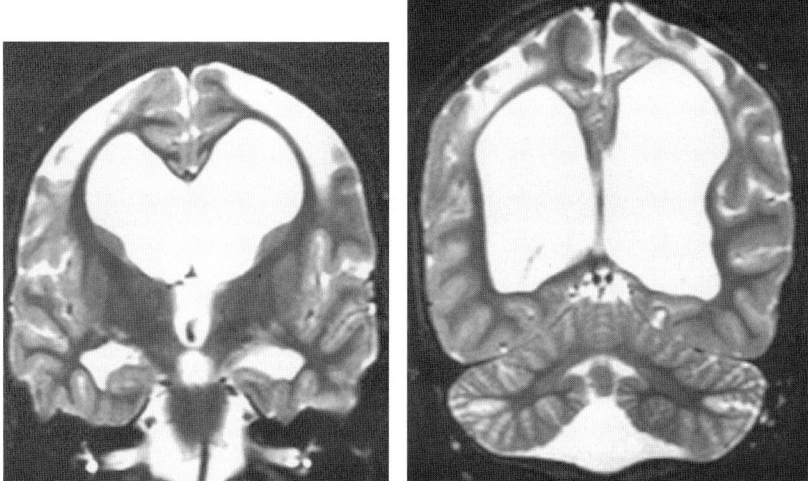

Figure 11. Long standing effect of hypoxia/ischemia in the watershed distribution resulting in gliosis.

signal on T1 weighted images and high signal on T2. Due to the lack of myelin in the neonatal period, the white matter edema is more apparent on the T1 weighted images. These regions evolve with time, demonstrating volume loss with cortical thinning and diminution of the underlying white matter in the parasagittal watershed territory. The greater involvement of the deep portions of the gyri than the superficial portion results in mushroom-shaped cortical gyri, also known as ulegyria (33). There may be ex-vacuo dilatation of the trigones and occipital horns of the lateral ventricles.

CONCLUSION

The pattern of injury depends on the gestational age and the severity of injury. In preterm infants, hypoxia/ischemia results in periventricular white matter damage. This contrasts with the basal ganglia, thalamic, and parasagittal involvement in term infants. Currently, ultrasound remains the imaging modality of choice in the evaluation of acute hypoxia/ischemia. MR imaging plays a more significant role in the imaging of those with long-term sequelae of hypoxia/ischemia, particularly those with cerebral palsy.

REFERENCES

1. Truwit CL, Barkovich AJ, Koch TK, Ferriero DM. Cerebral palsy: MR findings in 40 patients. AJNR Am J Neuroradiol 1992; 13:67–78.
2. Surveillance of Cerebral Palsy in Europe (SCPE). Surveillance of cerebral palsy in Europe: a collaboration of cerebral palsy surveys and registers. Dev Med Child Neurol 2000; 42:816–824.
3. Wood E, Rosenbaum P. The gross motor function classification system for cerebral palsy: A study of reliability and stability over time. Dev Med Child Neurol 20;42:292–296.
4. Hagberg B, Hagberg G. Dyskinetic and dystonic cerebral palsy and birth. Acta Paediatr 1992; 81:93–94.
5. Neville B. The Worster-Drought syndrome: a severe test of paediatric neurodisability services? Dev Med Child Neurol 1997; 39:982–984.
6. Stanley FJ, Blair E, Alberman E. How common are the cerebral palsies?. In: Stanley F, Blair E, Alberman E, eds. Cerebral Palsies: Epidemiology and Causal Pathways. London: Mac Keith Press/Cambridge University Press, 2000:22–39.
7. Kuban KCK, Leviton A. Cerebral palsy. N Engl J Med 1994; 330:188–195.
8. Little WJ. On the influence of abnormal parturition, labour, premature birth and asphyxia neonatorum on the mental and physical condition of the child especially in relation to deformities. Trans Obstet Soc Lond 1862; 3:293–344 (reprinted Cerebral Paly Bulletin 1958;1:5-36).
9. Nelson KB, Ellenberg JH. Antecedents of cerebral palsy: multivariate analysis of risk. N Engl J Med 1986; 315:81–86.
10. Blair E, Stanley FJ. Intrapartum asphyxia: a rare cause of cerebral palsy. J Pediatr 1988; 112:515–519.
11. Torfs CP, van der Berg BJ, Oechsli FW. Prenatal and perinatal factors in the etiology of cerebral palsy. J Pediatr 1990; 116:615–619.
12. Pschirrer ER, Yeomans ER. Does asphyxia cause cerebral palsy? Semin Perinatol 2000; 24:215–220.
13. Nelson KB, Elenberg JH. Antecedents of cerebral palsy I. univariate analysis of risk. Am J Dis Child 1985; 139:1031–1038.
14. Nelson KB, Elenberg JH. Obstetric complications as risk factors for cerebral palsy or seizure disorder. JAMA 1984; 251:1843–1848.
15. Freeman JM, Nelson KB. Intrapartum asphyxia and cerebral palsy. Pediatrics 1988; 82:240–249.
16. Forfar JO, Hume R, McPhial FM, et al. Low birth weight: a 10 year outcome study of the continuum of reproductive casualty. Dev Med Child Neurol 1994; 36:1037–1048.
17. Volpe JJ. 4th ed Neurology of the newborn. Philadelphia: W.B. Saunders, 2001.
18. American College of Obstetricians and Gynecologists. Fetal and neonatal neurologic injury. ACOG technical bulletin no. 163. Washington: American College of Obstetricians and Gynecologists, 1992:1–5.
19. MacLennan A. A template for defining a causal relation between acute intrapartum events and cerebral palsy: International consensus statement. BMJ 1999; 319:1054–1059.
20. American College of Obstetricians and Gynecologists' Task Force on Neonatal Encephalopathy and cerebral palsy: Defining the pathogenesis and pathophysiology. Washington: American College of Obstetricians and Gynecologists, 2003.
21. Hankins GDV, Speer M. Defining the pathogenesis and pathophysiology of neonatal encephalopathy and cerebral palsy. Obstet Gynecol 2003; 102:628–636.
22. Nelson KB, Dambrosia JM, Grether JK, Phillips TM. Neonatal cytokines and coagulation factors in children with cerebral palsy. Ann Neurol 1998; 44:665–675.
23. Grether JK, Nelson KB. Maternal infection and cerebral palsy in infants of normal birth weight. JAMA 1997; 278:207–211.
24. Nelson KB, Ellenberg JH. Apgar scores as predictors of chronic neurologic disability. Pediatrics 1981; 68:36–44.

25. Hankins GDV, Koen S, Gei AF, Lopez SM, Van Hook JW, Anderson GD. Neonatal organ system injury in acute birth asphyxia sufficient to result in neonatal encephalopahty. Obstet Gynecol 2002; 99:688–691.
26. Barkovich AJ, Truwit CL. Brain damage from perinatal asphyxia: correlation of MR findings with gestational age. Am J Neuroradiol 1990; 11:1087–1096.
27. Rayband C. Destructive lesions of the brain. Neuroradiology 1983; 25:265–291.
28. DeReuck J. The human periventricular arterial blood supply and the anatomy of cerebral infarctions. Eur Neurol 1971; 5:321–334.
29. Takashima S, Tanaka K. Development of the cerebrovascular architecture and its relationship of periventricular leukomalacia. Arch Neurol 1978; 35:11–16.
30. Takashima S, Tanaka K. Subcortical leukomalacia, relationship to development of the cerebral sulcus, and its vascular supply. Arch Neurol 1978; 35:470–476.
31. Mayer PL, Kier EL. The controversy of the periventricular white matter circulation: a review of the anatomic literature. Am J Neuroradiol 1991; 12:223–228.
32. Nelson MD, Jr., Gonzalez-Gomex I, Gilles FH. The search for human telencephalic ventriculofugal arteries. AJNR Am J Neuroradiol 1991; 12:215–222.
33. Barkovich AJ. Brain and spine injuries. 3rd ed. Pediatric Neuroimaging. Philadelphia: Lippincott Williams and Wilkins, 2000 pp. 168–208.
34. Oka A, Belliveau MJ, Rosenberg PA, Vople JJ. Vulnerability of oligodendroglia to glutamate: pharmacology, mechanisms and prevention. J Neurosci 1993; 13:1441–1453.
35. Back SA, Gan X, Li Y, Rosenberg PA, Volpe JJ. Maturation-dependent vulnerability of oligodendrocytes to oxidative stress-induced death caused by glutathione depletion. J Neurosci 1998; 18:6241–6253.
36. Ness JK, Romanko MJ, Rothstein RP, Wood TL, Levison SW. Perinatal hypoxia-ischemia induces apoptotic and excitotoxic death of periventricular white matter oligodendrocyte progenitors. Dev Neurosci 2001; 23:203–208.
37. Levison SW, Rothstein RP, Romanko MJ, Snyder MJ, Meyers RL, Vannucci SJ. Hypoxia/ischaemia depletes the rat perinatal subventricular zone of oligodendrocyte progenitors and neural stem cells. Dev Neurosci 2001; 23:234–247.
38. Nelson KB, Grether JK. Potentially asphyxiating conditions and spastic cerebral palsy in infants of normal birth weight. Am J Obstet Gynecol 1998; 179:507–513.
39. Zupan V, Gonzalez P, Lacaze-Masmonteil T, et al. Periventricular leukomalacia: risk factors revisited. Dev Med Child Neurol 1996; 38:1961–1967.
40. Baud O, Emilie D, Pelletier E, et al. Amniotic fluid concentrations of interleukin-1 beta, interleukin-6 and TNF-alpha in chorioamnionitis before 32 weeks of gestation: histological associations and neonatal outcome. Br J Obstet Gynaecol 1999; 106:72–77.
41. Yoon BH, Jun JK, Romero R, et al. Amniotic fluid inflammatory cytokines (interleukin-6, interleukin-1β, and tumour necrosis factor-α), neonatal brain white matter lesions, and cerebral palsy. Am J Obstet Gynecol 1997; 177:19–26.
42. Yoon BH, Romero R, Yang SH, et al. Interleukin-6 concentrations in umbilical cord plasma are elevated in neonates with white matter lesions associated with periventricular leukomalacia. Am J Obstet Gynecol 1996; 174:1433–1440.
43. Bejar R, Wozniak P, Allard M, et al. Antenatal origin of neurologic damage in newborn infants I. Preterm infants. Am J Obstet Gynecol 1988; 159:357–363.
44. Cai Z, Pan ZL, Pang Y, Evans OB, Rhodes PG. Cytokine induction in fetal rat brains and brain injury in neonatal rats after maternal lipopolysaccharide administration. Pediatr Res 2000; 47:64–72.
45. Yoon BH, Romero R, Kim CJ, et al. Experimentally induced intrauterine infection causes fetal brain white matter lesions in rabbits. Am J Obstet Gynecol 1997; 177:797–802.
46. Savman K, Blennow M, Gustafson K, et al. Cytokine response in cerebrospinal fluid after birth asphyxia. Pediatr Res 1998; 43:746–751.
47. Baud O, Foix-L'Helias L, Kaminski M, et al. Antenatal glucocorticoid treatment and cystic periventricular leukomalacia in very premature infants. N Engl J Med 1999; 341:1190–1196.
48. Kadhim H, Tabarki B, Verellen G, De Prez C, Rona AM, Sébire G. Inflammatory cytokines in the pathogenesis of periventricular leukomalacia. Neurology 2001; 56:1278–1284.
49. Aloisi F, Ria F, Adorini L. Regulation of T-cell responses by CNS antigen-presenting cells: different roles for microglia and astrocytes. Immunol Today 2000; 21:141–147.
50. Lanzi G, Fazzi E, Uggetti C, et al. Cerebral visual impairment in periventricular leukomalacia. Neuropediatrics 1998; 29:145–150.

51. Pinto-Martin JA, Dobson V, Cnaan A, Zhao H, Paneth NS. Vision outcome at age 2 years in a low birth weight population. Pediatr Neurol 1996; 14:281–287.

52. Schenk-Rootlieb AJ, van Nieuwenhuizen O, van der Graaf Y, Wittebol-Post D, Willemse J. The prevalence of cerebral visual disturbance in children with cerebral palsy. Dev Med Child Neurol 1992; 34:473–480.

53. Uggetti C, Egitto ME, Fazzi E, et al. Cerebral visual impairment in periventricular leukomalacia: MR correlation. AJNR Am J Neuroradiol 1996; 17:979–985.

54. Cioni G, Fazzi B, Ipata AE, et al. Correlation between cerebral visual impairment and magnetic resonance imaging in children with neonatal encephalopathy. Dev Med Child Neurol 1996; 38:120–132.

55. Eken P, de Vries LS, van Nieuwenhuizen O, et al. Early predictors of cerebral visual impairment in infants with cystic leukomalacia. Neuropediatrics 1996; 27:16–25.

56. Dubowitz LMS, Bydder GM, Mushin J. Developmental sequence of periventricular leukomalacia: correlation of ultrasound, clinical, and nuclear magnetic resonance functions. Arch Dis Child 1985; 60:349–355.

57. De Vries LS, Eken P, Dubowitz LMS. The spectrum of leukomalacia using cranial ultrasound. Beh Brain Res 1992; 49:1–6.

58. Carson SC, Hertzberg BS, Bowie JD, Burger PC. Value of sonography in the diagnosis of intracranial hemorrhage and periventricular leukomalacia: a postmortem study of 35 cases. AJNR Am J Neuroradiol 1990; 155:595–601.

59. Adcock LM, Moore PJ, Schlesinger AE, Armstrong DL. Correlation of ultrasound with postmortem neuropathologic studies in neonates. Pediatr Neurol 1998; 19:263–271.

60. Inder TE, Anderson NJ, Spencer C, Wells S, Volpe JJ. White matter injury in the premature infant: a comparison between serial cranial sonographic and MR findings at term. AJNR Am J Neuroradiol 2003; 24:805–809.

61. Inder T, Huppi PS, Zientara GP, et al. Early detection of periventricular leukomalacia by diffusion-weighted magnetic resonance imaging techniques. J Pediatr 1999; 134:631–634.

62. Robertson N, Kuint J, Counsell SJ, et al. Characterization of cerebral white matter damage in preterm infants using 1H and 31P magnetic resonance spectroscopy. J Cereb Blood Flow Metab 2000; 20:1446–1456.

63. Van de Bor M, Guit GL, Schreuder AM, et al. Does very preterm birth impair myelination of the central nervous system? Neuropediatrics 1990; 21:37–39.

64. Van de Bor M, Guit GL, Schreuder A, Wondergem J, Vielvoye GJ. Early detection of delayed myelination in preterm infants. Pediatrics 1989; 84:407–411.

65. Skranes J, Vik T, Nilsen G, et al. Cerebral magnetic resonance imaging and mental and motor function of very low birth weight infants at one year of corrected age. Neuropediatrics 1993; 24:256–262.

66. Mercuri E, Jongmans M, Henderson S, et al. Evaluation of the corpus callosum in clumsy children born prematurely: a functional and morphological study. Neuropediatrics 1996; 27:317–322.

67. Sugita K, Takeuchi A, Iai M, et al. Neurologic sequelae and MRI in low-birth weight patients. Paediatr Neurol 1989; 5:365–369.

68. Yokochi K, Aiba K, Horie M, et al. Magnetic resonance imaging in children with spastic diplegia: correlation with the severity of their motor and mental abnormality. Dev Med Child Neurol 1991; 33:18–25.

69. Vannucci RC. Experimental biology o fcerebral hypoxia-ischemia: relation to perinatal brain damage. Pediatr Res 1990; 27:317–326.

70. Johnston MV, Trescher WH, Taylor GA. Hypoxic and ischemic central nervous system disorders in infants and children. Adv Pediatr 1995; 42:1–5.

71. Azzarelli B, Caldemeyer KS, Phillips JP, DeMyer WE. Hypoxic-ischemic encephalopathy in areas of primary myelination: a neuroimaging and PET study. Pediatr Neurol 1996; 14:108–116.

72. Barkovich AJ. MR and CT evaluation of profound neonatal and infantile asphyxia. AJNR Am J Neuroradiol 1992; 13:959–972.

73. Rademaker RP, van der Knapp MS, Verbeeten B, Jr., et al. Central cortico-subcortical involvement: a distinct pattern of brain damage caused by perinatal and postnatal asphyxia in term infants. J Comput Assist Tomogr 1995; 19:252–263.

74. Roland EH, Hill A, Norman MG, et al. Selective brainstem injury in an asphyxiated newborn. Ann Neurol 1988; 23:89–92.

75. Roland EH, Poskett K, Rodriguez E, Lupton BA, Hill A. Perinatal hypoxic-ischemic thalamic injury: clinical features and neuroimaging. Ann Neurol 1998; 44:161–166.

76. Menkes J, Curran JG. Clinical and magnetic resonance imaging correlates in children with extrapyramidal cerebral palsy. Am J Neuroradiol 1994; 15:451–457.

77. Hayashi M, Satoh J, Sakamoto K, Morimatsu Y. Clinical and neuropathological findings in severe athetoid cerebral palsy: a comparative study of globo-luysian and thalamo-putaminal groups. Brain Dev 1991; 13:47–51.

78. Burke RE, Fahn S, Gold AP. Delayed-onset dystonia in patients with "static" encephalopathy. J Neurol Neurosurg Psychiatry 1980; 43:789–797.

79. Saint-Hilaire MH, Burke RE, Bressman SB, et al. Delayed-onset dystonia due to perinatal or early childhood asphyxia. Neurology 1991; 41:216–221.

80. Chugani HT, Phelps ME. Maturational changes in cerebral function in infants determined by 18 FDG positron emission tomography. Science 1986; 231:840–843.

81. Barks JD, Silverstein FS, Sims K, Greenmayre JT, Johnston MV. Glutamate recognition sites in human fetal brain. Neurosci Lett 1988; 84:131–136.

82. MacDonald JW, Johnston MV. Physiological and pathophysiological roles in excitatory amino acids during central nervous system development. Brain Res Rev 1990; 15:41–70.

83. Silverstein FS, Torke L, Barks J, Johnston MV. Hypoxia-ischemia produces focal disruption of glutamate receptors in developing brain. Dev Brain Res 1987; 34:33–39.

84. Ankarcrona M, Dypbukt JM, Bonfoco E, et al. Glutamate-induced neuronal death: a succession of necrosis or apoptosis depending on mitochondrial function. Neuron 1995; 15:961–973.

85. Abe K, Aoki M, Kawagoe J, et al. Ischaemic delayed neuronal death, a mitochondrial hypothesis. Stroke 1995; 26:1478–1489.

86. Gilland E, Puka-Sundvall M, Hillered L, Hagberg H. Mitochondrial function and energy metabolism after hypoxia-ischemia in the immature brain: involvement of NMDA receptors. J Cereb Blood Flow Metab 1998; 18:297–304.

87. Cheng Y, Deshmukh M, D'Costa A, et al. Caspase inhibitor affords neuroprotection after delayed administration in a rat model of neonatal hypoxic-ischemic brain injury. J Clin Invest 1998; 101:1992–1999.

88. Banasiak KJ, Xia Y, Haddad GG. Mechanisms underlying hypoxia-induced neuronal apoptosis. Prog Neurobiol 2000; 62:215–249.

89. Schulz JB, Weller M, Moskowitz MA. Caspases as treatment targets in stroke and neurodegenerative diseases. Ann Neurol 1999; 45:421–429.

90. Cheng Y, Gidday JM, Yan Q, Shah AR, Holtzman DM. Marked age-dependent neuroprotection by BDNF against neonatal hypoxic-ischemic brain injury. Ann Neurol 1997; 41:521–529.

91. Johnston MV, Trescher WH, Ishida A, Nakajima W. Neurobiology of hypoxic-ischemic injury in the developing brain. Pediatr Res 2001; 49:735–741.

92. Hossain MA, Fielding KE, Trescher WH, Ho T, Wilson MA, Laterra J. Human FGF-1 gene delivery protects against quinolinate-induced striatal and hippocampal injury in neonatal rats. Eur J Neurosci 1998; 10:2490–2499.

93. Johnston BM, Mallard EC, Williams CE, Gluckman PD. Insulin-like growth factor-1 is a potent neuronal rescue agent after hypoxic-ischemic injury in fetal lamb. J Clin Invest 1996; 97:300–308.

94. Gustafson K, Hagberg H, Bengtsson BA, Brantsing C, Isgaard J. Possible protective role of growth hormone in hyhpoxia-ischemia. Pediatr Res 1999; 45:318–323.

95. Holtzman DM, Sheldon RA, Jaffe W, Cheng Y, Ferriero DM. Nerve growth factor protects the neonatal brain against hypoxic-ischemic injury. Ann Neurol 1996; 39:114–122.

96. Bona E, Hagberg H, Loberg EM, Bagenhoolm R, Thoresen M. Protective effects of moderate hypothermia after neonatal hypoxia-ischemia: short- and long-term outcome. Pediatr Res 1998; 43:738–745.

97. Gunn AJ, Gunn TR, Guming MI, Williams CE, Gluckman PD. Neuroprotection with prolonged head cooling started before postischemic seizures in fetal sheep. Pediatrics 1998; 102:1098–1106.

98. Guan J, Gunn AJ, Sirimanne ES, et al. The window of opportunity for neuronal rescue with insulin-like growth factor-1 after hypoxia-ischemia in rats is critically modulated by cerebral temperatures during recovery. J Cereb Blood Flow Metab 2000; 20:513–519.

99. Volpe JJ, Herscovitch P, Perlman JM, et al. Positron emission tomography in the asphyxiated term newborn: parasagittal impairment of cerebral blood flow. Ann Neurol 1985; 17:287–296.

100. Pryds O, Greisen G, Lou H, Friis-Hansen B. Vasoparalysis associated with brain damage in asphyxiated term infants. J Pediatr 1990; 117:119–125.

101. Volpe JJ. Value of MR in definition of the neuropathology of cerebral palsy in vivo. AJNR Am J Neuroradiol 1992; 13:79–83.

102. Connolly B, Kelehan P, O'Brien N, et al. The echogenic thalamus in hypoxic ischaemic encephalopathy. Pediatr Radiol 1994; 24:268–271.

103. Allison JW, Seibert JJ. Transcranial Doppler in the newborn with asphyxia. Neuroimaging Clin N Am 1999; 9:11–16.

104. Gray PH, Tudehope DI, Masel JP, et al. Perinatal hypoxic-ischaemic brain injury: prediction of outcome. Dev Med Child Neurol 1993; 35:965–973.

105. Kuenzle BC, Baenziger O, Martin E, et al. Prognostic value of early MR imaging in term infants with severe perinatal asphyxia. Neuropediatrics 1994; 25:191–200.

106. Rutherford MA. The asphyxiated term infant. In: Rutherford MA, ed. MR of the Neonatal Brain. Philadelphia: Elsevier Science, 2002:99–128.

107. Barkovich AJ, Westmark K, Partridge C, Sola A, Ferriero DM. Perinatal asphyxia: MR findings in the first 10 days. AJNR Am J Neuroradiol 1995; 16:427–438.

108. Connolly DJA, Widjaja E, Griffiths PD. Involvement of the anterior lobe of the cerebellar vermis in perinatal profound hypoxia. Br Soc Neuroradiol 2003 (conference abstract).

109. Barkovich AJ, Westmark KD, Bedi HS, Partridge JC, Ferriero DM, Vigneron DB. Proton spectroscopy and diffusion imaging on the first day of life after perinatal asphyxia: preliminary report. AJNR Am J Neuroradiol 2001; 22:1786–1794.

110. Robertson RL, Ben-Sira L, Barnes PD, et al. MR line-scan diffusion-weighted imaging of term neonates with perinatal brain ischemia. AJNR Am J Neuroradiol 1999; 20:1658–1670.

111. McKinstry RC, Miller JH, Snyder AZ, et al. A prospective longitudinal diffusion tensor imaging study of brain injury in newborns. Neurology 2002; 59:824–833.

112. Penrice J, Cady EB, Lorek A, et al. Proton magnetic resonance spectroscopy of the brain in normal preterm and term infants and early changes after perinatal hypoxia-ischemia. Pediatr Res 1996; 40:6–14.

113. Shu SK, Ashwal S, Holshouser BA, Nystrom G, Hinshaw DB, Jr. Prognostic value of 1-H MRS in perinatal CNS insults. Pediatr Neurol 1997; 17:309–318.

114. Hanrahan JD, Sargentoni J, Azzopardi D, et al. Cerebral metabolism within 18 hours of birth asphyxia: a proton magnetic resonance spectroscopy study. Pediatr Res 1996; 39:584–590.

115. Barkovich AJ, Baranski K, Vigneron D, et al. Proton MR spectroscopy for the evaluation of brain injury in asphyxiated, term neonates. Am J Neuroradiol 1999; 20:1399–1405.

116. Zarifi MK, Astrakas LG, Poussaint TY, Plessis AdA, Zurakowski D, Tzika AA. Prediction of adverse outcome with cerebral lactate level and apparent diffusion coefficient in infants with perinatal asphyxia. Radiology 2002; 225:859–870.

117. Cappellini M, Rapisardi G, Cioni ML, Fonda C. Acute hypoxic encephalopathy in the full-term newborn: correlation between Magnetic Resonance Spectroscopy and neurological evaluation at short and long term. Radiol Med 2002; 104:332–340.

3.4

Imaging Intracranial Hemorrhage in the Neonate and Infant

Paul D. Griffiths and Elysa Widjaja
Academic Unit of Radiology, University of Sheffield, Sheffield, U.K.

Alan Sprigg
Sheffield NHS Trust, Sheffield, U.K.

ANATOMY OF INTRACRANIAL HEMORRHAGE

It is important to be accurate with anatomical descriptions of intracranial hemorrhage (ICH) at any patient age. The correct delineation of the compartment(s) confining the hemorrhage may give an indicator to the underlying cause and provide the neurosurgeon with vital information if intervention is required. The classical anatomical descriptions of ICH are (from superficial to deep) extradural, subdural, subarachnoid, parenchymal, and intraventricular and these can be found in isolation or in combination. Hematoma is the term used radiologically if the collection of blood is comparatively focal and has mass effect. Hemorrhage is usually used to describe more diffuse collections of blood, for example, many bleeds into the subarachnoid space. Knowledge of the anatomical compartments is vital for interpretation of imaging ICH and forming a usable differential diagnosis.

EXTRA-AXIAL HEMORRHAGE

The brain is sometimes referred to as part of the neuraxis, therefore 'extra-axial' is used to define intra-cranial lesions that do not involve the brain, i.e., related to the meninges or ependyma. The meninges are the key to defining hemorrhages on the surface of the brain and consist of the pia, arachnoid, and dura mater (Fig. 1). The pia mater consists of a thin sheet of only a few cells thickness and is firmly adherent to the brain substance, and it is comparatively unusual for blood to separate the pia from the underlying cortex. Superficial to the pia is the arachnoid mater that consists of fairly tough fibrous components throughout its extent and forms the subarachnoid space (between arachnoid and pia). This space is usually filled with cerebrospinal fluid circulating over the brain. In some regions at the base of the brain the spaces become capacious and these are called the basal cisterns. This is the site of subarachnoid hemorrhage, which is the commonest site for bleeding when aneurysms rupture (very uncommon in neonates and infants) because the major large calibre arteries supplying the brain occupy that space.

The dura mater (pachymeninges) are the thickest and most resilient of the meninges and the space between them and the arachnoid mater is called the subdural space; it is only a potential space. The dura mater has two components, an outer (periosteal) portion that is firmly attached to the skull and an inner (meningeal) portion. This creates another potential compartment, the extradural space (misnamed as it should be the intradural space). This is a common site for hematoma following trauma and skull fractures

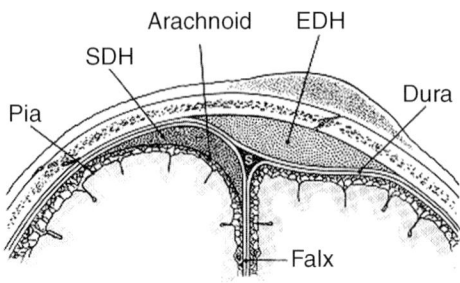

Figure 1. Diagram showing the anatomy of the meninges and the site of the common extra-axial hematoma in the coronal plane. *Abbreviations*: SDH, sub-dural hematoma; EDH, extra-dural hematoma. *Source*: Modified from Ref. 1.

in adults (extradural hematoma) but is very uncommon in neonates. The exact cause for the rarity of extradural hematoma in neonates is not known, but the leaves of the periosteal and meningeal dura are firmly attached in early childhood by interleaving fibrous structures.

The anatomy of the meninges can be used to explain the characteristic appearances of extra-axial hemorrhages on cross sectional imaging.

Subarachnoid Hemorrhage

The anatomy of the subarachnoid space that confines this type of hemorrhage explains the radiological features on cross sectional imaging. Blood is directly in contact with the pia mater and therefore tracks into the depths of cortical sulci rather than staying on the surface of the hemisphere, as in subdural and extradural hemorrhages. The subarachnoid space is expanded at several sites at the base of the brain (the basal cisterns) and blood tends to accumulate and be most visible at those sites. Over a period of time some blood may redistribute into the ventricular system, apparently against the overall direction of bulk flow of CSF.

Subdural Hematoma

These are much more frequently seen in neonates and infants when compared to extradural hematoma. The hemorrhage is confined to the space between the dura and arachnoid mater and is therefore not confined by the sutures of the skull. The shape of the acute hematoma is most frequently concentric and spreads out over the surface of the hemisphere. Fractures are less common with subdural hematoma and often are venous in origin, arising from disruption of small bridging veins.

Extradural Hematoma

As already stated, hemorrhage into this compartment is rare in the infant and exceptionally unusual in the neonate. This type of hematoma is confined by the skull sutures because of the anatomy of the pachymeninges. This gives the salient anatomical features on cross sectional imaging. The hematoma tends to be lens-shaped, its edges tapering as they approach the suture lines that are not crossed. Skull fractures are found in the majority of cases and the bleeding is usually arterial in nature, arising from branches of the external carotid or vertebral systems.

PARENCHYMAL HEMORRHAGE

Hemorrhage into the brain substance itself is frequently called parenchymal hemorrhage or intra-axial. It should be appreciated, however, that hemorrhage into different compartments in the same patient is common and in many cases parenchymal hemorrhage extends into the ventricular system. In most situations it is best to describe these lesions with reference to where the hemorrhage is centered anatomically as described in Table 1, however, it is occasionally more useful to describe the vascular territory involved, for example, when there has been hemorrhagic change into an area of arterial infarction. Alternatively the pattern of hemorrhage may fit with a known venous drainage territory, often representing venous infarction from sinus or cortical venous thrombosis.

Table 1. Anatomical Descriptors of Fetal/Neonatal Parenchymal Hemorrhage

Age specific location
 Germinal matrix hemorrhage
General locations
 (a) Infratentorial
      Brainstem—medulla, pons or midbrain
      Cerebellar—vermis or hemisphere
 (b) Supratentorial
      Lobar—frontal, parietal, temporal or occipital
      Ganglionic—putamen, caudate, globus pallidus
      Thalamic

IMAGING METHODS

In older patients the mainstay of imaging ICH is x-ray computed tomography (CT) to confirm hemorrhage and catheter angiography to confirm or refute the presence of a macroscopic vascular abnormality. Both of these do have a role in the investigation of some neonates with ICH but many are investigated by other methods. The reasons for this are complicated but are designed not to expose the young child to unnecessary risk. Both CT and catheter angiography use ionizing radiation and the use of this should be kept to a minimum in young children. CT and catheter angiography are mandatory however, if a treatable vascular abnormalities such as aneurysm or arterio-venous malformations (AVM) are suspected. Fortunately, ruptured vascular abnormalities are rare at this age and it is more likely that the cause of the ICH will not have an abnormality detectable on catheter angiography.

The favored approach in most centers is to use cranial ultrasound as the first diagnostic method and in many cases serial ultrasound examinations are all that is used (see below). CT is used to provide more detailed anatomical information and is vital for the confident diagnosis of subdural hematoma. MRI is not used a great deal in many institutions for a number of reasons including access, the need to use general anesthesia (GA) or sedation, and the perceived inability to detect acute ICH by MRI. However there are many advantages in using a combination of MRI techniques (see below).

X-Ray Computed Tomography

CT is considered to be the most accurate imaging method of detecting ICH in any compartment in the first few days after the hemorrhage and this has to do with the physical principles that produce tissue contrast and the biological process of clot formation and maturation. CT, like all x-ray based imaging methods, produces images depending on how much of the incident x-rays is stopped (attenuated) by a volume of tissue.

CT images display pixels of different intensity depending on the x-ray attenuation value of the tissue in the voxel. It is the electron density of the tissue that determines the attenuation and this rises as a clot matures in the acute phase due to hemo-concentration. CT is the most reliable method for detecting ICH in the acute timescale (0–7 days) and hemorrhage/hematoma will appear "whiter" than the lipid-rich brain parenchyma. With time, phagocytes lyse the hematoma and the attenuation falls, reducing the sensitivity of CT. The CT systems in use now can image the brain very quickly, usually obviating the need for sedation or GA.

Conventional Catheter Angiography

Conventional catheter angiography is the reference standard for imaging high flow vascular malformations (aneurysms and AVM). Modern angiographic equipment can produce images with a matrix size of 1024×1024, giving pixel sizes of the order of 0.2 mm. Images with a temporal resolution of up to 25 Hz can be obtained, giving detailed information of flow patterns. This combination of spatial and temporal resolution is not currently possible with any other method of vascular imaging. Catheter angiography can be a technically difficult procedure in neonates and infants because of the small size of the arteries, which can give problems for arterial access and for catheterizing the cranio-cervical vessels. In less experienced hands there is a significant risk of complications including death or permanent neurological deficits from neuro-complications, and reduced limb growth from damage to the femoral artery.

Cranial Ultrasonography

This is most commonly used in infants when the fontanels can provide an acoustic window to visualize the intracranial compartments. As described below it has been used extensively to study the hemorrhagic complications of prematurity and is well suited to detect and monitor intraparenchymal and intraventricular hemorrhage, although the posterior fossa structures may present diagnostic problems.

Ultrasound methods, however, do have significant problems in detecting hemorrhage on the surface of the brain and close to the skull. Ultrasound is very poor at detecting subarachnoid hemorrhage, though this is not usually of major clinical relevance in neonatal practice, but subdural hemorrhage/hematomas are important and ultrasound has a low sensitivity for showing that pathology when compared to CT or MRI.

Magnetic Resonance Imaging and Angiography

MR imaging has the advantage over CT that it can readily produce multiplanar images, allowing anatomical appreciation of the hematoma itself and its complications such as compartmental herniations and ischemic damage. MRI has many disadvantages, however, including lack of access, problems in monitoring, and long acquisitions that often require anesthesia or sedation.

Theoretically MR imaging would not be expected to show acute hemorrage well because the signal from fresh blood is often close to that from normal brain tissue on routine spin echo and fast spin echo T1 and T2 weighted images. If the hematoma has mass effect, however, detection is not usually a problem, but the detection of SAH and thin subdural hematomas may be difficult. There is extensive evidence from the adult literature that the use of other sequences such as FLAIR and gradient echo T2* images can significantly improve the detection of acute and subacute hemorrhage. These issues have not been completely addressed in neonatal imaging and one cannot expect complete similarities between the behavior of hematoma evolution in neonates when compared to adults.

The ability to image the intracranial vessels specifically by MRI is exceptionally useful because of the problems of performing catheter angiography in neonates. There are several forms of MRI angiography, including Time of Flight (TOF), phase contrast, and black blood imaging. These can be used to delineate either the arterial or venous side of the circulation as appropriate clinically. The most widely employed technique for imaging the cerebral circulation clinically is TOF MR angiography, which utilizes flow related signal enhancement of a gradient echo sequence with a short TR. The shorter the TR, the greater the background signal suppression but the faster the flow of incoming unsaturated spins that is required to obtain the maximum flow-related enhancement.

TOF angiography may be performed either in 2D or 3D mode. The 2D TOF is composed of many thin sections usually acquired one after the other. To maximize inflow of unsaturated spins these sections are oriented at right angles to the direction of flow in the vessels to be imaged. The 3D TOF, as with any other 3D sequence, has multiple partitions that are typically very thin (≈ 1 mm) and are contiguous with no inter-slice gap. This increases resolution at the penalty of increasing exposure of the incoming spins to the saturation effects of the RF at each TR, thus limiting the volume that can be covered. This problem has been overcome by using multiple overlapping thin slab acquisition (MOTSA). This utilizes multiple overlapping volumes that are a few millimeters or less thick, and that are stacked together to increase anatomical coverage. This has been our approach to produce static MRI angiographic examinations with the added refinement of using SLINKY, a method that improves signal/noise ratios and minimizes the "venetian blind" artifacts from routine MOTSA methods.

One of the most exciting advances in MRI angiography is the capacity to produce time resolved methods with frame rates of one per second or better. These involve the injection of MRI contrast agents (gadolinium chelates) into a peripheral vein and acquiring projectional data in multiple planes (2). We have applied this technique extensively in the neonatal and pediatric population for both head and neck (3) and intracranial vascular abnormalities.

EXAMPLES OF THE APPLICATION OF DIFFERENT IMAGING METHODS IN NEONATAL INTRACRANIAL HEMORRHAGE

Parenchymal Hemorrhage in Premature Babies

Cranial ultrasound can assess the presence of intra-parenchymal hemorrhage in the baby born prematurely. Scans are performed rapidly via the anterior fontanelle, although this is dependent on operator skill and there is some variability between operator performance and image interpretation. Scans are acquired in sagittal and coronal planes, but the anatomical planes are not directly comparable to those seen in CT and MR imaging. Ultrasound may suggest extra-axial hemorrhage (e.g., subdural) but assesses those with more difficulty.

The region of the germinal matrix (in the caudothalmic notch) is easy to assess by a trans-fontanelle ultrasound. This is a very vascular area and hemorrhage initially appears bright but subsequently resolves with time to form a cystic structure that often resolves ultimately on ultrasound, although gliosis can be detected on MR imaging. This is termed subependymal hemorrhage (Grade I) and is not usually associated with neurological deficit. True subependymal cysts can be seen anterior to the caudothalamic notch in anterior ventricular coaptation—which is a normal variant. These are different than more posteriorly sited subependymal cysts which may be associated with sepsis (TORCH) or calcified subependymal lesions (casting an acoustic shadow) that may be seen with tuberous sclerosis.

Traditionally ultrasonic assessment of ICH has been graded I–IV as listed below in Table 2. In reality, there is a spectrum of hemorrhage, and an accurate description of the ultrasound findings with a hard copy image record is more useful than a "grading." So-called grade IV hemorrhage was initially thought to be caused by intraventricular hemorrhage extending into the brain substance, but may be due to segmental ischemia related to venous infarction.

Table 2. Grading System Used to Classify Neonatal Intracranial Hemorrhage

Grade I	Subependymal hemorrhage at the caudothalmic notch
Grade II	Intraventricular hemorrhage without ventricular dilatation
Grade III	Intraventricular hemorrhage with ventricular dilatation
Grade IV	Parenchymal hemorrhage

Source: From Ref. 4.

On ultrasound a parasagittal view shows that the choroid plexus is widest in the ventricular atrium. The normal choroid plexus does not extend anterior to the caudothalmic notch—hence any area of brightness (hemorrhage) within the ventricular system anterior to the caudothalmic notch must be due to intraventricular hemorrhage and is not due to normal choroid plexus. Separating small amounts of intraventricular hemorrhage (bright) from the choroid plexus (also bright) can be difficult. If the baby is lying supine the hemorrhage tends to gravitate posteriorly into the occipital horn of the lateral ventricle, a region that should be checked for hemorrhage on ultrasound (as on CT) and showing a blood-CSF fluid level. Major intraventricular hemorrhage is assessed easily with ultrasound.

Very acute hemorrhage may not be clotted and may appear only as a faint echogenicity throughout the ventricles until it clots several hours later and appears white. CT is more sensitive in detecting early degrees of intraventricular hemorrhage than US, but this usually means moving a sick neonate from the neonatal unit to the radiology department. Ultrasound can be used to refer follow-up complications of intraventricular hemorrhage (development of hydrocephalus), monitor treatment (ventricular decompression following shunt placement and evaluation of shunt tip position), and show the resolution of parenchymal hemorrhage (porencephalic cyst development and resolution).

Intraparenchymal Hematoma in Neonates and Infants

The previous section dealt with germinal matrix hemorrhage with or without extension into the brain and its association with prematurity. Here we deal with parenchymal hemorrhage of the term delivery and older infant (Fig. 2). The commonest causes of parenchymal hemorrhage around the time of birth are mechanical birth trauma and clotting disturbances, both of which may be exacerbated by hypoxia/ischemia.

Thrombosis of the intracranial dural sinuses and/or veins is an uncommon cause of ICH in older children but is widely held to be an under-diagnosed condition in the newborn. Birth asphyxia, birth trauma, dehydration, and infections separately or in combination can account for the increased risk of venous thrombosis in the neonate. By and large, the clinical condition and outcomes are related to the extent and site of the thrombosis. Two patterns of involvement are described, namely "superficial" and "deep" depending on the dural/venous system involved. Superficial venous thrombosis involves the superior sagittal sinus, transverse sinus, sigmoid sinus, or cortical veins. This tends to produce venous infarction and hemorrhage in the cerebral white matter that is frequently bilateral if the sagittal sinus is involved. The gray matter of the cerebral cortex is often spared because it has an alternative route of drainage via the meninges. Deep venous thrombosis usually involves the straight sinus, vein of Galen, or its tributaries, and often produces bilateral hemorrhage in the thalami and posterior portions of the basal ganglia. This is the frequently cited mechanism of primary thalamo-ventricular hemorrhage (Fig. 3) (5).

In older neonates and infants ruptured aneurysms or arteriovenous malformations are rare causes of parenchymal hemorrhage (Fig. 4).

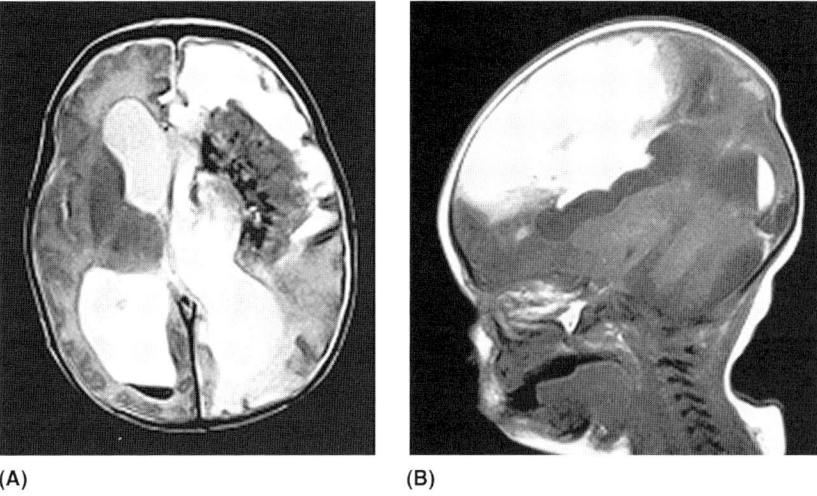

(A)   **(B)**

Figure 2. Unilateral grade 4 intraventricular hemorrhage in a premature baby shown by MRI. Axial T2-weighted (**A**) and parasagittal T1-weighted (**B**) imaging shows a large subacute hematoma in the vicinity of the left basal ganglia and thalamus. There is significant mass effect and hydrocephalus. Note the intraventricular blood in the right occipital horn.

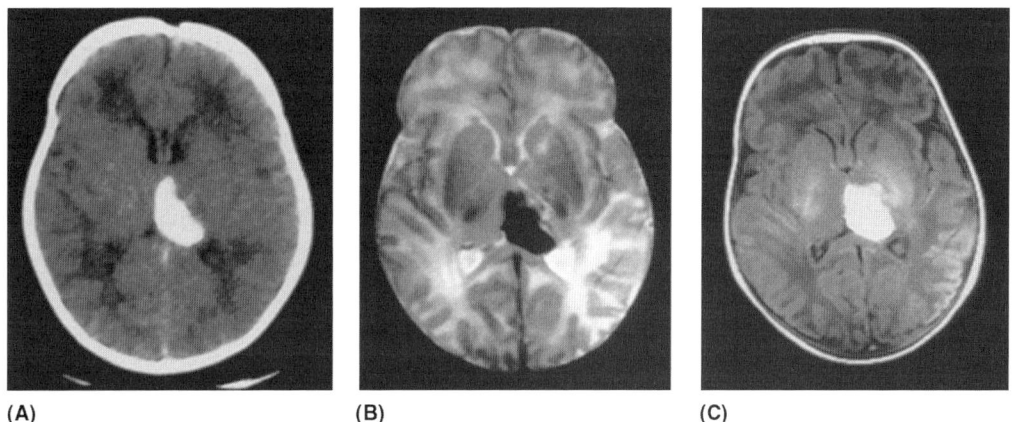

(A)   **(B)**   **(C)**

Figure 3. A 5-day-old child presented with irritability and seizures. Axial nonenhanced CT (**A**) showed acute hemorrhage into the left thalamus. Axial T2-weighted MRI (**B**) and T1-weighted (**C**) image confirmed hemorrhage and showed edema or possibly early ischemic changes in the left temporal lobe. No vascular abnormality on either the arterial or venous system was shown on MRI or catheter angiography.

Subarachnoid Hemorrhage in Neonates and Infants

Govaert considers subarachnoid hemorrhage (SAH) to be the commonest ICH in the term newborn (6) with estimates of frequency in the order of 1–2% of live births, rising to about 6% of instrumental deliveries (7,8). Most are thought to be due to damaged arachnoid veins and compounded by venous congestion as may occur in hypoxia/ischemia.

SAH due to ruptured intracranial aneurysm is recognized in the neonate and infant but is exceptionally rare (Fig. 5). The distribution and morphology of aneurysms

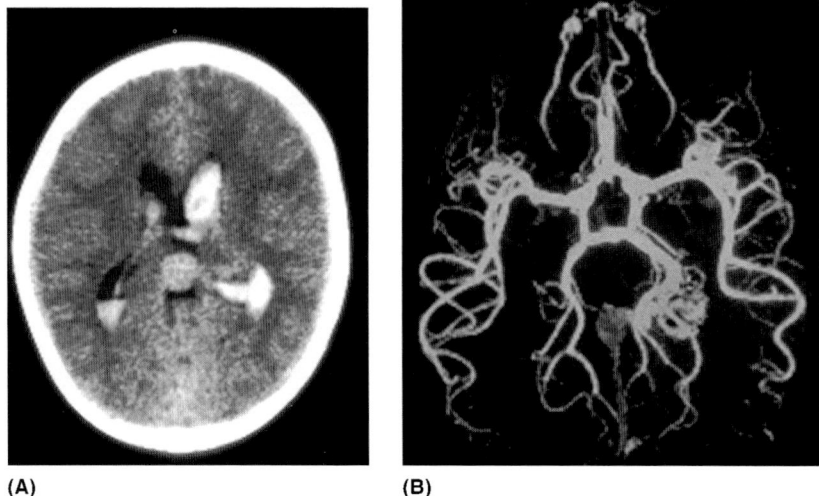

(A) **(B)**

Figure 4. A 2-year-old child presented with sudden loss of consciousness. Axial non-enhanced CT (**A**) showed intraventricular hemorrhage and a small peritrigonal parenchymal hematoma adjacent to the left trigone on the left. Note the enlarged vein of Galen. A collapsed axial projection of the MRI angiographic data set (**B**) showed a small peritrigonal arteriovenous malformation draining into the deep venous system.

in this patient group is not the same as in adults with ruptured "berry" aneurysms. In contrast to the "proximal" predilection for adult berry aneurysms (anterior communicating artery, posterior communicating artery, middle cerebral artery bi/ trifurcation, and basilar tip) neonatal aneurysms tend to on peripheral branches. In addition, the neonatal aneurysms tend to be large and irregular. These features suggest that neonatal aneurysms are fundamentally different from adult berry aneurysms and at least a proportion may be infective in origin. Aneurysms presenting in infancy are often found in children with other conditions (usually syndromic).

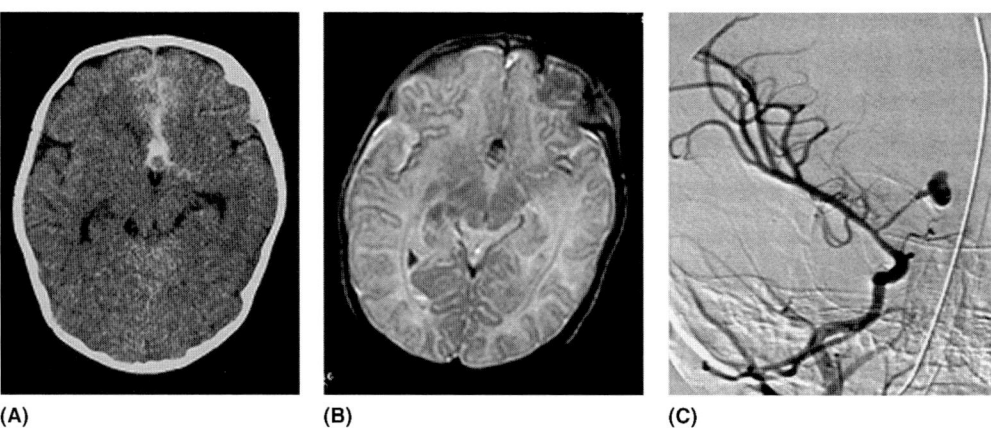

(A) **(B)** **(C)**

Figure 5. A 6-week-old child presented with seizures and signs of raised intracranial pressure. Axial nonenhanced CT (**A**) showed subarachnoid hemorrhage in the interhemispheric fissure with an outline of an aneurysm seen in relief. T2-weighted MRI confirmed localized acute clot (**B**) and an aneurysm was shown on catheter angiography (**C**).

Subdural Hematoma in Neonates and Infants

The vast majority of subdural hematoma found in older children and adults are due to trauma, and "trauma" in its various forms appears to account for a significant proportion of subdural hematoma in the neonatal period and early infancy. Non-accidental injury (NAI) should be considered in an infant with unexplained subdural hematoma, although it is thought to be relatively uncommon in children within 2 months of birth. In the authors' medico-legal experience most successful prosecutions for cranial NAI occur in children who were injured between 2–6 months of age. Ninty-five percent of cases of severe head injury in the first year of life are due to inflicted injury.

The majority of children with intracranial manifestations of NAI seen within a hospital environment present with either encephalopathy (with or without external signs of trauma) or as children being investigated for non-specific presentations (e.g., abnormal head growth, developmental problems, suspected meningitis). Subsequent investigations reveal unexpected and unexplained findings such as bloodstained CSF, retinal hemorrhages, and/or intracranial lesions (usually subdural hematomas) on scanning. The craniocerebral manifestations of cranial non-accidental head injury are listed in Table 3. It is obvious from the wide range of pathologies that no one imaging method has the overall advantage in assessing these children and a combined approach is needed. The interested reader is directed to a recent review of about imaging in these cases (9).

Skull Radiography

Plain films are the best method to assess skull vault fractures and the primary indication for skull radiographs is forensic; it should be appreciated that no information about the state of the intracranial contents can be made from plain films. Fractures of the skull base usually require CT for diagnosis and description of extent.

Table 3. Head and Spine Imaging Findings in Non-Accidental Trauma

1. Extracranial
   Scalp lacerations, abrasions or bruising
2. Cranial
   Fractures of the skull and skull base; sutural disruption
3. Intracranial–hemorrhagic
   Subdural hematoma
   Subarachnoid hemorrhage
   Intraventricular hemorrhage
   Parenchymal hemorrhage (particularly contusions, less commonly gray-white matter shear injuries)
4. Intracranial–non-hemorrhagic
   Mechanical—lobar disruption; cerebral lacerations; disruption of the cerebral falx or septum pellucidum
   Macroscopic damage to the intracranial or cervical vessels, e.g., dissection, pseudo-aneurysm
   Secondary—cerebral edema; hypoxia–ischemia; infarction
5. Spinal
   Vertebral fractures
   Spinal cord or extramedullary (subdural) hematomas
6. Late sequelae
   Hydrocephalus (communicating or obstructive)
   Atrophy
   Gliosis/encephalomalacia
   Growing fractures (leptomeningeal cysts)
   Impaired skull growth

Ultrasound

Cranial ultrasound has a limited role in the evaluation of head injury in general and cranial NAI in particular, primarily due to the low sensitivity of detecting extra-axial hemorrhage and complex brain injury which is considerably inferior to CT and MRI. However, it has been shown that contusional tears are shown by ultrasound but frequently not by other methods (10).

CT Imaging

CT is the primary imaging tool in the evaluation of cranio-cerebral NAI, having a number of practical advantages over MRI. In the acute phase, CT is useful because of its high sensitivity in detecting bone trauma, hemorrhage, edema, and hypoxic–ischemic injury. The rate of transition between the appearances of acute hematomas (high density), subacute hematomas (isodense), and chronic hematomas (low density) is difficult to predict with accuracy. Standard descriptions of the maturing appearances of SDH's describe the collections as being of high density within 7 days of hemorrhage, becoming isodense between 7–21 days, and hypodense after 21 days. These parameters were, however, based upon older generation CT scan studies performed on older children and adults (11). It is increasingly apparent that there is a much more complex spectrum of appearances of ICH in infants as demonstrated by CT and, in particular, MRI (12). Caution should thus be taken when attempting to estimate the timing of intracranial hematomas. Cerebral edema and hypoxic–ischemic injury are well demonstrated by CT, the high water content of the early infant brain tending to make their evaluation difficult employing standard MRI sequences.

MR Imaging

MRI is more difficult to perform in infants compared with CT because of the length of the procedure, the need for specialized monitoring equipment, and general anaesthesia in many cases. It is recommended, however, in the assessment of children with cranial NAI

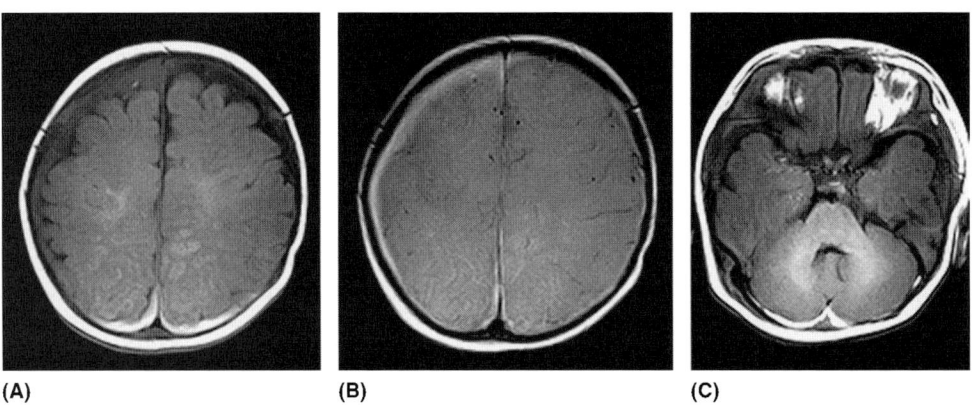

(A) (B) (C)

Figure 6. Nonaccidental injury. A 3-month-old child presented with encephalopathy and external signs of unexplained trauma. Axial T1-weighted image close to the vertex (**A**) shows high signal subdural collections overlying the pariteal lobes on both sides, indicative of relatively recent hemorrhage. The subdural space anteriorly on the right is wider than the left and shows slightly increased signal compared to the CSF containing structures. That region has high signal on proton density-weighted MRI (**B**) indicating an older hematoma. An axial T1-weighted image through the posterior fossa showed recent subdural hematoma over both cerebellar hemispheres (**C**).

because the extra information gained from MRI in cases of NAI is vital for clinical and medico-legal decision making. An example is shown in Figure. 6. MRI is the most sensitive modality for detecting early ischemic changes if diffusion weighted imaging is used.

Major arterial trauma is rarely encountered but may be evaluated by MRI angiography. A particular advantage of MRI angiography is the ability to image the cervical spine as well, because of the perceived high association of brain and cervical spine/cord trauma.

One common defense put forward in cases of suspected cranial NAI is that the subdural hematoma was the result of a difficult birth which lead to hemorrhagic complication not related to intentional physical abuse. Our work in this area has been published elsewhere and is summarized in chap. 3.2 of this book.

CONCLUSIONS

ICH is comparatively common in the newborn and is frequently related to the delivery process itself. Brain hemorrhage frequently occurs in the background of prematurity and low birth weight children and both of those groups are most appropriately imaged usually by ultrasound alone. In older infants non-traumatic ICH is considerably less common and most cases will be due to covert, inflicted damage. CT and MRI and angiography play a major role and in some cases catheter angiography may be required.

REFERENCES

1. Gean AD. In: Gean AD, ed. Imaging of Head Trauma. New York: Raven Press, 1994:76.
2. Griffiths PD, Hoggard N, Warren DJ, Wilkinson ID, Anderson B, Romanowski CA. Dynamic MR Digital subtraction angiography: Assessment of brain arteriovenous malformations. Am J Neurorad. 2000; 21:1892–1899.
3. Chooi WK, Woodhouse N, Coley SC, Griffiths PD. Pediatric head and neck lesions: Assessment of vascularity by MR digital subtraction angiography. Am J Neurorad 2004; 25:1251–1255.
4. Stewart AL, Reynolds EOR, Hope PL, et al. Probability of neurodevelopmental disorders estimated from ultrasound appearance of brains of very pre-term infants. Developmental Medicine and Child Neurology 1987; 29:3–11.
5. Govaert P, Achten E, Vanhausebrouck P, De Praeter C, Van Damme J. Deep cerebral venous thrombosis in thalamo-ventricular hemorrhage of the term newborn. Pediatric Radiology 1992; 22:123–127.
6. Govaert P. In: Govaert P, ed. Cranial hemorrhage in the term newborn infant. London: Mac Keith Press, 1994:16–83.
7. Brand M, Saling E. Obstetrical factors and intracranial hemorrhage. In: Kubli F, Patel N, Schmidt W, Linderkamp O, eds. Perinatal events and brain damage in surviving children. Berlin: Springer-Verlag, 1988:216–227.
8. Blennow G, Svenningsen NW, Gustafsson B, Sunden B, Cronquist S. Neonatal and prospective follow up study of infants delivered by vacuum extraction. Acta Obstetricia et Gynaecologica Scandinavica 1977; 56:189–192.
9. Jaspan T, Griffiths PD, McConachie NS, Punt JAG. Neuroimaging for non-accidental head injury in childhood: a proposed protocol. Clin Radiol 2003; 58:44–53.
10. Jaspan T, Narborough G, Punt JAG, Lowe J. Cerebral contusional tears as a marker of child abuse—detection by cranial sonography. Pediatr Radiol 1992; 22:237–245.
11. Scotti G, Terbrugge K, Melancon D, Belanger G. Evaluation of the age of subdural haematomas by computerized tomography. J Neurosurg 1977; 47:311–315.
12. Kleinman PK. Head trauma. In: Kleinman PK, ed. Diagnostic Imaging of Child Abuse. 2nd ed. St Louis, U.S.A.: Mosby, 1998:285–342.

SECTION 4

New Horizons

4.1

Advances in Fetal Ultrasound

Pam Loughna
Academic Division of Obstetrics and Gynaecology, Nottingham City Hospital, Nottingham, U.K.

Since ultrasound was introduced as an imaging technique in obstetrics, there has been significant improvement in the quality and resolution of images obtained. The early static scans permitted the detection of gross lesions, such as anencephaly. The introduction of real time (B mode) imaging with increased resolution has permitted fetal anatomy to be examined in greater detail and with considerable accuracy such that ultrasound has replaced maternal serum alphafetoprotein measurement as the screening test of choice for neural tube defects in England.

However, there are limitations to fetal ultrasound, particularly relating to fetal position, gestation, and maternal body habitus. Recent advances such as native tissue harmonics have increased the penetration and resolution of ultrasound in difficult cases, e.g., maternal obesity and oligohydramnios, and such techniques are increasingly available on standard ultrasound machines. Despite these advances, there are some situations where ultrasound is extremely limited as a diagnostic tool.

Three-dimensional ultrasound has attracted considerable interest in the past few years. Initial limitations related to the inability to create real-time 3-D images, but this has been overcome in the last two or three years. Real-time, or 4-D, imaging relies on a tissue fluid interface, which does not exist in terms of imaging the fetal central nervous system. While it is possible to create three-dimensional images of internal body structures, this cannot be done in real time and requires high quality two-dimensional images taken from a still object. The sweep of the transducer over the object to be imaged needs to be standardized as far as possible. The need for this, and the object of interest not to move, limits the day to day application of 3-D ultrasound in the investigation of internal fetal organs. In situations where 4-D ultrasound has been used in clinical situations, there is limited international experience but this is growing.

Early experience with three- and four-dimensional ultrasound has been primarily in the investigation of the facial abnormalities, volume assessment, and fetal echocardiology. However, there is growing experience of these ultrasound modalities in imaging the CNS. This relates both to structure (1,2) and circulation, where detailed information concerning the vascular connections of vascular anomalies such as the vein of Galen can be obtained with 3-D power Doppler (3). The addition of 3-D ultrasound may improve the characterization of spinal lesions including spina bifida, with greater accuracy of assessment of the segments involved (1).

Further developments in ultrasound will continue to improve fetal imaging, permitting a greater degree of accuracy in the diagnosis of anomalies of the central nervous system. However, there will remain a significant number of anomalies for which prenatal ultrasound is not the modality of choice and for which other imaging modalities such as MRI will be invaluable.

REFERENCES

1. Lee W, Chaiworapongsa T, Romero R, et al. A diagnostic approach for the evaluation of spina bifida by three-dimensional ultrasonography. J Ultrasound Med 2002; 21:619–626.
2. Xu H, Zhang Q, Lu MD, Xiao XT. Comparison of two-dimensional and three-dimensional sonography in evaluating fetal malformations. J Clin Ultrasound 2002; 30:515–525.
3. Ruano R, Benachi A, Aubry MC, et al. Perinatal three-dimensional color power Doppler ultrasonography of vein of Galen aneurysms. J Ultrasound Med 2003; 22:12357–12362.

4.2

Expected Developments in In Utero Magnetic Resonance Imaging of the Fetal Central Nervous System

Elspeth H. Whitby
Academic Unit of Radiology, University of Sheffield, Sheffield, U.K.

EXPECTED DEVELOPMENTS

The interest in in utero magnetic resonance imaging (MRI) is rapidly increasing and several centers throughout the world have active research programs in various aspects of this technique. Other centers are using the technique in a clinical environment despite their limited experience. Most of this work relates to the fetal central nervous system (CNS) and structural imaging. The main thrust of the work is to provide diagnostic and prognostic information on the fetus for the parents.

The increasing availability of fast imaging sequences on MRI scanners from all manufacturers has made the use of the technique possible. The limiting factors are now scanning time and radiologist experience. Recently there have been a few dedicated courses on fetal imaging helping educate radiologists for this role.

The mainstay of in utero MRI is ultrafast sequences that provide heavily T2 weighted images in three orthogonal planes. These are supplemented by T1 weighted images (Fig. 1A) however these sequences are longer and usually only really successful in the third trimester. They are useful earlier in pregnancy to delineate other body areas, e.g., liver, bowel, lung (Fig. 1B). The use in the CNS is mainly for hemorrhage and myelination. They provide important information on the developing gray and white matter, but until the third trimester there is little myelination, so they are of limited use in early pregnancy.

As the fetus develops rapidly and the composition of the brain changes it is becoming evident that sequence parameters need to be changed and adjusted for gestational age.

Diffusion Weighted Imaging (DWI)

DWI can be used to demonstrate white matter maturation and early cortical maturation (Fig. 2). Diffusion anisotropy of white matter tracts increases with increasing gestational age, allowing visualization of the maturing tracts before there is signal change on T1 and T2 weighted images. DWI used in cases with hydrocephalus has lead to the suggestion that areas of high signal may indicate that the surrounding brain tissue is under pressure. When there is ventriculomegaly due to brain loss the signal on the DWI is not increased. DWI can also contribute to the assessment of brain maturation (1). See also chap. 2.3.

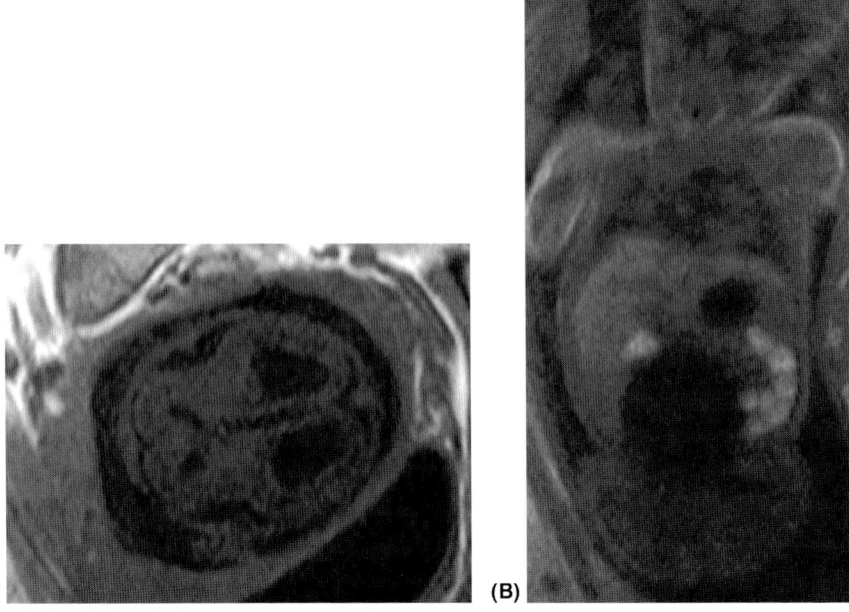

(A)   **(B)**

Figure 1. (**A**) T1-weighted image of the fetal brain apial at 24 weeks gestational age. Axial section. (**B**) T1-weighted image of the fetal body. Note the high signal from liver and bowel.

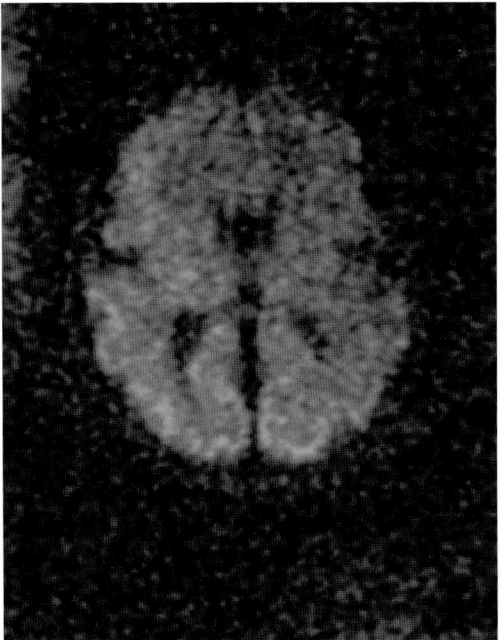

Figure 2. Diffusion weighted image of the fetal brain, axial section. Normal appearance at 36 weeks gestation.

Functional MRI

Most of this work has been done in Nottingham. They have looked at both auditory (2,3) and visual stimulation (4) in the third trimester of pregnancy and have detected responses to visual stimuli in approximately 50% of the fetuses studied. Visual stimulation appears to activate the frontal regions of the brain rather than the expected visual cortex. They have not seen the negative BOLD response that has been reported in neonates (5), but the traditional positive response similar to that in adults although slightly delayed. Auditory responses are detected in the temporal lobes in 25% of the fetuses examined. This work is still in its infancy but holds promise for assessing brain development, especially in babies with intrauterine growth restriction (IUGR).

Spectroscopy has been done in normal and abnormal neonates mainly in France and Holland. There is increasing data on normal spectroscopy (Fig. 3) in the third trimester from the Dutch workers (6,7). They have chosen the third trimester as the fetus is engaged and movement is restricted. The technique used takes 30 minutes and includes structural imaging at the beginning and the end to ensure that the information obtained is not from fetal movement. As yet unpublished work from Girad et al. in France includes normative data from a wider range of gestational ages and is essential

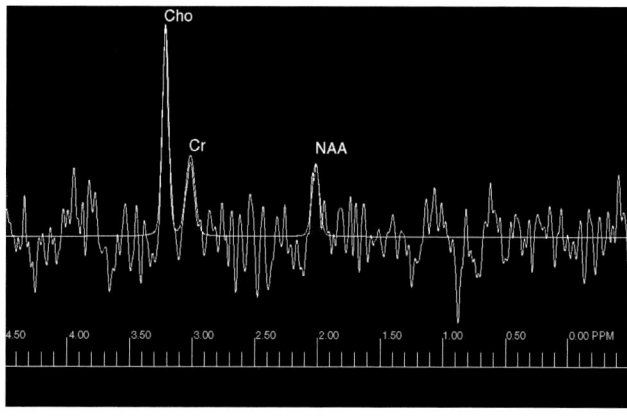

Figure 3. Brain spectroscopy at 29 weeks gestation.

to establish a normal database from which to develop the technique for detection of abnormalities. Additional information is available in chap. 2.3.

Spinal Abnormalities

There is little published on in utero MRI for spinal abnormalities but this is an area where MRI can add information to the ultrasound. With the increasing interest in in utero surgery MRI has a pivotal role in patient selection and follow up. This is predominantly for cases of open spina bifida at present and in utero MRI defines the anatomy prior to surgery both at the spinal level (Fig. 4A) and in the brain (Fig. 4B and Fig. 5).

Spina Bifida

There have been over 200 spina bifida cases operated on in utero in the USA but the true benefits remain uncertain. The selection criteria are becoming tighter and late gestation surgery is no longer an option. It is thought that there is a reduction in the degree of the Chiari 2 malformation post operation and that less of these babies require shunting in later life. It is thought that as the pregnancy progresses the exposed neural tissue is affected by amniotic fluid, meconium, or even trauma, e.g., as the baby hits the uterine wall. A prospective randomized controlled trial is currently ongoing to provide the vital answers.

It has been noted that cases with a myelomeningocele have a small posterior fossa, chiari 2, and no extra axial CSF space and these cases usually develop hydrocephalus.

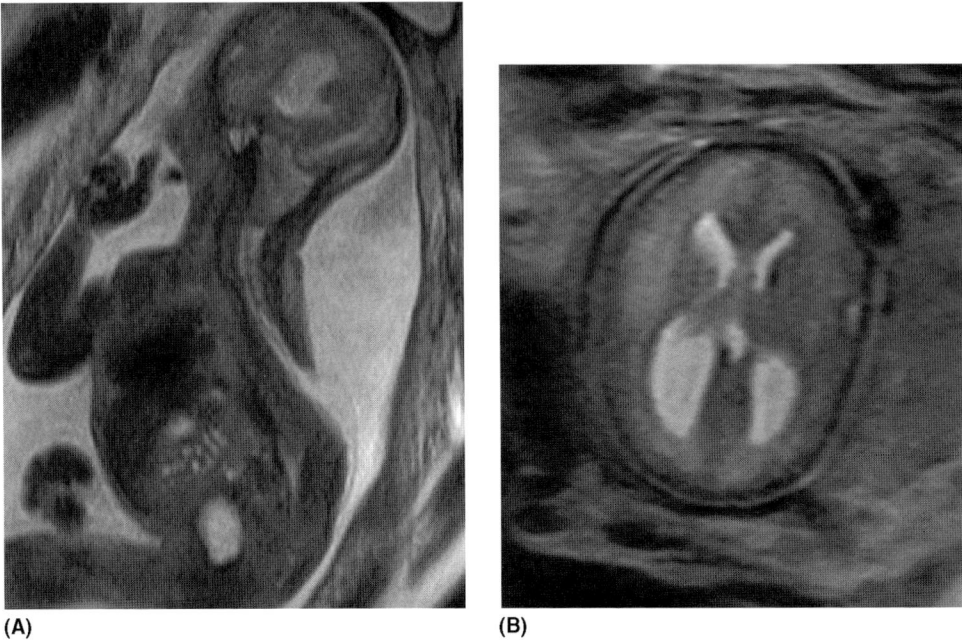

(A)   (B)

Figure 4. A fetus with (**A**) large thoracic myelomeningocele and (**B**) Chiari 2 malformation in the brain.

Closed spinal dygraphisms do not have loss of the extra axial CSF space, do not develop hydrocephalus, and do not have hindbrain herniation (Chiari 2). Fetal MRI allows differentiation of the two types (8). Our work has shown that the lack of extra axial CSF space occurred in all cases of spina bifida where there was a Chiari 2 malformation

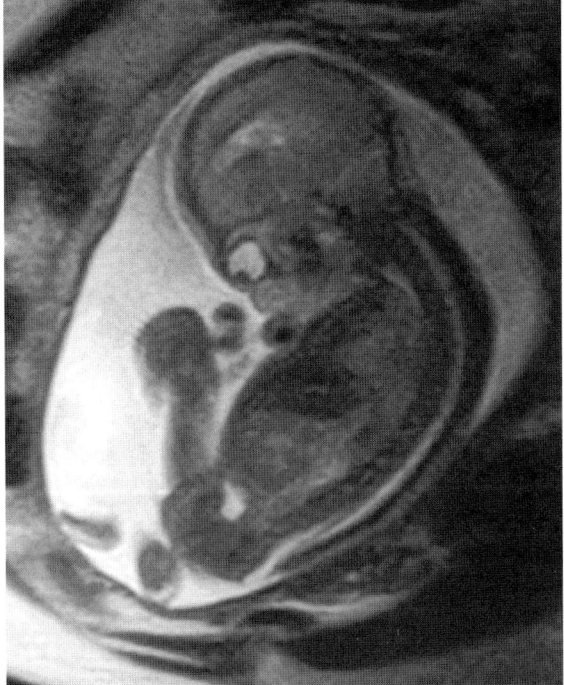

Figure 5. 26-weeks gestational age. Note the Chiari 2 malformation, lack of extra axial CSF, and open myelomeningocele.

(Fig. 5). We also had cases where there was a lack of extra axial CSF space but no tonsillar decent. We postulate that this is a preceding stage and these cases develop a Chiari 2 malformation later in gestation. Currently the natural history of the development of the Chiari 2 in utero is not clear and further prospective studies are required (9).

Diastomatomyelia

MRI aids in location of the lesion and determining its type. If isolated with a common thecal sac and no bony spur, the outlook is good; if it is associated with other abnormalities, e.g., renal, genital tract, the prognosis is more guarded. If separate thecal sacs and a bony spur are present, complications can occur in later life as a syrinx tends to develop and growth of the cord is restricted. In utero MRI demonstrates the

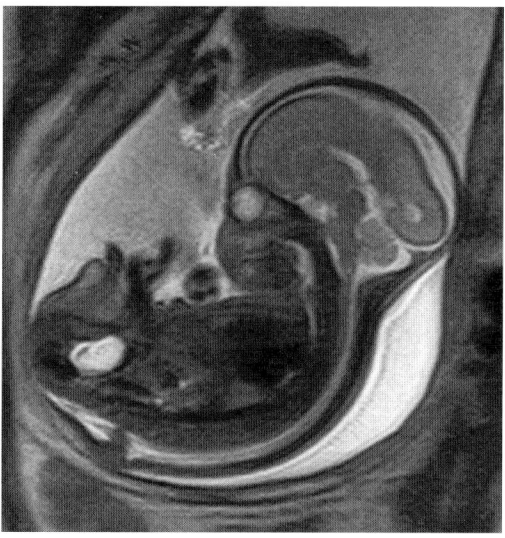

Figure 6. Diastomatomyelia. Large dumbbell shaped bony spur splitting the spinal cord.

anatomical abnormality (Fig. 6) and any syrinx. The level of the filum and any tethering of the cord can also be identified.

Abnormal Sulcation and Gyration

There is increasing interest in in utero MRI for cases of abnormal sulcation and gyration. Knowledge of normal patterns of sulcation and gyration is increasing (10) but as yet, little knowledge of how early and how accurate the detection of abnormalities is. The sensitivity and specificity are as yet unknown and future work is essential.

3-D MRI

Using a three dimensional gradient echo sequence in a 3-D acquisition a slab of tissue is excited, giving a 3-D image, but this is prone to motion artifact and although it can give an "overview" of the fetus, adds little if anything to the ultrasound and has high SAR values. However 3-D images of the fetal brain show great potential for imaging sulcation and gyration and also for imaging complex malformations (15). See also chap. 2.3.

Angiography

MRI angiography is particularly useful for demonstrating vascular abnormalities of the central nervous system. There are several case reports on the detection and diagnosis of a vein of Galen malformation in utero (11–13) and other vascular abnormalities (14).

Placental MRI

Placental MRI has great promise but currently the data is limited. The initial report dates from 1988 (16) but the majority of work since has concentrated on placental abnormalities such as placenta accreta (17–19) and retained products of conception. Imaging of the placenta during pregnancy as a tool to assess fetal well being is slowly evolving as the normal MRI characteristics of the placenta are being established (20–22). Placental changes could help identify the fetus at risk of growth retardation or cerebral hypoxia.

It is hoped that by imaging blood flow it may be possible to detect the failing placenta. Structural information has been obtained using Gadolinium-enhanced imaging, but this provides little if any information on placental function (23). Echo planar imaging can assess the flow in the utero-placental unit and may be exploited to assess function as more detail becomes available (21). If the blood flow pattern in the placenta of twins can be delineated it will aid in the determination of chorionicity, especially in those patients that present late with a twin pregnancy. It will also help in the management of the fetus with intrauterine growth restriction (IUGR) or those of diabetic mothers.

Invasive MRI

Will it be possible in the future to do invasive testing of the fetus under MRI guidance?

REFERENCES

1. Prayer DBP, Mittermayer C. Assessment of intrauterine brain maturation using diffusion weighted imaging. Ultrasound Obstet Gynaecol 2003; 22:3.
2. Moore RJ, Vadeyar S, Fulford J, et al. Antenatal determination of fetal brain activity in response to an acoustic stimulus using functional magnetic resonance imaging. Hum Brain Mapp 2001; 12:94–99.
3. Fulford J, Vadeyar SH, Dodampahala SH, et al. Fetal brain activity and hemodynamic response to a vibroacoustic stimulus. Hum Brain Mapp 2004; 22:116–121.
4. Fulford J, Vadeyar SH, Dodampahala SH, et al. Fetal brain activity in response to a visual stimulus. Hum Brain Mapp 2003; 20:239–245.
5. Martin E. Imaging of brain function during early human development. In: Rutherford M, ed. MRI of the Neonatal Brain. London: WB Saunders, 2002.
6. Kok RD, van den Berg PP, van den Bergh AJ, Nijland R, Heerschap A. Maturation of the human fetal brain as observed by 1H MR spectroscopy. Magn Reson Med 2002; 48:611–616.
7. Kok RD, van den Berg PP, van den Bergh AJ, Nijland R, Heerschap A. MR spectroscopy in the human fetus. Radiology 2002; 223:584 author reply 584-585.
8. Brugger P, Dietrich W, Mittermayer C, Prayer D. Magnetic resonance imaging of the fetus with spina bifida. ISUOG, Paris, France 2003:2.
9. Whitby EH, Capener D, Griffiths PD. Magnetic resonance imaging of the fetal spine. ECR, Vienna, Austria 2004: 298.
10. Garel C. 1st ed MRI of the Fetal Brain. New York: Springer, 2004.
11. Campi A, Scotti G, Filippi M, Gerevini S, Strigimi F, Lasjaunias P. Antenatal diagnosis of vein of Galen aneurysmal malformation: MR study of fetal brain and postnatal follow-up. Neuroradiology 1996; 38:87–90.
12. Kurihara N, Tokieda K, Ikeda K, et al. Prenatal MR findings in a case of aneurysm of the vein of Galen. Pediatr Radiol 2001; 31:160–162.

13. Maheshwari PR, Pungavkar SA, Narkhede P, Patkar DP. Images in radiology. Vein of Galen aneurysmal malformation: antenatal MRI. J Postgrad Med 2003; 49:350–351.
14. Roche CJ, Pilling DW, Walkinshaw SA, May PL. Extracranial vascular malformation: value of antenatal and postnatal MRI in management. Pediatr Radiol 2001; 31:706–708.
15. Schierlitz L, Dumanli H, Robinson JN, et al. Three-dimensional magnetic resonance imaging of fetal brains. Lancet 2001; 357:1177–1178.
16. Mattison DR, Kay HH, Miller RK, Angtuaco T. Magnetic resonance imaging: a noninvasive tool for fetal and placental physiology. Biol Reprod 1988; 38:39–49.
17. Thorp JM, Jr., Councell RB, Sandridge DA, Wiest HH. Antepartum diagnosis of placenta previa percreta by magnetic resonance imaging. Obstet Gynecol 1992; 80:506–508.
18. Entel RJ, Kane JA, Weiss BR. Postpartum magnetic resonance imaging in a case of placenta accreta with intrauterine abscess formation. Arch Gynecol Obstet 1998; 262:91–94.
19. Maldjian C, Adam R, Pelosi M, Pelosi M, III, Rudelli RD, Maldjian J. MRI appearance of placenta percreta and placenta accreta. Magn Reson Imaging 1999; 17:965–971.
20. Kubik-Huch RA, Wildermuth S, Cettuzzi L, et al. Fetus and uteroplacental unit: fast MR imaging with three-dimensional reconstruction and volumetry–feasibility study. Radiology 2001; 219:567–573.
21. Duncan KR. Fetal and placental volumetric and functional analysis using echo-planar imaging. Top Magn Reson Imaging 2001; 12:52–66.
22. Ong SS, Tyler DJ, Moore RJ, et al. Functional magnetic resonance imaging (magnetization transfer) and stereological analysis of human placentae in normal pregnancy and in pre-eclampsia and intrauterine growth restriction. Placenta 2004; 25:408–412.
23. Marcos HB, Semelka RC, Worawattanakul S. Normal placenta: gadolinium-enhanced dynamic MR imaging. Radiology 1997; 205:493–496.

4.3

Emerging Options for Imaging Neonatal Anatomy and Function

Martyn N. J. Paley and Elspeth H. Whitby
Academic Unit of Radiology, University of Sheffield, Sheffield, U.K.

Pamela Ohadike and Michael Smith
Department of Neonatology, Neonatal Intensive Care Unit, Sheffield Teaching Hospitals, Sheffield, U.K.

INTRODUCTION

Ultrasound has been the mainstay of neonatal imaging over the past two decades. However, there are a number of complementary approaches now emerging which include both dedicated magnetic resonance imaging (MRI) systems located on the intensive care unit and MRI- compatible transport incubators used in conjunction with conventional high field MRI- systems. Following a short review of "conventional" MRI of neonates, the next two chapters discuss some of the system development issues and the likely future clinical role of these two new options together with descriptions of several advanced MRI techniques for neonatal imaging which are currently emerging. Combination of MRI with in-magnet Ultrasound could lead to new ways to diagnose and perform image-guided interventions in neonates in future, taking advantage of the strengths of both modalities. Our initial experience with these combined modalities is described. Imaging studies of neonatal lungs have so far been very difficult to achieve, but in future this could be changed radically through use of hyperpolarized gas MRI which is producing revolutionary results in adults and is briefly reviewed here. The possible role of near infra-red (NIR) optical spectroscopy and an attempt to establish this method for measurement of brain function in neonates in our unit is also discussed.

REVIEW OF NEONATAL MRI USING CONVENTIONAL MRI SYSTEMS

Although MRI is less frequently used in neonates than adults, many research studies have been performed using conventional MR imaging equipment linked to specialized neonatal MRI-compatible monitoring equipment. Many studies on neonates have concentrated on brain development including white matter myelination and normal gray matter development (1–11). Most of these studies have taken place at a field strength of 1.5T using conventional superconducting magnets, although some of the earlier studies were completed at field strengths of 0.15T or 0.6T. Babies have either been sedated or placed under full anesthesia for many of these studies. A more limited number of studies have investigated the neonatal spine (12,13) and the neonatal lungs (14,15). MR imaging of neonatal lungs is particularly difficult (unless they contain fluid), due to their small size and the high susceptibility artifacts encountered.

The new technique of hyperpolarized 3-He gas imaging may overcome this problem in future and is described further below.

In terms of neonatal pathology, many MRI studies have addressed the effects of birth asphyxia and hypoxic ischemic encephalopathy (HIE) which is one of the most common problems encountered in the neonatal brain (16–49). Neonatal stroke has also been extensively studied using MRI methods (50–54). Neonatal tumors are relatively infrequent but can be effectively studied using MRI techniques in the neonate (55–57). As tumors can have devastating effects on developing neural systems, it is vital that they are rapidly diagnosed and treated in neonates.

Development of therapeutic techniques to alleviate the effects of birth asphyxia or to overcome congenital disorders is becoming of great interest, including the use of scalp cooling (30). Increasing use of minimally invasive surgical methods may place increasing demands on neonatal MRI systems in future and a combination of a dedicated MRI system and ultrasound for interventional monitoring is discussed further below.

Angiographic MRI methods are now routinely applied in neonates, as they can be performed without the use of exogenous contrast agents, although some studies do now in fact use contrast agents to obtain improved delineation of the very small intracranial vessels found in neonates (58–60). Development of specific MR contrast agents for use in neonates has not really been addressed by the pharmaceutical companies and many standard agents are currently used off-label under ethical review for neonatal studies.

As many of the problems encountered with prematurity are of a metabolic nature, it is natural that MR spectroscopy should be studied in neonates. Many early studies concentrated on 31-P spectroscopy but more recently, proton spectroscopy has become the most commonly practiced method due to its ease of implementation and the extra information which it provides on neuronal integrity and the production of lactate after brain injury (61–80). The N-acetyl Aspartate (NA) to Creatine (Cr) ratio has been established as a useful marker of neuronal function in both adults and neonates. Also, use of the Lactate/Creatine (Lac/Cr) ratio as a surrogate marker has found some success in predicting neonatal outcome after birth asphyxia.

A number of studies have concentrated on using MRI to measure brain or lung volumes in neonates (81–84), relying on the high dimensional accuracy and large number of acquired pixels to obtain normal developmental changes or changes with pathology.

As ultrasound is still the mainstay of neonatal imaging on the wards, it is not surprising that many studies have compared the results of MRI with ultrasound (85–89). While ultrasound is a very convenient tool, the extra diagnostic capability of MRI, especially for the central nervous system, means that it is often the method of choice if the logistical difficulties of scanning the neonate on a central facility whole body MRI system can be overcome.

Diffusion weighted imaging has become a very popular technique for neonatal imaging due to the sensitivity to intra- and extra-cellular dimensional changes which occur rapidly during development and with many pathologies of the neonatal brain (90–101). More recently, diffusion tensor imaging has been used to investigate the development of white matter tracts (90–101) and will grow in importance as the technique becomes more widely available for neonatal imaging studies, where it has great potential for following the maturation of white matter tracts.

Functional MRI is difficult to perform in neonates, mainly because the level of compliance of the neonate with the stimulation paradigm is not always clear. However, with carefully designed studies it has been possible to investigate function of the visual and auditory systems (102–103). It has been reported that the BOLD effect is often negative in neonates, implying that the vascular response to demands for oxygenation has not yet developed fully. Also, in some studies, the location of the BOLD response has been found in different locations from adults which suggests that it may be possible to observe the development of neuronal networks and connections over time with suitable experimental designs.

THE ROLE OF DEDICATED MRI SYSTEMS LOCATED ON THE INTENSIVE CARE UNIT

Although many successful studies have been performed, MRI scanning has not been used as extensively for imaging neonates as for adults due to the considerable difficulties associated with transporting patients to centrally located MRI facilities. Support personnel trained in neonatal care need to leave the neonatal unit and accompany the infant, which can pose significant logistical difficulties. One option is to site the MRI scanner directly on the neonatal ward, where support staff should always be available in an emergency. Conventional superconducting MRI systems (>1T field strength) are not really suitable for siting in the intensive care unit environment due to the large space requirement, need for cryogen fills, and the magnetic projectile hazard associated with the large fringe field. High field systems can potentially pose additional safety hazards including the effects of high RF energy deposition and acoustic noise. It is also relatively difficult to observe and monitor a baby properly within a long super-conducting magnet tunnel unless special MRI-compatible life support equipment is made available.

As neonates are so much smaller than adults, compact dedicated MRI systems can be designed to site in a much smaller area than conventional large super-conducting magnets. In designing an MRI system for use in neonatal applications, first a complete analysis of safety hazards is needed. A number of advantages are obtained for neonatal scanning if the MR magnet is designed to operate at modest field strength, e.g., 0.2–0.3 T. Acoustic noise and RF energy deposition are reduced significantly with low field systems and operation within regulatory safety guidelines is possible, for extended periods, for both patients and staff. For these reasons, we decided to design a low field MRI system specifically for imaging neonates in the supportive environment of the neonatal intensive care unit. As well as safe operation, excellent image quality is a pre-requisite. Scanning neonates is more difficult than adults due to the long MR relaxation times found, especially in the neonatal brain. Changes to the imaging sequences to take account of this are discussed further below. One advantage of the compact magnet size is that the cost of the system can be made dramatically lower than a conventional system, thus putting less pressure for the system to be used with a full scan list, instead allowing imaging to be based around the needs of the baby.

DEDICATED NEONATAL MRI SYSTEM DESIGN CONSIDERATIONS

The size of the uniform imaging volume provides the key physical design specification for a dedicated MRI system, ultimately defining the overall system size, weight and cost. The initial design goal for our dedicated neonatal imager was to enable scanning of the entire body of neonates up to the age of 3 months. After detailed analysis, it was decided that a uniform spherical field of 160 mm diameter would satisfy this requirement. An elliptical "racetrack" design was chosen which provides good mechanical, thermal, and magnetic flux stability. It was felt important that the imaging volume was uncluttered and clinically compatible. To achieve this, flat printed circuit board gradient and radiofrequency coils were located within a recess on the magnet pole face behind easily cleaned covers. This allowed the overall horizontal aperture to be kept to 200 mm. The vertical aperture of the magnet was set at 750 mm (even larger than conventional whole body magnets which typically have a 600 mm diameter bore) to provide good visibility and easy access to the baby in case of emergency (Fig. 1).

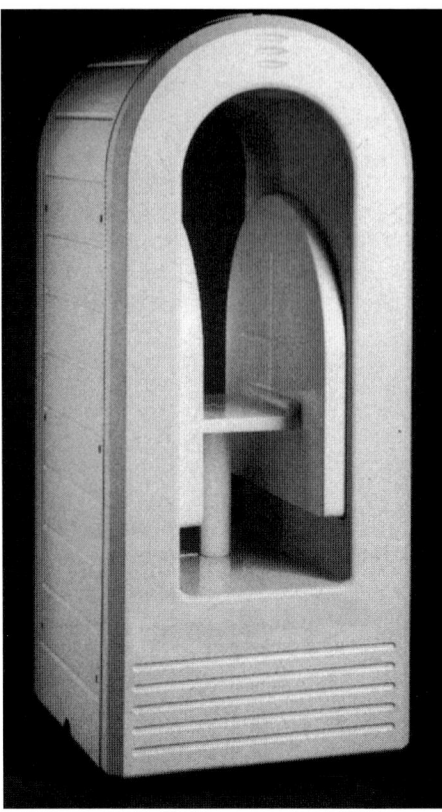

Figure 1. Dedicated MRI system showing the compact but open design of the Neodymium Boron Iron 0.2T magnet. The large aperture provides excellent access for monitoring the patient and for rapid removal in the case of emergency.

The short length of the magnet set at 530 mm means the baby is easily visible and accessible at all times (Fig. 1).

The final magnet design resulted in a fringe field (0.5 mT) within 300 mm, which meant that the magnet could be made entirely safe by housing it within a small radiofrequency-shielded enclosure with a footprint of 2.5×1.5 m. The completed magnet weighed 500 Kg and so could be easily moved and installed on the neonatal ward using a standard supplies lift.

Systems designed for use within a non-specialist MRI environment should have simple software operation. As most people are now familiar with the personal computer and Windows operating system, it was decided to base the system around this ubiquitous platform. Dedicated digital signal processing and acquisition hardware were used to enhance the ability of the PC to control the MRI system. The radiofrequency system uses a low cost direct digital synthesizer which provides a very accurate phase coherent frequency source. In addition, a digital quadrature detection system provides good stability without the high costs traditionally associated with analogue RF systems. Radiofrequency coils were developed especially for neonatal imaging, including a 15 cm diameter loop coil and a 15 cm diameter volume coil which can accept the entire neonatal body. A perspex "pod" was also developed to safely hold the babies and restrict motion within the radiofrequency coils (Fig. 2).

The dedicated MRI system has a very modest power requirement due to use of low power gradient (1 KW) and radiofrequency (100 W) amplifiers. No additional power or cryogens are required for the permanent magnet, which results in considerable economic and operational advantage over resistive or superconducting magnets.

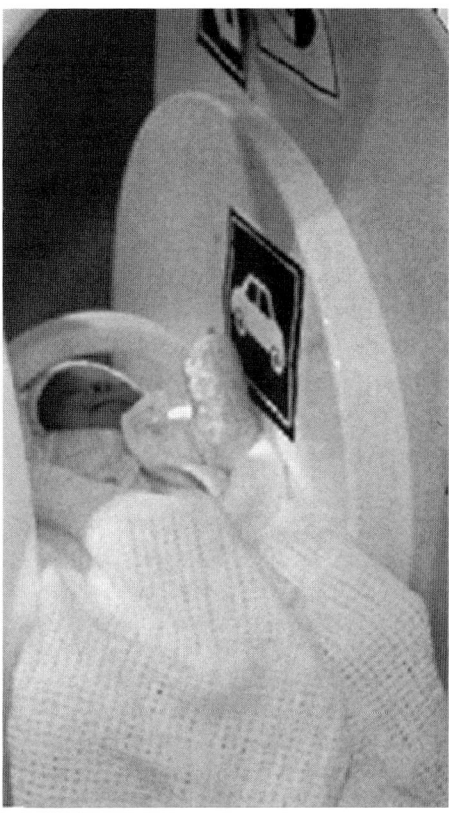

Figure 2. Baby in place in the magnet in the 150 mm diameter loop coil showing excellent visibility for monitoring.

NEONATAL IMAGING SEQUENCE CONSIDERATIONS

Low field imaging requires some rework from conventional high field operation in terms of imaging sequences. This is due to:

1. Shorter T1 and higher T1 contrast (although neonates have much longer T1s than adults at all field strengths)
2. Reduced chemical shift artifact
3. Lower artifacts due to motion
4. Reduced signal-to-noise ratio (SNR).

The fourth factor, which is crucial in terms of image quality, can be improved at low field through a number of techniques including extended sampling time sequences, low resistance coils (including cooled copper or High Temperature Superconducting Conductor coils), signal averaging with reduced repeat time, image processing, and the appropriate use of contrast agents. It is possible to provide most of the sequences currently employed at high field. Spin echo, field echo, and inversion recovery in their various guises and fast imaging sequences are all possible on a specialized scanner. Chemical shift fat suppression sequences are also possible at low field although they are, in general, less successful due to the much reduced chemical shift. The Short Tau Inversion Recovery sequence can be used as an effective alternative in most cases. A typical examination on the dedicated MRI system includes axial and coronal T1 weighted scans with TR=600 ms, TE=20 ms, slice thickness=5 mm, FOV=160 mm, matrix=160×256, NEX=3, Acquisition time 4.8 mins and a coronal T2 weighted sequence TR=3000 ms, TE=120 ms, slice thickness=5 mm, FOV=160 mm, matrix=128×256, NEX=1, Acquisition time 6.4 minutes. Additional (optional) sequences include gradient echo and diffusion weighted imaging. Specific Absorption Rate is typically a factor of at least ten lower than the National Radiological Radiofrequency Protection Board guidelines. Measured acoustic noise levels for the T1 weighted sequence is less than 65 dBA. Figure 3 shows T1 weighted images from the brain of a normal baby and from a baby with profound hypoxic ischemic encephalopathy (HIE) imaged 5 days after birth. Bright signal can be seen in the motor tract and basal ganglia consistent with HIE.

A number of advances in volumetric acquisition rate have recently been introduced including methods which collect data for several slices simultaneously and also reduce scan time by collecting data from several parallel receiver channels, reducing the required number of phase encode steps by using sensitivity encoding (104,105). These advanced methods can potentially play a significant role in speeding up image acquisition rates which is, of course, essential for non-sedated neonatal imaging.

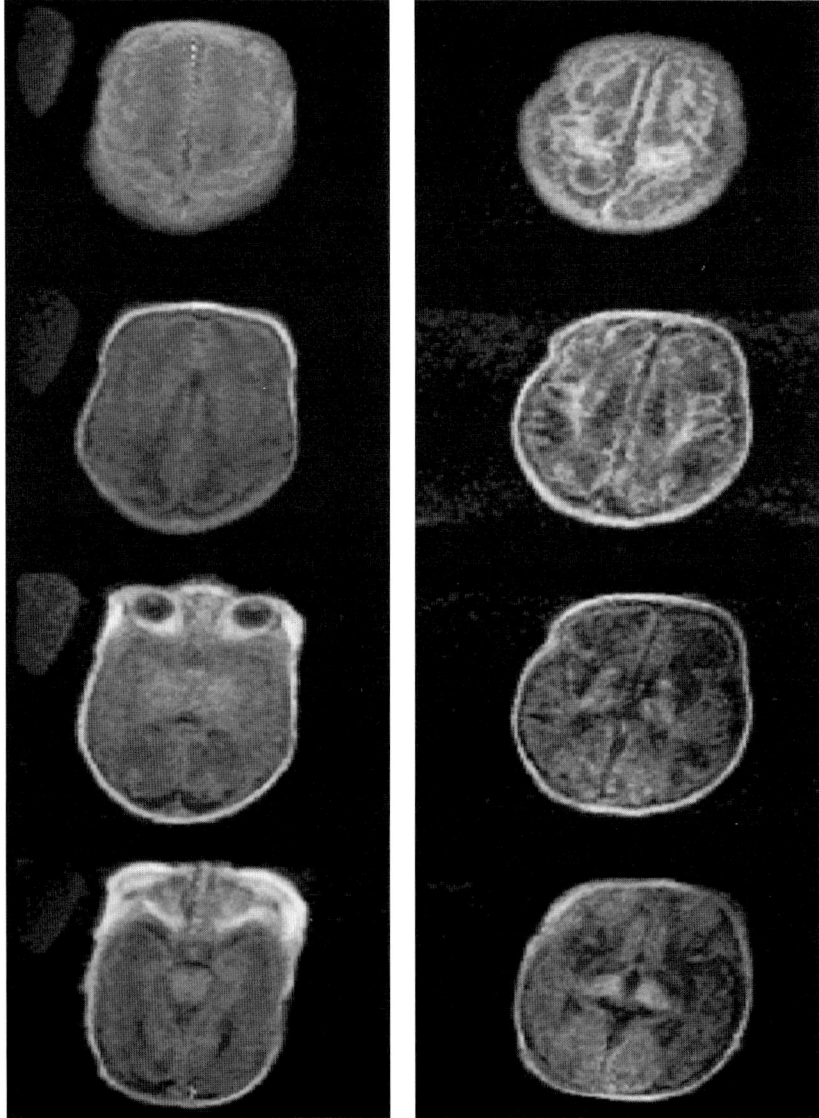

Figure 3. T1-weighted images from the brain of a normal baby (left) and from a baby with profound hypoxic ischemic encephalopathy (HIE) (right) imaged 5 days after birth. Bright signal can be seen in the motor tract and basal ganglia consistent with HIE.

NEONATAL MEDICATION AND MONITORING FOR DEDICATED MRI SYSTEMS

Approval from the local ethics committee and informed parental consent is essential before any neonatal MRI studies are carried out. It was decided as a policy decision that no sedation or anesthesia would be used for the MRI scanning to reduce the requirement for support staff and to avoid the associated risks. Of course, this means that extra effort must be made in terms of careful patient handling and that extra time must be allocated for the procedure to ensure the baby settles before scanning. A major requirement is that all necessary medical treatment can be maintained during scanning and the baby can be fully monitored. Ability to site non-MRI compatible equipment, such as a Resuscitaire, close to the system without a safety hazard is an advantage over high field imaging equipment where expensive MRI compatible equipment is required and in some cases may not even be available. MRI compatible pulse Oximetry (MR 3500, MR Resources Inc., U.S.A.) is integrated with the MRI system to enable assessment of blood oxygen saturation and pulse rate through an infrared probe taped to the babies foot. All monitoring equipment leads are fed through waveguides into the radiofrequency enclosure.

PRACTICAL ASPECTS OF NEONATAL IMAGING WITH A DEDICATED MRI SYSTEM

We have now performed scans on over 600 neonates safely using the dedicated MRI system and have found improved detection of pathology when compared to ultrasound (106–108). The ability of MRI to visualize the posterior fossa and superficial areas of the brain is a major clinical advantage over ultrasound. In addition, hypoxic changes are detected earlier with MRI compared to ultrasound. Figure 4 shows a T1 weighted spin echo image from a term baby and Figure 5 shows similar images from a term baby who suffered an infarct inutero. Figure 6 shows T1 weighted coronal spin echo images of the abdomen of a baby showing low motion artifact due to rapid breathing rate, although the intestines are distended with air trapping which is also reducing motional effects. The liver can be clearly seen on these images. The lungs appear dark due to susceptibility artifacts. However, use of ultra-short TE radial imaging and hyperpolarized gases promises to open up a new method of investigation for the neonatal lungs in the near future. Figure 7 shows coronal T1 weighted spin echo images of a baby who was still-born and who was found to have a large teratoma in the abdomen on post-mortem MR imaging. The lungs can be seen filled with fluid on this image.

NOVEL TECHNIQUE DEVELOPMENTS FOR NEONATAL IMAGING AND SPECTROSCOPY

Parallel MRI

One of the greatest challenges facing neonatal imaging is acquiring images without motion artifact. In recent years, numerous methods have been developed to reduce overall scan time which should find great applicability in neonatal imaging in future when the required radiofrequency and magnetic field coil hardware has been fully developed for neonatal imaging.

Current parallel imaging methods can be broken down into two major categories:

1. Methods such as SMASH and SENSE (104,105) which reduce the number of phase encode steps required by using information from multiple receiver coils to remove the effects of aliasing which would otherwise occur. These methods typically reduce scan times in the range R=2–4 with a decrease in SNR which is greater than the square root of R.

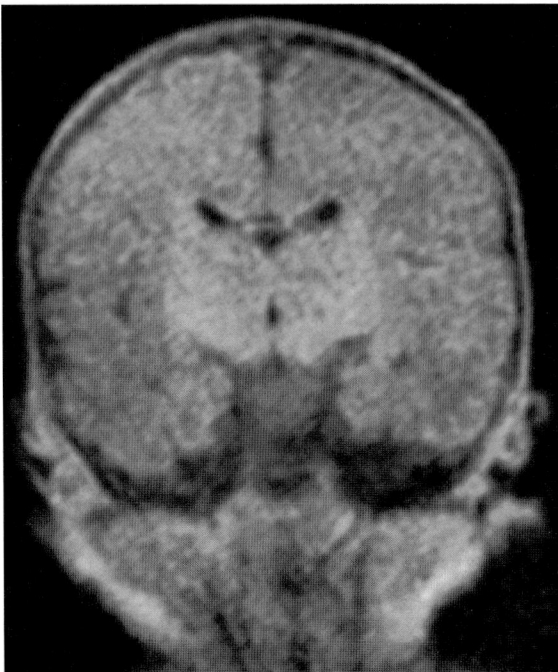

Figure 4. T1 weighted spin echo image from a term baby.

2. Methods which excite several slices in parallel. These can either be extensions to SMASH or SENSE using sets of receiver coils for each slice (109) or methods which enable multiple slices to be acquired without aliasing in a single excitation such as the Multiple Acquisition Micro B0 Array Coil (MAMBA) technique or the SPIRIT method (110,111) which are discussed further below.

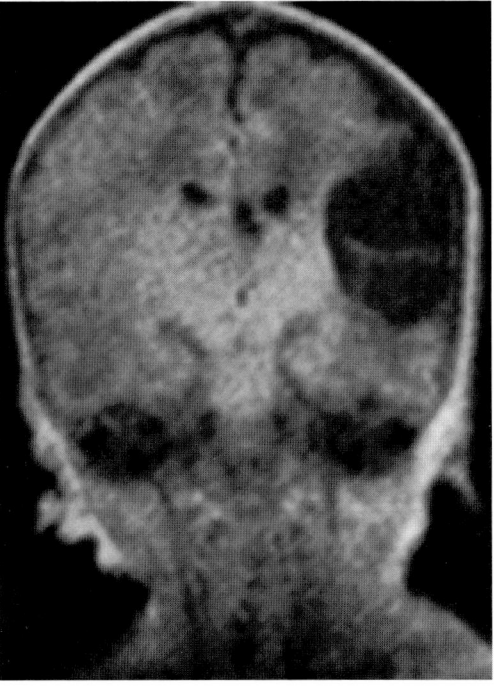

Figure 5. Similar images from a term baby who suffered an infarct in utero.

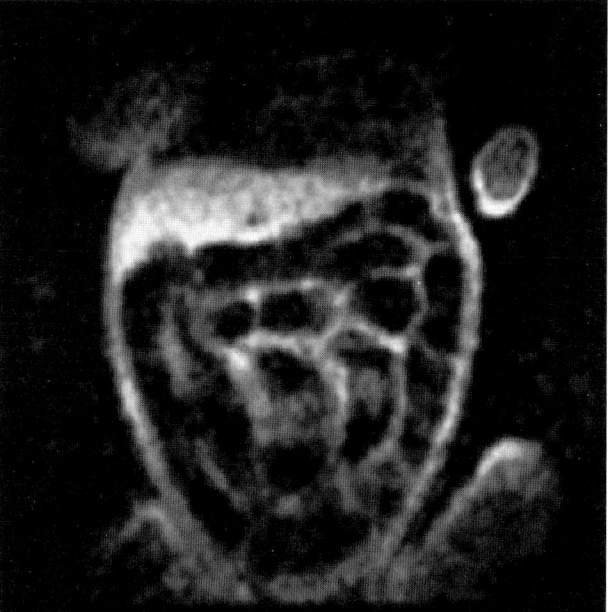

Figure 6. T1 weighted coronal spin echo images of the abdomen of a baby showing low motion artifact due to rapid breathing rate, although the intestines are distended with air trapping which is also reducing motional effects. The liver can be clearly seen on these images. The lungs appear dark due to susceptibility artifacts. However, use of ultra-short TE radial imaging and hyperpolarized gases promises to open up a new method of investigation for the neonatal lungs in the near future.

A MAMBA coil is designed to produce a number of uniform field steps within the main MR magnet so that images from different slices are acquired in separate regions of the imaging frequency bandwidth (110). Without the field step, images from all the slices would overlap (alias). Two or more slices are simultaneously excited using a cosine modulated RF pulse with an appropriate frequency separation. A simpler method to produce parallel images with a very high acceleration factor is known as SPIRIT and uses only standard MR imaging gradients to prevent aliasing. Slices are simultaneously excited in combination with SENSE which reduces the number of phase

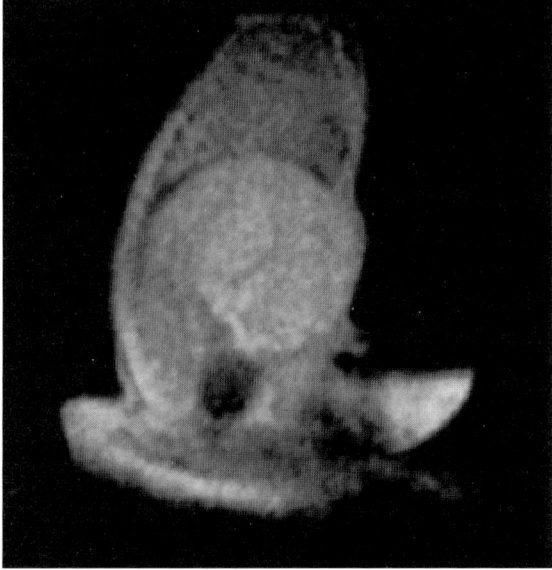

Figure 7. Coronal T1-weighted spin echo images of a baby who was stillborn and who was found to have a large teratoma in the abdomen on post-mortem MRI. The lungs can be seen filled with fluid on this image.

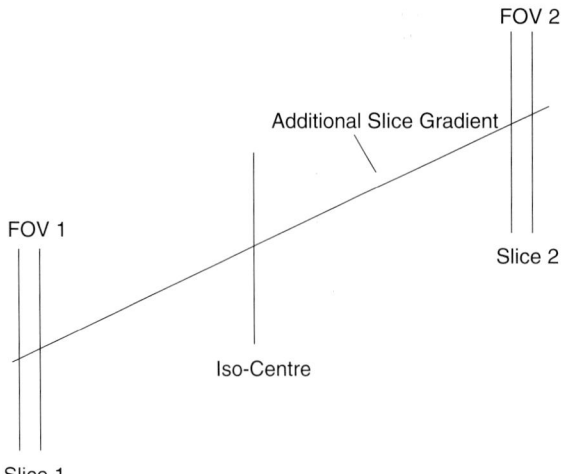

Figure 8. Schematic diagram of the SPIRIT parallel imaging process.

encode steps required, resulting in a multiplicative reduction in the time required to scan an MR volume by a factor up to ×8 or more (Figs. 8 and 9) (111).

SPIRIT should be very useful for neonatal imaging including whole body screening applications where acceleration factors up to x16 are anticipated; this technique is currently under development for the Niche dedicated neonatal MRI system.

Combined Ultrasound and MRI for Interventional Procedures in Neonates

In future, minimally invasive procedures may play an important role in correcting pathology found at birth. Combining ultrasound and MRI for interventional procedure monitoring offers a number of possible advantages for neonatal applications. MRI provides high intrinsic contrast but lacks the flexibility of ultrasound for real-time imaging. Ultrasound has rapid dynamic update and flow imaging capability but lacks the sophisticated soft tissue contrast capability of MRI.

To investigate the combination of technologies, the ability to perform ultrasound within the low-field Niche magnet has been assessed. A standard ultrasound machine (Accuson, Ca, USA) was located immediately outside the screened room and the probe located at the center of the magnet at the edge of a neonatal head/wrist imaging coil shown in Figure 10. The ultrasound system was operated while the Niche MRI system acquired an image from a quality assurance phantom and then from a wrist. Following this the ultrasound system was switched into standby mode and an MR image (spin echo, TR/TE=500/20, Slt=5 mm, spatial resolution=1 mm) was acquired with the ultrasound probe still in position immediately adjacent to the RF coil. MR and ultrasound images were assessed for artifacts.

Ultrasound images suffered no degradation as compared to operation outside the magnet. When the RF from the MRI system pulsed, a brief high intensity radial line was observed on the ultrasound system which did not interfere with operation. The MRI system could not operate with the ultrasound system in active mode due to broad band interference. However, with the ultrasound probe (general purpose) in position, it was possible to acquire MR images and both imaging systems could easily visualize standard MRI-compatible biopsy needles. A combination of gated low field MRI and gated ultrasound may in future provide an optimal solution to the problem of visualization and tracking of interventional instruments for minimally-invasive procedures in neonates.

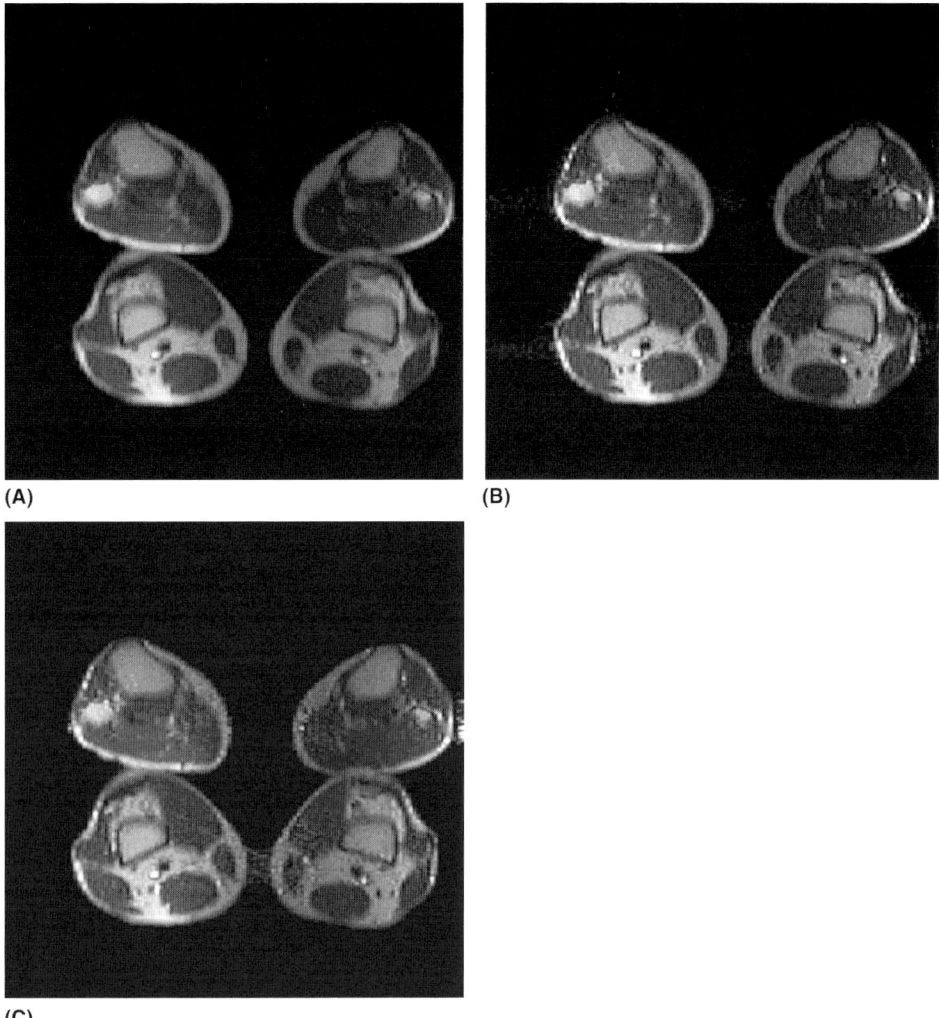

(A)

(B)

(C)

Figure 9. Images from two slices of the lower limb of an adult volunteer acquired ×2 (**A**), ×4 (**B**) and ×8 (**C**) faster than normal using the SPIRIT parallel MRI technique (111).

There is also the possibility that ultrasound may be useful for dynamically modifying the contrast in MRI through its interaction with the "lattice" when driven at the MR frequency which can potentially alter the MR relaxation times. An MRI-compatible probe tuned to the Larmor frequency will allow this exciting prospect to be studied in future.

Lung Imaging in Neonates—Hyperpolarized 3-He MRI

Hyperpolarized gases have recently revolutionized imaging of the ventilation of lungs in animal models and in human adults (112–116), although so far they have not yet been applied to imaging of the neonatal lung. As immaturity of the lungs and the clinical sequelae give rise to major complications in cases of premature birth, it is expected that 3-He imaging of the neonatal lungs will eventually be developed as a very useful tool for the neonatologist. 4-He and oxygen mixtures have previously been frequently used in treatment regimens for neonates and so there should be no real safety obstacles to this development. The Niche dedicated neonatal MRI system is

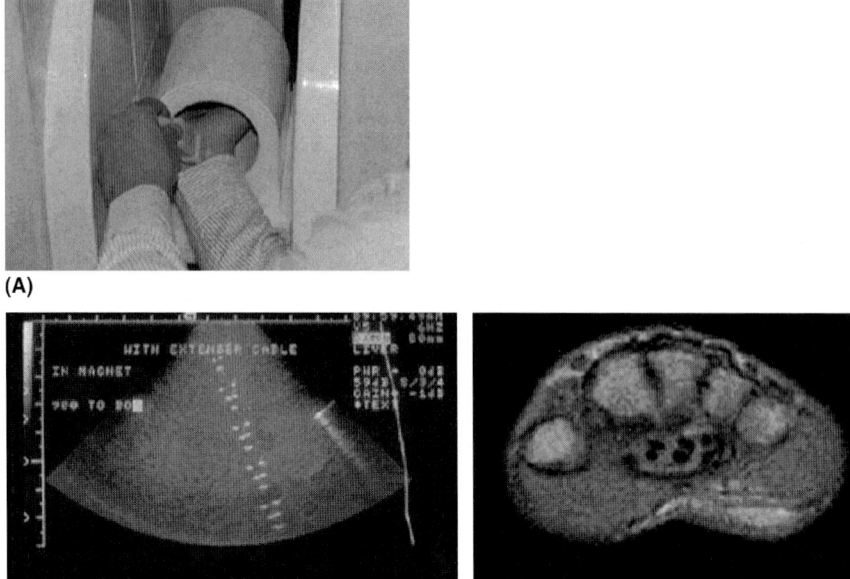

(A)

(B)   (C)

Figure 10. Ultrasound probe in operation within the Niche magnet (**A**). Image of ultrasound resolution phantom acquired inside the magnet showing no image distortion by the magnetic field (**B**). Image of wrist acquired with ultrasound probe adjacent to the imaging coil showing no distortion by the ultrasound probe (**C**). These images show the potential for combining MR and ultrasound for neonatal imaging.

currently being adapted for rapid imaging of 3-He using a novel multi-frequency, multi-channel transceiver design (117). Figure 11 shows coronal 3-He breath-hold image of the lungs of an adult patient with chronic obstructive pulmonary disease acquired at 1.5T on a whole body MRI system (courtesy of Dr. Jim Wild and Prof. Edwin van Beek, University of Sheffield, Sheffield, U.K.).

Low field imaging is actually advantageous for Helium imaging of the lungs as the susceptibility artifacts normally encountered at high field which destroy the MR signal are much less. The signal strength in hyperpolarized gas imaging is governed by intense laser polarization outside the magnet rather than the normal weak polarization achieved through the magnetic field.

Optical Spectroscopy

Since the pioneering studies of Jobsis (118), near infrared (NIR) spectroscopy has been extensively developed and now systems are widely available commercially for a range of neonatal monitoring tasks. However, the study of brain function using NIR has only recently commenced (119–157) in human adults, although animal experiments have been underway for several years.

Very premature babies have quite transparent skin and skulls and, despite limited spatial penetration of light, combining both visible and NIR spectroscopy may provide additional information for functional studies of the brain due to the high absorption of visible light by oxy/deoxyhemoglobin. Our initial experience in setting up a neonatal optical spectroscopy system to study brain function is described below.

A real time (3 ms minimum) optical reflectance spectrometer (350–950 nm, Ocean Optics, FL) calibrated against a white traceable standard was connected to a co-axial transmit-receive fiber optic to acquire data in the visible (VIS) and NIR. Spectra were analysed using spectral fitting in the visible region of the spectrum with the algorithm

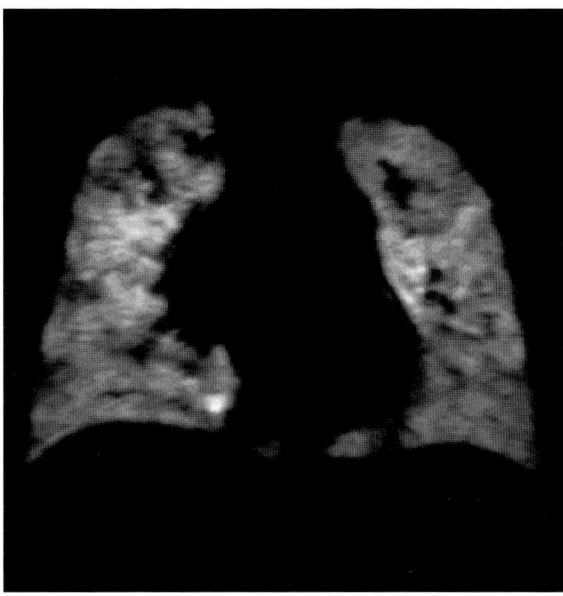

Figure 11. Coronal 3-He breath-hold image of the lungs of an adult patient with chronic obstructive pulmonary disease acquired at 1.5T on a whole body MRI system. *Source*: Courtesy of Dr. Jim Wild and Prof. Edwin van Beek, University of Sheffield, Sheffield, U.K.

of Kohl et al. (153) and using the UCL6 algorithm (124) in the NIR. Prior to undertaking studies in neonates, the system was calibrated using data from adults. Figure 12 shows spectra (red) acquired from the index finger of an adult volunteer with application of a pressure cuff to the forearm. Overlaid on the spectra is a fit of a composite spectrum from oxy- and deoxy-hemoglobin adjusted to provide the best (least-squares) fit to the data.

The pressure cuff was applied to the forearm at time-point 180 and switched off at time-point 360. Figures 13 and 14 show the data for specific wavelengths in the visible and NIR regions. Large signal changes can be seen in both the visible and NIR reflectance time series due to the restriction of blood flow to the finger through the tourniquet effect of the pressure cuff.

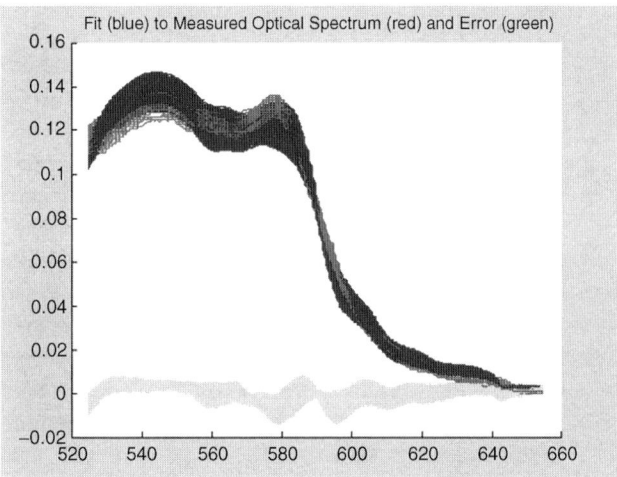

Figure 12. Spectra (black) acquired from the index finger of an adult volunteer with application of a pressure cuff to the forearm. Overlaid on the spectra is a fit of a composite spectrum from oxy- and deoxy-hemoglobin adjusted to provide the best (least-squares) fit to the data (mid-gray). The residual error from the (it is shown at the bottom light gray)

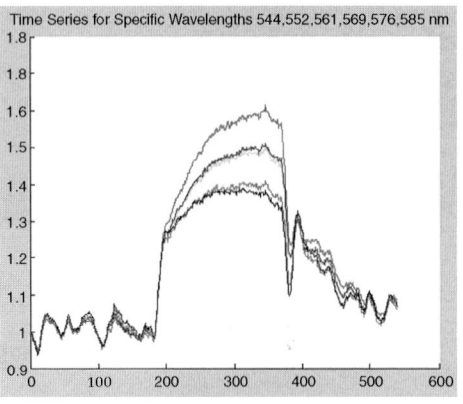

Figure 13. The data for specific wavelengths in the visible regions. Large signal changes can be seen in both the visible and NIR reflectance time series due to the restriction of blood flow to the finger through the tourniquet effect of the pressure cuff.

In order to collect meaningful data from neonatal brains, it is essential to minimize all motion between the optical probe and the brain. In our studies, the reflectance probe was located 20 mm from the occiput of the neonate using a custom foam holder which also restrained the neonatal head from moving. With careful preparation, optical spectra could be acquired from neonates with good stability over periods of up to three minutes without sedation or anesthesia as shown in Figure 15.

However, spectral quality is often confounded by gross head motion, hair, and skin pigmentation, resulting in an overall low experimental success ratio (~20% in our experience). Preliminary evidence for functional changes has been obtained in both visible and NIR spectra in several studies, although much further work remains to make this a robust functional technique in infants. There is also some evidence that it may be possible to detect much more rapid changes in optical spectra, related more directly to the effects of neuronal firing (157). This effect is thought to be mediated by the effects on cell dimensions due to opening and closing of ion channels during action potentials. Such rapid changes due to neuronal firing may now also have been observed using MRI through the effects of the magnetic fields associated with the ion channel currents directly modulating the MRI signal (158).

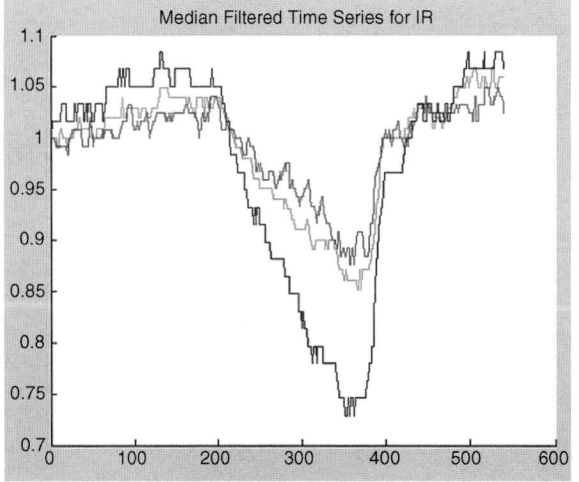

Figure 14. The data for specific wavelengths in the NIR regions. Large signal changes can be seen in both the visible and NIR reflectance time series due to the restriction of blood flow to the finger through the tourniquet effect of the pressure cuff.

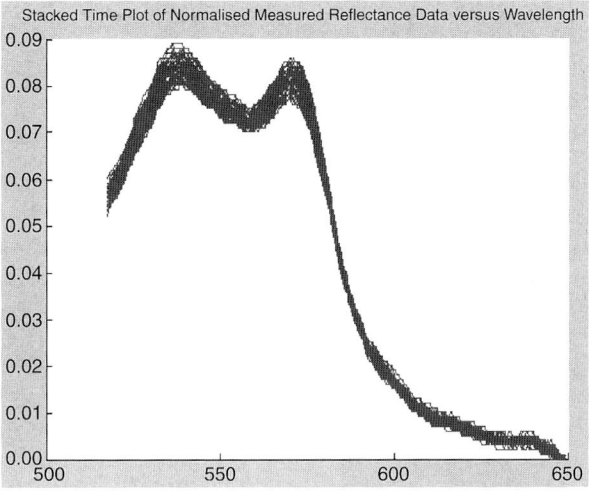

Figure 15. In order to collect meaningful data from neonatal brains, it is essential to minimize all motion between the optical probe and the brain. In our studies, the reflectance probe was located 20 mm from the occiput of the neonate using a custom foam holder which also restrained the neonatal head from moving. With careful preparation, optical spectra could be acquired from neonates with good stability over periods of up to three minutes without sedation or anesthesia.

The promise of a simple, non-invasive, MRI-compatible and inexpensive real time monitor of brain function suggests that visible and NIR optical spectroscopy is a useful research topic to pursue, although the difficulties associated with tomographic implementations may mean that a multi-channel topographic array of probes may be a more practical alternative for functional studies of the developing cortex in the neonate.

SUMMARY

We are entering an exciting era for the study of neonates in situ on the Neonatal Intensive Care Unit by safe and novel imaging and spectroscopic methods. A dedicated MRI unit located on the NICU means that fully trained staff can constantly monitor and care for the neonate during imaging procedures with full clinical backup in case of an emergency. So far we have safely imaged over 600 neonates using dedicated MRI without a serious incident. A range of advanced rapid parallel MRI acquisition methods such as SPIRIT will in future reduce the problems associated with patient motion and allow improved contrast between normal and pathological tissues. Strategic combinations of non-invasive diagnostic technologies such as MRI, Ultrasound and Near Infra Red promise the early diagnosis of functional deficits in the central nervous system such as those found in the visual, auditory, or motor systems. New possibilities for monitoring early therapeutic interventions will also be provided. Other important organ systems can be studied in function throughout the body, including the neonatal lungs which play a vital role in the successful development of a premature baby, and will soon be visualized using hyperpolarized gas MR imaging on the NICU.

REFERENCES

1. Whitby EH, Griffiths PD, Lonneker-Lammers T, et al. Ultrafast magnetic resonance imaging of the neonate in a magnetic resonance-compatible incubator with a built-in coil. Pediatrics 2004; 113:150–152.
2. Morgan B, Finan A, Yarnold R, et al. Assessment of infant physiology and neuronal development using magnetic resonance imaging. Child Care Health Dev 2002; 28:7–10.
3. Ruoss K, Lovblad K, Schroth G, Moessinger AC, Fusch C. Brain development (sulci and gyri) as assessed by early postnatal MR imaging in preterm and term newborn infants. Neuropediatrics 2001; 32:69–74.
4. Huppi PS, Inder TE. Magnetic resonance techniques in the evaluation of the perinatal brain: recent advances and future directions. Semin Neonatol 2001; 6:195–210.

5. Rivkin MJ. Developmental neuroimaging of children using magnetic resonance techniques. Ment Retard Dev Disabil Res Rev 2000; 6:68–80.

6. Hoon AH, Jr., Melhem ER. Neuroimaging: applications in disorders of early brain development. J Dev Behav Pediatr 2000; 21:291–302.

7. Maalouf EF, Counsell S, Battin M, Cowan FM. Magnetic resonance imaging of the neonatal brain. Hosp Med 1998; 59:41–45.

8. Yamada H, Sadato N, Konishi Y, et al. A rapid brain metabolic change in infants detected by fMRI. Neuroreport 1997; 8:3775–3778.

9. Huppi PS, Schuknecht B, Boesch C, et al. Structural and neurobehavioral delay in postnatal brain development of preterm infants. Pediatr Res 1996; 39:895–901.

10. Allen RJ, Brunberg J, Schwartz E, Schaefer AM, Jackson G. MRI characterization of cerebral dysgenesis in maternal PKU. Acta Paediatr Suppl 1994; 407:83–85.

11. Barkovich AJ, Kjos BO, Jackson DE, Jr., Norman D. Normal maturation of the neonatal and infant brain: MR imaging at 1.5 T. Radiology 1988; 166:173–180.

12. Rypens F, Avni EF, Matos C, Pardou A, Struyven J. Atypical and equivocal sonographic features of the spinal cord in neonates. Pediatr Radiol 1995; 25:429–432.

13. Fotter R, Sorantin E, Schneider U, Ranner G, Fast C, Schober P. Ultrasound diagnosis of birth-related spinal cord trauma: neonatal diagnosis and follow-up and correlation with MRI. Pediatr Radiol 1994; 24:241–244.

14. Mahieu-Caputo D, Sonigo P, Dommergues M, et al. Fetal lung volume measurement by magnetic resonance imaging in congenital diaphragmatic hernia. BJOG 2001; 108:863–868.

15. Kuwashima S, Nishimura G, Iimura F, et al. Low-intensity fetal lungs on MRI may suggest the diagnosis of pulmonary hypoplasia. Pediatr Radiol 2001; 31:669–672.

16. Kaufman SA, Miller SP, Ferriero DM, Glidden DH, Barkovich AJ, Partridge JC. Encephalopathy as a predictor of magnetic resonance imaging abnormalities in asphyxiated newborns. Pediatr Neurol 2003; 28:342–346.

17. Fan G, Wu Z, Chen L, Guo Q, Ye B, Mao J. Hypoxia-ischemic encephalopathy in full-term neonate: correlation proton MR spectroscopy with MR imaging. Eur J Radiol 2003; 45:91–98.

18. Cowan F, Rutherford M, Groenendaal F, et al. Origin and timing of brain lesions in term infants with neonatal encephalopathy. Lancet 2003; 361:736–742.

19. Counsell SJ, Rutherford MA, Cowan FM, Edwards AD. Magnetic resonance imaging of preterm brain injury. Arch Dis Child Fetal Neonatal Ed 2003; 88:F269–F274.

20. Mercuri E, Rutherford M, Barnett A, et al. MRI lesions and infants with neonatal encephalopathy. Is the Apgar score predictive? Neuropediatrics 2002; 33:150–156.

21. Malik GK, Pandey M, Kumar R, Chawla S, Rathi B, Gupta RK. MR imaging and in vivo proton spectroscopy of the brain in neonates with hypoxic ischemic encephalopathy. Eur J Radiol 2002; 43:6–13.

22. Cappellini M, Rapisardi G, Cioni ML, Fonda C. Acute hypoxic encephalopathy in the full-term newborn: correlation between magnetic resonance spectroscopy and neurological evaluation at short and long term. Radiol Med (Torino) 2002; 104:332–340.

23. Maneru C, Junque C, Bargallo N, et al. (1)H-MR spectroscopy is sensitive to subtle effects of perinatal asphyxia. Neurology 2001; 57:1115–1118.

24. Coskun A, Lequin M, Segal M, Vigneron DB, Ferriero DM, Barkovich AJ. Quantitative analysis of MR images in asphyxiated neonates: correlation with neurodevelopmental outcome. AJNR Am J Neuroradiol 2001; 22:400–405.

25. Barkovich AJ, Westmark KD, Bedi HS, Partridge JC, Ferriero DM, Vigneron DB. Proton spectroscopy and diffusion imaging on the first day of life after perinatal asphyxia: preliminary report. AJNR Am J Neuroradiol 2001; 22:1786–1794.

26. Sie LT, Barkhof F, Lafeber HN, Valk J, van der Knaap MS. Value of fluid-attenuated inversion recovery sequences in early MRI of the brain in neonates with a perinatal hypoxic-ischemic encephalopathy. Eur Radiol 2000; 10:1594–1601.

27. Heinz ER, Barkovich AJ. MR and CT evaluation of profound neonatal and infantile asphyxia. AJNR Am J Neuroradiol 1992; 13:959–972. Heinz ER, Barkovich AJ. MR and CT evaluation of profound neonatal and infantile asphyxia. AJNR Am J Neuroradiol 2000; 21:979–981.

28. Forbes KP, Pipe JG, Bird R. Neonatal hypoxic-ischemic encephalopathy: detection with diffusion-weighted MR imaging. AJNR Am J Neuroradiol 2000; 21:1490–1496.

29. Cowan F. Outcome after intrapartum asphyxia in term infants. Semin Neonatol 2000; 5:127–140.

30. Azzopardi D, Robertson NJ, Cowan FM, Rutherford MA, Rampling M, Edwards AD. Pilot study of treatment with whole body hypothermia for neonatal encephalopathy. Pediatrics 2000; 106:684–694.
31. Robertson RL, Ben-Sira L, Barnes PD, et al. MR line-scan diffusion-weighted imaging of term neonates with perinatal brain ischemia. AJNR Am J Neuroradiol 1999; 20:1658–1670.
32. Mercuri E, Haataja L, Guzzetta A, et al. Visual function in term infants with hypoxic-ischaemic insults: correlation with neurodevelopment at 2 years of age. Arch Dis Child Fetal Neonatal Ed 1999; 80:F99–F104.
33. Barkovich AJ, Baranski K, Vigneron D, et al. Proton MR spectroscopy for the evaluation of brain injury in asphyxiated, term neonates. AJNR Am J Neuroradiol 1999; 20:1399–1405.
34. Amess PN, Penrice J, Wylezinska M, et al. Early brain proton magnetic resonance spectroscopy and neonatal neurology related to neurodevelopmental outcome at 1 year in term infants after presumed hypoxic-ischaemic brain injury. Dev Med Child Neurol 1999; 41:436–445.
35. Aida N, Nishimura G, Hachiya Y, Matsui K, Takeuchi M, Itani Y. MR imaging of perinatal brain damage: comparison of clinical outcome with initial and follow-up MR findings. AJNR Am J Neuroradiol 1998; 19:1909–1921.
36. Thornton JS, Ordidge RJ, Penrice J, et al. Anisotropic water diffusion in white and gray matter of the neonatal piglet brain before and after transient hypoxia-ischaemia. Magn Reson Imaging 1997; 15:433–440.
37. Yokochi K, Fujimoto S. Magnetic resonance imaging in children with neonatal asphyxia: correlation with developmental sequelae. Acta Paediatr 1996; 85:88–95.
38. Nakai T, Rhine WD, Enzmann DR, Stevenson DK, Spielman DM. A model for detecting early metabolic changes in neonatal asphyxia by 1H-MRS. J Magn Reson Imaging 1996; 6:445–452.
39. Cioni G, Fazzi B, Ipata AE, Canapicchi R, van Hof-van Duin J. Correlation between cerebral visual impairment and magnetic resonance imaging in children with neonatal encephalopathy. Dev Med Child Neurol 1996; 38:120–132.
40. Rutherford MA, Pennock JM, Schwieso JE, Cowan FM, Dubowitz LM. Hypoxic ischaemic encephalopathy: early magnetic resonance imaging findings and their evolution. Neuropediatrics 1995; 26:183–191.
41. Mercuri E, Cowan F, Rutherford M, Acolet D, Pennock J, Dubowitz L. Ischaemic and haemorrhagic brain lesions in newborns with seizures and normal Apgar scores. Arch Dis Child Fetal Neonatal Ed 1995; 73:F67–F74.
42. Barkovich AJ, Westmark K, Partridge C, Sola A, Ferriero DM. Perinatal asphyxia: MR findings in the first 10 days. AJNR Am J Neuroradiol 1995; 16:427–438.
43. Rutherford MA, Pennock JM, Dubowitz LM. Cranial ultrasound and magnetic resonance imaging in hypoxic-ischaemic encephalopathy: a comparison with outcome. Dev Med Child Neurol 1994; 36:813–825.
44. Kuenzle C, Baenziger O, Martin E, et al. Prognostic value of early MR imaging in term infants with severe perinatal asphyxia. Neuropediatrics 1994; 25:191–200.
45. Cowan FM, Pennock JM, Hanrahan JD, Manji KP, Edwards AD. Early detection of cerebral infarction and hypoxic ischemic encephalopathy in neonates using diffusion-weighted magnetic resonance imaging. Neuropediatrics 1994; 25:172–175.
46. Goplerud JM, Delivoria-Papadopoulos M. Nuclear magnetic resonance imaging and spectroscopy following asphyxia. Clin Perinatol 1993; 20:345–367.
47. Barkovich AJ. MR and CT evaluation of profound neonatal and infantile asphyxia. AJNR Am J Neuroradiol 1992; 13:959–972 discussion 955–973.
48. Nalin A, Frigieri G, Caggia P, Vezzalini S. State of the art of magnetic resonance (MR) in neonatal hypoxic-ischemic encephalopathy. Childs Nerv Syst 1989; 5:350–355.
49. Barkovich AJ, Truwit CL. Brain Damage from Perinatal Asphyxia: correlation of MR findings with gestational age. AJNR 1990; 11:1087–1096.
50. Mader I, Schoning M, Klose U, Kuker W. Neonatal cerebral infarction diagnosed by diffusion-weighted MRI: pseudonormalization occurs early. Stroke 2002; 33:1142–1145.
51. Groenendaal F, van der Grond J, Witkamp TD, de Vries LS. Proton magnetic resonance spectroscopic imaging in neonatal stroke. Neuropediatrics 1995; 26:243–248.
52. Koelfen W, Freund M, Konig S, Varnholt V, Rohr H, Schultze C. Results of parenchymal and angiographic magnetic resonance imaging and neuropsychological testing of children after stroke as neonates. Eur J Pediatr 1993; 152:1030–1035.

53. Smith CD, Baumann RJ. Clinical features and magnetic resonance imaging in congenital and childhood stroke. J Child Neurol 1991; 6:263–272.

54. Amato M, Huppi P, Herschkowitz N, Huber P. Prenatal stroke suggested by intrauterine ultrasound and confirmed by magnetic resonance imaging. Neuropediatrics 1991; 22:100–102.

55. Hanquinet S, Christophe C, Rummens E, et al. Ultrasound, computed tomography and magnetic resonance of a neonatal ganglioglioma of the brain. Pediatr Radiol 1986; 16:501–503.

56. Radkowski MA, Naidich TP, Tomita T, Byrd SE, McLone DG. Neonatal brain tumors: CT and MR findings. J Comput Assist Tomogr 1988; 12:10–20.

57. Lee MJ, Cairns RA, Munk PL, Poon PY. Congenital-infantile fibrosarcoma: magnetic resonance imaging findings. Can Assoc Radiol J 1996; 47:121–125.

58. Peng SS, Li YW, Chang MH, Ni YH, Su CT. Magnetic resonance cholangiography for evaluation of cholestatic jaundice in neonates and infants. J Formos Med Assoc 1998; 97:698–703.

59. Guibaud L, Lachaud A, Touraine R, et al. MR cholangiography in neonates and infants: feasibility and preliminary applications. AJR Am J Roentgenol 1998; 170:27–31.

60. Lago P, Rebsamen S, Clancy RR, et al. MRI, MRA, and neurodevelopmental outcome following neonatal ECMO. Pediatr Neurol 1995; 12:294–304.

61. Kugel H, Roth B, Pillekamp F, et al. Proton spectroscopic metabolite signal relaxation times in preterm infants: a prerequisite for quantitative spectroscopy in infant brain. J Magn Reson Imaging 2003; 17:634–640.

62. Jan W, Zimmerman RA, Wang ZJ, Berry GT, Kaplan PB, Kaye EM. MR diffusion imaging and MR spectroscopy of maple syrup urine disease during acute metabolic decompensation. Neuroradiology 2003; 45:393–399.

63. Fan G, Wu Z, Chen L, Guo Q, Ye B, Mao J. Hypoxia-ischemic encephalopathy in full-term neonate: correlation proton MR spectroscopy with MR imaging. Eur J Radiol 2003; 45:91–98.

64. Kreis R, Hofmann L, Kuhlmann B, Boesch C, Bossi E, Huppi PS. Brain metabolite composition during early human brain development as measured by quantitative in vivo 1H magnetic resonance spectroscopy. Magn Reson Med 2002; 48:949–958.

65. Robertson NJ, Lewis RH, Cowan FM, et al. Early increases in brain myo-inositol measured by proton magnetic resonance spectroscopy in term infants with neonatal encephalopathy. Pediatr Res 2001; 50:692–700.

66. Robertson NJ, Kuint J, Counsell TJ, et al. Characterization of cerebral white matter damage in preterm infants using 1H and 31P magnetic resonance spectroscopy. J Cereb Blood Flow Metab 2000; 20:1446–1456.

67. Holshouser BA, Ashwal S, Shu S, Hinshaw DB, Jr. Proton MR spectroscopy in children with acute brain injury: comparison of short and long echo time acquisitions. J Magn Reson Imaging 2000; 11:9–19.

68. Cooper CE, Wyatt JS. NMR spectroscopy and imaging of the neonatal brain. Biochem Soc Trans 2000; 28:121–126.

69. Thomas EL, Hanrahan JD, Ala-Korpela M, et al. Noninvasive characterization of neonatal adipose tissue by 13C magnetic resonance spectroscopy. Lipids 1997; 32:645–651.

70. Ordidge R, Thornton J, Clemence M, et al. NMR studies of hypoxic-ischaemic injury in neonatal brain using imaging and spectroscopy. Adv Exp Med Biol 1997; 428:539–544.

71. Holshouser BA, Ashwal S, Luh GY, et al. Proton MR spectroscopy after acute central nervous system injury: outcome prediction in neonates, infants, and children. Radiology 1997; 202:487–496.

72. Kimura H, Fujii Y, Itoh S, et al. Metabolic alterations in the neonate and infant brain during development: evaluation with proton MR spectroscopy. Radiology 1995; 194:483–489.

73. Toft PB, Leth H, Lou HC, Pryds O, Henriksen O. Metabolite concentrations in the developing brain estimated with proton MR spectroscopy. J Magn Reson Imaging 1994; 4:674–680.

74. Toft PB, Christiansen P, Pryds O, Lou HC, Henriksen O. T1, T2, and concentrations of brain metabolites in neonates and adolescents estimated with H-1 MR spectroscopy. J Magn Reson Imaging 1994; 4:1–5.

75. Cortey A, Jarvik JG, Lenkinski RE, Grossman RI, Frank I, Delivoria-Papadopoulos M. Proton MR spectroscopy of brain abnormalities in neonates born to HIV-positive mothers. AJNR Am J Neuroradiol 1994; 15:1853–1859.

76. Tzika AA, Vigneron DB, Ball WS, Jr., Dunn RS, Kirks DR. Localized proton MR spectroscopy of the brain in children. J Magn Reson Imaging 1993; 3:719–729.

77. Terk MR, Gober JR, DeGiorgio C, Wu P, Colletti PM. Brain death in the neonate: assessment with P-31 MR spectroscopy. Radiology 1992; 182:582–583.

78. Peden CJ, Cowan FM, Bryant DJ, et al. Proton MR spectroscopy of the brain in infants. J Comput Assist Tomogr 1990; 14:886–894.

79. Martin E, Grutter R, Boesch C. In vivo NMR spectroscopy: investigation of brain metabolism in neonates and infants. Pediatrie 1990; 45:677–682.

80. Boesch C, Martin E. Combined application of MR imaging and spectroscopy in neonates and children: installation and operation of a 2.35-T system in a clinical setting. Radiology 1988; 168:481–488.

81. Hunt RW, Warfield SK, Wang H, Kean M, Volpe JJ, Inder TE. Assessment of the impact of the removal of cerebrospinal fluid on cerebral tissue volumes by advanced volumetric 3D-MRI in posthaemorrhagic hydrocephalus in a premature infant. J Neurol Neurosurg Psychiatry 2003; 74:658–660.

82. Murphy BP, Inder TE, Huppi PS, et al. Impaired cerebral cortical gray matter growth after treatment with dexamethasone for neonatal chronic lung disease. Pediatrics 2001; 107:217–221.

83. Duncan KR, Gowland PA, Moore RJ, Baker PN, Johnson IR. Assessment of fetal lung growth in utero with echo-planar MR imaging. Radiology 1999; 210:197–200.

84. Toft PB, Leth H, Ring PB, Peitersen B, Lou HC, Henriksen O. Volumetric analysis of the normal infant brain and in intrauterine growth retardation. Early Hum Dev 1995; 43:15–29.

85. Auriemma A, Agostinis C, Bianchi P, et al. Hemimegalencephaly in hypomelanosis of Ito: early sonographic pattern and peculiar MR findings in a newborn. Eur J Ultrasound 2000; 12:61–67.

86. van Wezel-Meijler G, van der Knaap MS, Sie LT, et al. Magnetic resonance imaging of the brain in premature infants during the neonatal period. Normal phenomena and reflection of mild ultrasound abnormalities. Neuropediatrics 1998; 29:89–96.

87. Naidich TP, Grant JL, Altman N, et al. The developing cerebral surface. Preliminary report on the patterns of sulcal and gyral maturation—anatomy, ultrasound, and magnetic resonance imaging. Neuroimaging Clin N Am 1994; 4:201–240.

88. Bouza H, Dubowitz LM, Rutherford M, Cowan F, Pennock JM. Late magnetic resonance imaging and clinical findings in neonates with unilateral lesions on cranial ultrasound. Dev Med Child Neurol 1994; 36:951–964.

89. de Vries LS, Eken P, Groenendaal F, van Haastert IC, Meiners LC. Correlation between the degree of periventricular leukomalacia diagnosed using cranial ultrasound and MRI later in infancy in children with cerebral palsy. Neuropediatrics 1993; 24:263–268.

90. Schneider JF, Il'yasov KA, Hennig J, Martin E. Fast quantitative diffusion-tensor imaging of cerebral white matter from the neonatal period to adolescence. Neuroradiology 2004.

91. Khong PL, Lam BC, Chung BH, Wong KY, Ooi GC. Diffusion-weighted MR imaging in neonatal nonketotic hyperglycinemia. AJNR Am J Neuroradiol 2003; 24:1181–1183.

92. Arzoumanian Y, Mirmiran M, Barnes PD, et al. Diffusion tensor brain imaging findings at term-equivalent age may predict neurologic abnormalities in low birth weight preterm infants. AJNR Am J Neuroradiol 2003; 24:1646–1653.

93. Melhem ER. Time-course of apparent diffusion coefficient in neonatal brain injury: the first piece of the puzzle. Neurology 2002; 59:798–799.

94. McKinstry RC, Miller JH, Snyder AZ, et al. A prospective, longitudinal diffusion tensor imaging study of brain injury in newborns. Neurology 2002; 59:824–833.

95. Roelants-van Rijn AM, Nikkels PG, Groenendaal F, et al. Neonatal diffusion-weighted MR imaging: relation with histopathology or follow-up MR examination. Neuropediatrics 2001; 32:286–294.

96. Huppi PS, Murphy B, Maier SE, et al. Microstructural brain development after perinatal cerebral white matter injury assessed by diffusion tensor magnetic resonance imaging. Pediatrics 2001; 107:455–460.

97. Bydder GM, Rutherford MA, Cowan FM. Diffusion-weighted imaging in neonates. Childs Nerv Syst 2001; 17:190–194.

98. Tanner SF, Ramenghi LA, Ridgway JP, et al. Quantitative comparison of intrabrain diffusion in adults and preterm and term neonates and infants. AJR Am J Roentgenol 2000; 174:1643–1649.

99. Krishnamoorthy KS, Soman TB, Takeoka M, Schaefer PW. Diffusion-weighted imaging in neonatal cerebral infarction: clinical utility and follow-up. J Child Neurol 2000; 15:592–602.

100. Sakuma H, Nomura Y, Takeda K, et al. Adult and neonatal human brain: diffusional anisotropy and myelination with diffusion-weighted MR imaging. Radiology 1991; 180:229–233.

101. Rutherford MA, Cowan FM, Manzur AY, et al. MR imaging of anisotropically restricted diffusion in the brain of neonates and infants. J Comput Assist Tomogr 1991; 15:188–198.

102. Anderson AW, Marois R, Colson ER, et al. Neonatal auditory activation detected by functional magnetic resonance imaging. Magn Reson Imaging 2001; 19:1–5.

103. Yamada H, Sadato N, Konishi Y, et al. A rapid brain metabolic change in infants detected by fMRI. Neuroreport 1997; 8:3775–3778.

104. Pruessmann KP, Weiger M, Scheidegger MB, Boesiger P. SENSE: sensitivity encoding for fast MRI. Magn Reson Med 1999; 42:952–962.

105. Sodickson DK, Manning WJ. Simultaneous acquisition of spatial harmonics (SMASH): fast imaging with radiofrequency coil arrays. Magn Reson Med 1997; 38:591–603.

106. Paley MNJ, McGinley JVM. Specialised MRI systems: design, operation and economics, developments in magnetic resonance, 1995; 1:48–52.

107. Whitby EH, Paley MNJ, Smith MF, Teasdale K, Darwent G, Griffiths PD. Magnetic Resonance Imaging in the Pre-term Neonate using a 0.2 Tesla dedicated MR scanner: Comparison with Ultrasound. Seventh Meeting of the International Society for Magnetic Resonance in Medicine, Philadelphia, Pennsylvania, U.S.A., 22–28 May 1999.

108. Whitby EH, Paley MNJ, Smith MF, Sprigg A, Woodhouse N, Griffiths PD. Low field strength magnetic resonance imaging of the neonatal brain, Archives of childhood diseases. Fetal Neonatal Ed 2003; 88:F203–F208.

109. Larkman DJ, Hajnal JV, Herlihy AH, Coutts GA, Young IR, Ehnholm G. Use of multicoil arrays for separation of signal from multiple slices simultaneously excited. J Magn Reson Imaging 2001; 13:313–317.

110. Paley MNJ, Lee KJ, Wild JM, et al. B1AC-MAMBA: B1 array combined with multiple acquisition micro B_0 array parallel magnetic resonance imaging. Magn Reson Med 2003; 49:1196–1200.

111. Paley MNJ, Lee KJ, Wild JM, Griffiths PD, Whitby EH. SPIRIT: simultaneous parallel inclined readout image technique, Proc UKRC 2004, 1100, Manchester, June 2004.

112. Albert MS, Cates GD, Driehuys B, et al. Biological magnetic resonance imaging using laser-polarized 129Xe. Nature 1994; 370:199–201.

113. Middleton H, Black RD, Saam B, et al. MR imaging with hyperpolarized 3He gas. Magn Reson Med 1995; 33:271–275.

114. Wild JM, Paley MNJ, Kasuboski L, et al. Dynamic radial projection MRI of inhaled hyperpolarized 3He gas. Magn Reson Med 2003; 49:991–997.

115. Wild JM, Schmiedeskamp J, Paley MNJ, et al. MR imaging of the lungs with hyperpolarized helium-3 gas transported by air. Phys Med Biol 2002; 47:N185–N190.

116. Kauczor HU, Hanke A, Van Beek EJ. Assessment of lung ventilation by MR imaging: current status and future perspectives. Eur Radiol 2002; 12:1962–1970.

117. Paley MNJ, Whitby EH, Wild JM, van Beek E, Smith M, Griffiths PD. Development of a flexible multi-channel, multi-frequency transceiver for a dedicated neonatal MR system. Proc Int Soc Mag Reson Med 2002; 10:909.

118. Jobsis FF. Non-invasive, infra-red monitoring of cerebral O2 sufficiency, bloodvolume, HbO2-Hb shifts and bloodflow. Acta Neurol Scand Suppl 1977; 64:452–453.

119. Maki A, Yamashita Y, Ito Y, Watanabe E, Mayanagi Y, Koizumi H. Spatial and temporal analysis of human motor activity using noninvasive NIR topography. Med Phys 1995; 22:1997–2005.

120. Firbank M, Elwell CE, Cooper CE, Delpy DT. Experimental and theoretical comparison of NIR spectroscopy measurements of cerebral hemoglobin changes. J Appl Physiol 1998; 85:1915–1921.

121. Firbank M, Okada E, Delpy DT. A theoretical study of the signal contribution of regions of the adult head to near-infrared spectroscopy studies of visual evoked responses. Neuroimage 1998; 8:69–78.

122. Firbank M, Okada E, Delpy DT. Investigation of the effect of discrete absorbers upon the measurement of blood volume with near-infrared spectroscopy. Phys Med Biol 1997; 42:465–477.

123. Firbank M, Arridge SR, Schweiger M, Delpy DT. An investigation of light transport through scattering bodies with non-scattering regions. Phys Med Biol 1996; 41:767–783.

124. Matcher SJ, Elwell CE, Cooper CE, Cope M, Delpy DT. Performance comparison of several published tissue near-infrared spectroscopy algorithms. Anal Biochem 1995; 227:54–68.

125. Araki R, Nashimoto I. Near-infrared imaging in vivo (I): image restoration technique applicable to the NIR projection images. Adv Exp Med Biol 1992; 316:155–161.

126. Wyatt JS, Cope M, Delpy DT, et al. Quantitation of cerebral blood volume in human infants by near-infrared spectroscopy. J Appl Physiol 1990; 68:1086–1091.

127. Van der Zee P, Delpy DT. Simulation of the point spread function for light in tissue by a Monte Carlo method. Adv Exp Med Biol 1987; 215:179–191.

128. Wyatt JS, Cope M, Delpy DT, Wray S, Reynolds EO. Quantification of cerebral oxygenation and haemodynamics in sick newborn infants by near infrared spectrophotometry. Lancet 1986; 2:1063–1066.

129. van der Zee P, Cope M, Arridge SR, et al. Experimentally measured optical pathlengths for the adult head, calf and forearm and the head of the newborn infant as a function of inter optode spacing. Adv Exp Med Biol 1992; 316:143–153.

130. Leung TS, Aladangady N, Elwell CE, Delpy DT, Costeloe K. A new method for the measurement of cerebral blood volume and total circulating blood volume using near infrared spatially resolved spectroscopy and indocyanine green: application and validation in neonates. Pediatr Res 2004; 55:134–141.

131. Culver JP, Durduran T, Cheung C, Furuya D, Greenberg JH, Yodh AG. Diffuse optical measurement of hemoglobin and cerebral blood flow in rat brain during hypercapnia, hypoxia and cardiac arrest. Adv Exp Med Biol 2003; 510:293–297.

132. Zubritsky E. NIR observes infants' brains. Anal Chem 2001; 73:128A.

133. Rolfe P, Wickramasinghe YA, Thorniley MS, et al. Fetal and neonatal cerebral oxygen monitoring with NIRS: theory and practice. Early Hum Dev 1992; 29:269–273.

134. Faris F, Thorniley M, Wickramasinghe Y, et al. Non-invasive in vivo near-infrared optical measurement of the penetration depth in the neonatal head. Clin Phys Physiol Meas 1991; 12:353–358.

135. Ramanujam N, Vishnoi G, Hielscher A, Rode M, Forouzan I, Chance B. Photon migration through fetal head in utero using continuous wave, near infrared spectroscopy: clinical and experimental model studies. J Biomed Opt 2000; 5:173–184.

136. Zhang Q, Ma H, Nioka S, Chance B. Study of near infrared technology for intracranial hematoma detection. J Biomed Opt 2000; 5:206–213.

137. Ramanujam N, Long H, Rode M, Forouzan I, Morgan M, Chance B. Antepartum, transabdominal near infrared spectroscopy: feasibility of measuring photon migration through the fetal head in utero. J Matern Fetal Med 1999; 8:275–288.

138. Mancini DM, Bolinger L, Li H, Kendrick K, Chance B, Wilson JR. Validation of near-infrared spectroscopy in humans. J Appl Physiol 1994; 77:2740–2747.

139. Martindale J, Mayhew J, Berwick J, et al. The hemodynamic impulse response to a single neural event. J Cereb Blood Flow Metab 2003; 23:546–555.

140. Martin C, Berwick J, Johnston D, et al. Optical imaging spectroscopy in the unanaesthetised rat. J Neurosci Methods 2002; 120:25–34.

141. Berwick J, Martin C, Martindale J, et al. Hemodynamic response in the unanesthetized rat: intrinsic optical imaging and spectroscopy of the barrel cortex. J Cereb Blood Flow Metab 2002; 22:670–679.

142. Jones M, Berwick J, Mayhew J. Changes in blood flow, oxygenation, and volume following extended stimulation of rodent barrel cortex. Neuroimage 2002; 15:474–487.

143. Jones M, Berwick J, Johnston D, Mayhew J. Concurrent optical imaging spectroscopy and laser-Doppler flowmetry: the relationship between blood flow, oxygenation, and volume in rodent barrel cortex. Neuroimage 2001; 13:1002–1015.

144. Mayhew J, Johnston D, Martindale J, Jones M, Berwick J, Zheng Y. Increased oxygen consumption following activation of brain: theoretical footnotes using spectroscopic data from barrel cortex. Neuroimage 2001; 13:975–987.

145. Zheng Y, Johnston D, Berwick J, Mayhew J. Signal source separation in the analysis of neural activity in brain. Neuroimage 2001; 13:447–458.

146. Paley MNJ, Mayhew JE, Martindale AJ, et al. Design and initial evaluation of a low-cost 3-Tesla research system for combined optical and functional MR imaging with interventional capability. J Magn Reson Imaging 2001; 13:87–92.

147. Mayhew J, Johnston D, Berwick J, Jones M, Coffey P, Zheng Y. Spectroscopic analysis of neural activity in brain: increased oxygen consumption following activation of barrel cortex. Neuroimage 2000; 12:664–675.
148. Martindale J, Berwick J, Johnston D, et al. Pseudo-random procedures for rapid presentation rates using optical imaging and spectroscopy. Neuroreport 2000; 11:2247–2252.
149. Mayhew JE, Askew S, Zheng Y, et al. Cerebral vasomotion: a 0.1-Hz oscillation in reflected light imaging of neural activity. Neuroimage 1996; 4:183–193.
150. Obrig H, Villringer A. Beyond the visible—imaging the human brain with light. J Cereb Blood Flow Metab 2003; 23:1–18.
151. Obrig H, Wenzel R, Kohl M, et al. Near-infrared spectroscopy: does it function in functional activation studies of the adult brain? Int J Psychophysiol 2000; 35:125–142.
152. Heekeren HR, Kohl M, Obrig H, et al. Noninvasive assessment of changes in cytochrome-c oxidase oxidation in human subjects during visual stimulation. J Cereb Blood Flow Metab 1999; 19:592–603.
153. Kohl M, Nolte C, Heekeren HR, et al. Determination of the wavelength dependence of the differential pathlength factor from near-infrared pulse signals. Phys Med Biol 1998; 43:1771–1782.
154. Villringer A, Chance B. Non-invasive optical spectroscopy and imaging of human brain function. Trends Neurosci 1997; 20:435–442.
155. Hock C, Villringer K, Muller-Spahn F, et al. Decrease in parietal cerebral hemoglobin oxygenation during performance of a verbal fluency task in patients with Alzheimer's disease monitored by means of near-infrared spectroscopy (NIRS)—correlation with simultaneous rCBF-PET measurements. Brain Res 1997; 755:293–303.
156. Villringer K, Minoshima S, Hock C, et al. Assessment of local brain activation. A simultaneous PET and near-infrared spectroscopy study. Adv Exp Med Biol 1997; 413:149–153.
157. Gratton G, Fabiani M. Fast optical signals: principles, methods, and experimental results. In: Frostig R, ed. In Vivo Optical Imaging of Brain Function. Boca Raton: CRC Press, 2002:223.
158. Chow LS, Cook G, Whitby EH, Paley MNJ. Investigating direct detection of axonal firing in the adult human optic nerve using MRI, NeuroImage 2006, In Press.

4.4

Incubators for Magnetic Resonance Imaging Use

T. M. Bohnen
LMT Lammers Medical Technology GmbH, Luebeck, Germany

INCUBATORS FOR MRI USE

The utility of incubators in Neonatal Intensive Care Units is as undoubted as the usefulness of magnetic resonance imaging (MRI) is in Radiology. It is no wonder that the combination of those technologies is considered highly beneficial for the population of preterm babies born suffering from various diseases (1,2). The indication for use of a MRI-compatible incubator is evident in this book.

The following chapter discusses the technical aspects of neonatal intensive care inside the MRI environment. It starts with the basics of warming therapy and thermoregulation. The design considerations for a MRI-compatible incubator and suitable coils are outlined based on the requirements from the view of radiologists, neonatologists, and finally on the requirements the patients. A short note on regulatory aspects is also given. Finally, there is more needed besides the incubator to make a practical solution for clinical use and this is discussed under system considerations.

BASICS OF WARMING THERAPY

Effects of Cold Stress

A warm body is one of the basic needs of the human being. When adults feel uncomfortable about the temperature, immediate action is taken. Windows are closed, heaters are turned up, cardigans are pulled out. The newborn and especially the preterm is completely dependent on care as it requires experienced nurses and doctors to understand the communicated need and to react adequately and timely. Physiological reactions to cold stress that clearly show the significance of warming therapy are shown in Figure 1 (3).

There are four ways through which the human body loses heat:

1. Radiation: heat exchange with distant surfaces,
2. Conduction: heat exchange with surfaces in contact with the body,
3. Convection: losing heat to air flowing across the body and
4. Transepidermal evaporation: losing water (and thus energy) by evaporating water.

The aim of warming therapy is to decrease these heat exchanges to close to zero. The patient can then invest energy in healing and growing rather than maintaining body temperature. For preterms the natural protection against cold stress, the mothers womb, is not available anymore. However, this can be replaced by an artificial environment created by warming therapy devices. Closed warming therapy, namely incubators,

233

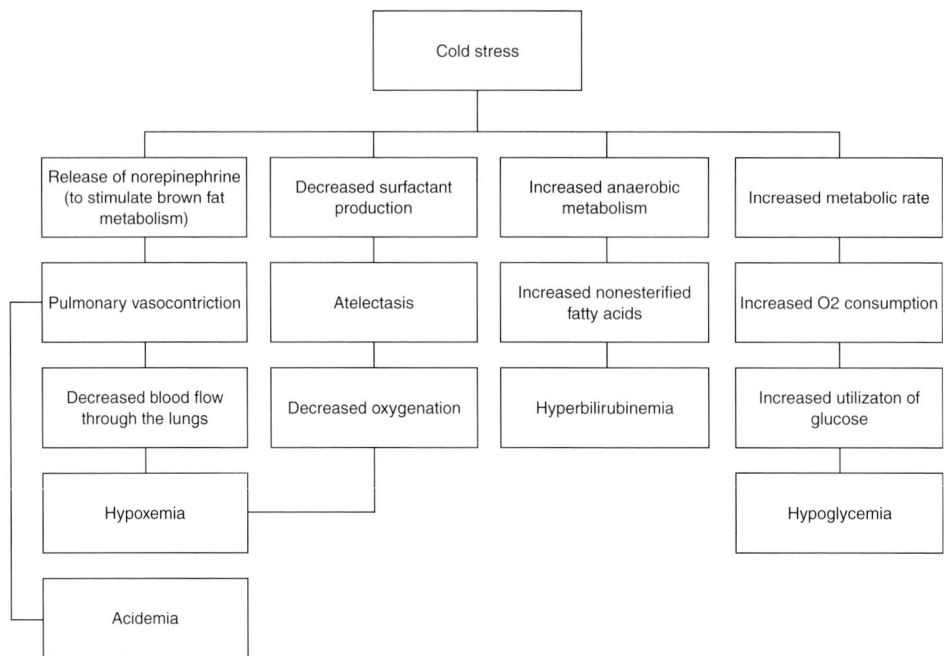

Figure 1. Routes of heat exchange in incubators.

focuses on low convective heat loss by providing warm air with low velocity around the patient's body. When humidification is used, the evaporative heat loss can be reduced to zero as everybody who has ever entered a humidified green house knows. Conductive heat loss is low, as the incubator mattress can be seen as nearly ideal insulation. Intensive care incubators are equipped with double walls that create a similar effect to double glazed windows, bringing the inner surface temperature closer to the air temperature inside. In this manner radiative heat loss is reduced but not eliminated.

With these measures thermal balance of the patient can be achieved. That means that heat production of the body is in equilibrium with the heat losses and in addition the required heat production is minimized. Whatever warming therapy device is used to keep the patient in thermal balance at the NICU, it cannot be interrupted without consequences when MR imaging is required. When no MRI-compatible incubator is available, it is a difficult decision whether the benefits of imaging will outweigh the consequences of cold stress.

REQUIREMENTS FOR A MRI-COMPATIBLE INCUBATOR

There are several aspects of MRI compatibility which have to be considered when designing a MRI-compatible incubator:

1. Magnetic forces: Every ferromagnetic part is attracted by the B_0 field of the scanner. This has resulted in an unfortunate history of more or less severe accidents and damage to equipment.
2. Immunity of incubator electronics: This aspect of electromagnetic compatibility (EMC) consideration ensures that no function of the incubator is influenced by the fields of the scanner.
3. The other aspect of EMC compatibility, i.e., emissions from the incubator, is less a safety aspect but of more vital interest to the radiologist, as they lead to decreased imaging quality.

4. The geometry of the incubator must reflect the top of the MRI table. It must fit on the table and into the bore of present standard scanners to be universally usable.
5. Finally, positioning of the MR imaging coil close to the patient's body must be possible as it is necessary to have the best conditions for imaging.

Besides the special characteristics of the MRI environment, simpler though not unimportant problems must be solved. Since the number of patients examined is crucial to economic efficiency, patients requiring use of an incubator should not disturb the routine procedures and schedules of the MRI site. The weight and geometry of the incubator should allow handling by two persons (e.g., shifting from the gurney to the patient scanner table).

Lastly the MRI-compatible incubator should serve as an intensive care incubator with all needed functions:

1. Air control temperature regulation with a defined degree of accuracy
2. Air flow patterns with minimum air speed inside the patient compartment
3. Bactericidal humidification for the benefit of the preterm
4. Other performance and safety parameters required by international standards.

MRI Safety

As well as MRI-compatibility there is the vital area of MRI safety. This means, among other things, that all devices or parts can be brought into the scanner room to their normal position of use without imposing any risk. However, they may have to be removed before imaging.

NOTE: There is not yet an internationally accepted definition or marking for MRI-compatibility or MRI safety either by the industry or by standardization bodies. However the ECRI (Emergency Care Research Institute, Plymouth Meeting, Pennsylvania, U.S.A, a non-profit organization) proposed a marking system in their journal recently (6).

The attractive force of the magnet results in two effects:

1. Acceleration of magnetic parts towards the isocenter of the magnet
2. Inertia caused by the reaction forces of induced eddy currents.

While the first imposes a risk to anybody inside the MRI room, the second point generates a handling problem when bodies do not react to moving forces as expected.

Accelerating forces are dependent on the following factors derived from physical formulae:

1. The B_0 (magnetic) field strength of the scanner
2. The local gradient of the field
3. The magnetic properties of the part in question, namely the susceptibility
4. The volume/mass of the magnetic object.

Practically there is more acceleration when you:

1. Have a 3T instead of a 1.5T scanner. This is very important due to the rapidly growing number of 3T scanners which are often installed side by side with 1.5T scanners
2. Get closer to the bore
3. Have a scanner without active shielding of the magnet and
4. Have devices or parts with steel instead of MRI-compatible devices made entirely of aluminium, brass, inox, and plastics.

Both acceleration and inertial effects have to be tested, after sufficient theoretical analysis, by slowly bringing the equipment into a scanner room under very controlled conditions. The incubator has to be put on top of the table of different MRI scanner models and then the table moved into the bore until the position of maximum insertion is reached. This should be clearly defined when there are limits to proper function of the device. The test must not show any movement of the incubator induced by magnetic forces.

When handling the incubator with the required number of persons, e.g., shifting from the gurney onto the table, no inertial forces should be detected. The moving masses should react as under normal conditions.

What applies to the whole incubator also applies for detachable parts of the device. Although it may not be intended that parts are detached during use at the MRI site, it is still likely to happen in clinical operation. No user-detachable parts or assemblies (e.g., covers, sealings) shall contain metal parts. There must be no risk associated with removing these parts from the incubator due to magnetic forces.

MRI Compatibility

As discussed under MRI Safety, the effects of the MRI scanner on the mechanical structures refers both to the attraction of ferromagnetic parts and to eddy current induced inertial forces. Both effects not only create a handling problem, but also influence the function of the scanner and the incubator.

1. Magnetic forces prevent ferromagnetic parts from moving (e.g., relays)
2. Magnetic fields prevent solenoids or electric motors from functioning
3. Eddy currents can decrease the imaging quality of the MRI in terms of signal to noise ratio's and distortion
4. Magnetic fields resulting from eddy currents of sufficient strength prevent conducting parts from moving.

An incubator consists of multiple components, some of which are factory designed, like the housing, and some which are catalogue parts which have to be purchased "as is." There are sometimes components which cannot be purchased in MRI- compatible fashion. The number and total mass of these has to be minimized and the distance to the magnet has to be maximized. If this is not sufficient, magnetic shielding has to be installed. Raising the total weight of the incubator to anchor it is not really an option due to handling requirements.

Eddy currents have to be avoided by minimizing the number and volume of parts made of conductive material. Even screws are preferably made of plastics. Unavoidable aluminium parts in the aggregate section like the heater body or electronic housings and some necessary brass screws can be designed not to have a significant negative influence on the SNR.

What must be avoided in any case are moving parts made of conductive material. The electromagnetic fields resulting from eddy currents induced into a rotating metal shaft are clearly visible in a MR image.

Image Quality (Emissions)

Every emission from the incubator, its parts and accessories that match the RF frequency of 64 MHz $\pm$ 1 MHz (for a 1.5T MRI) or multiples, may be visible on the acquired MR image. When developing any MRI accessory the aim must be uncompromised image quality.

These are typical image artifacts which can occur:

1. Geometric distortion: metal parts can distort the field of the scanner
2. Noise: an overall increase of noise, lowering the image contrast. This can be the result of wide band electromagnetic radiation

3. Ghosting: resulting, e.g., from vibration or parts containing water
4. Lack of uniformity: resulting, e.g., from RF-absorbing plastics or magnetic parts.

Despite the intended use in an MRI environment there are test procedures and requirements defined in the IEC 60601-1-2 applying to every medical device:

1. Conducted emission
2. Disturbing field measurement
3. Voltage fluctuation and flicker
4. Harmonic current emissions

These tests can be seen as a minimum requirement and practical tests have shown that an emission curve 10 dB below A-curve is a good entrance to the world of MRI-compatibility.

Besides the "active emission" of electronics there are "passive emissions" of parts triggered by the MRI sequence. The aim of the imaging sequences is to excite the proton in the nuclei of water molecules. Protons are not only present in water in the human body but also in many materials, e.g., Polymethylmetacrylat or acrylic glass (PMMA) is capable of absorbing 2% water at room temperature and even more at 39°C.

Some polymers and monomers also produce signals at the same resonance frequency as water. These components may show up in the image as ghosts.

Other material properties like heat resistance, strength, and biocompatibility are also very important when designing an incubator for use in on MR.

Incubator Function (Immunity)

It must not be forgotten that an MRI system acts as a large transmitting antenna which causes difficulties for any surrounding microelectronics. The incubator electronics and any other devices around the magnet must be immune to the fields generated by the MRI.

Again there are minimum requirements for medical devices in the IEC consisting of the following tests:

1. Immunity to electrical fast transient/burst
2. Immunity to conducted disturbances induced by RF fields: Frequency range: 150 kHz to 80 MHz
3. Immunity to voltage dips, short interruptions and voltage variations
4. Immunity to surge
5. Immunity to electrostatic discharge.

Where the first three tests refer to conducted disturbances via the mains supply, the "immunity to radiated RF electromagnetic fields" is very important in the MRI environment as the frequency band covers the Larmor frequencies of all standard MRI's in clinical use: 26 MHz to 2500 MHz (steps <1%).

The test "immunity to power frequency magnetic field" is not required because the magnetic field strength in the MRI room is much higher than the test level according to the applicable IEC standard.

The pass/fail criterion for the tests has to be defined in accordance with IEC 60601-1-2 clause 36.202.1 j. The "essential performance" as defined by the standard can be derived from a risk analysis, but it is better to consider the complete functional scope of the device. The following degradations are not allowed and are defined as a failure of the test:

1. Component failures
2. Changes in programmable parameters

3. Reset to factory defaults (manufacturer's presets)
4. Change of operating mode
5. False alarms
6. Cessation or interruption of any intended operation, even if accompanied by an alarm
7. Initiation of any unintended operation, including unintended or uncontrolled motion, even if accompanied by an alarm
8. Error of a displayed numerical value sufficiently large to affect diagnosis or treatment.

As already mentioned these tests define the entrance level for MRI compatibility and cannot replace in situ tests at the MRI site using the diagnostic tools incorporated into those parts of the scanner software which are only accessible by the original manufacturer.

To achieve MRI compatibility for the electronics three basic principles were applied in the design of the LMT nomag IC 1.5 incubator:

1. Shielding: The boards, sensors, and cables are completely shielded against high frequency by keeping a closed chain of shield around every component.
2. Grounding: All parts having a shield function are grounded to the protective earth potential of the mains plug which has to be connected (during scanning) to the same ground as the MRI scanner and cage.
3. Filtering: All lines of the cables are filtered to protect circuits from induced RF of the MRI scanner.

Basic Incubator Functions

The basic incubator function is to keep the patient in a warm and, when necessary, humidified environment separated from ambient conditions. The patient compartment with the patient bed, mattress, and coil interface is bordered by a transparent hood. Routine procedures of patient care require access to the patient provided by large flaps on the side or handports for minor handling procedures.

Although the hood is transparent, patient visibility is strictly limited when the incubator is inserted into the magnet. This can be improved by the geometry of the patient compartment providing at least a limited view of the patient. Alternatively this can be solved by a camera on top of the incubator.

Similar to standard NICU incubators, some tubing ports provide access to the patient compartment for, e.g., ECG lines, infusion lines, or a ventilation hose. These lines have to be routed and fixed carefully to protect the cables from unwanted hooking when the incubator is driven into the magnet.

The geometry of the patient compartment in general must reflect the dimensions of the magnet bore and the patient table. It is desirable to provide maximum space for the patient while still fitting into a maximum number of scanners. To get the best possible imaging, the imaging coil should be brought as close to the patient as possible. The design conclusion must be to bring dedicated neonatal coils inside the patient compartment. Design implications for the coil are discussed later.

The LMT nomag IC 1.5 provides a space of w:26 cm*l:70 cm*h:19 cm which is large enough for patients with a maximum body length of 55 cm and a maximum weight of 4500 g as defined in the intended use. This equals about the 90th percentile of the term infants.

Air Flow Circuit

Except for some older transport incubators, all incubators warm up the patient compartment by circulating heated air through a blower wheel. A certain amount (around 10%) of fresh air is mixed with this. Fresh air is aspirated via a bacteria filter through a low pressure device, e.g., generated by a venturi tube.

The heated and humidified air is guided through air channels in the housing below the patient compartment. From there, some slots allow the air to flow into the compartment. Somewhere in the patient compartment is an opening where the air is aspirated and circulated back to the blower wheel (Fig. 2).

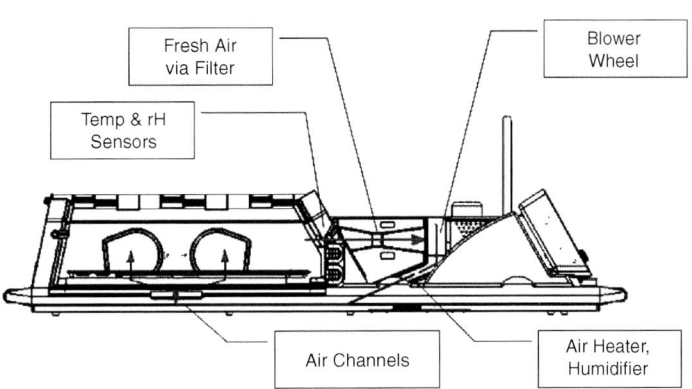

Figure 2. Picture shows air flow circuit of LMT nomag IC 1.5 (depicted without aggregate cover).

The contradicting design goals are to have a high amount of air exchanged in the patient compartment, to get the heat and fresh air in, and to get CO_2 out. On the other hand the patient must not experience drag, which is more difficult the smaller the patient compartment is.

The most hygienic way of humidifying circulating air is boiling demineralized water. Like the air heater, the water boiler is a small aluminium body heated by an electric resistor cartridge. Both units have a thermo-fuse attached to prevent damage if all other safety systems fail. In addition there is a switch closing a circuit at 115°C indicating that there is no water inside the pot. This triggers the low water alarm on the display.

The blower wheel drive is a very special design task as it naturally requires rotating parts which, as already mentioned, may not be made out of conducting material. Alternative drives for the air circulation using an injector proved to have a high consumption of compressed air, limiting the transportability.

The blower wheel of the LMT nomag IC 1.5 is driven by a special design DC motor with a special shield against magnetic fields. The motor is capable of turning at a field strength of nearly 0.5T which is present, e.g., at a distance of 1100 mm from isocenter and 100 mm above mattress of a Siemens Harmony 1.5T. This field strength is typical for actual 1.5T models of the big three manufacturers (Siemens, GE, Philips) with magnet lengths of approximately 1.6 m.

Air temperature and relative humidity are continuously measured in the air channel where the air is aspirated from the patient compartment. Due to the safety aspect, the temperature has to be measured with two sensors which have independent analogue and digital signal processing. A software PID controller activates the heater and the humidifier until set values are achieved.

Like any other incubator the revolutions of the blower wheel have to be monitored to ensure the air circulation. Additional safety features are a "temperature deviation alarm" and an "air overtemperature alarm."

Every software-controlled medical device has to run a self test during the boot sequence and after that periodically, e.g., every ten minutes. Other software-related functions must be checked more often, e.g., once a minute or once a second, depending on how critical the function is.

Among these functions are:

1. Supply voltages
2. Logical program monitoring
3. Program consistency EPROM
4. Heater control lines (solid state relais)
5. Analogue measurement circuits
6. Blower wheel rotation
7. Internal communication
8. Excess temperature channels.

In case of test values out of limits, the device must switch into a safe state, which means for an incubator that heater and humidifier are switched off and an audible and optical alarm is generated.

DESIGN CONSIDERATIONS: COILS

Incubator Safe Coil Design

Imaging neonates means imaging the most sensitive population in the hospital. Handling is minimized on the NICU and MRI diagnostics should work the same way. The requirements for a neonatal coil should reflect this fact. The geometry of the coil should support application with minimal interference with the patient.

When the LMT neonatal head coil is inserted through the rear flap of the incubator there are two rails that guide the coil around the narrow head section of the patient bed. Thus the head of the patient can be arranged on the head section of the patient bed in an appropriate way and the coil is positioned around it afterwards.

Finally, the patient's head and body can be fixed with Velcro straps to prevent movement during imaging. For this purpose straps and wedges of several thicknesses are supplied with the coil. The wedges also serve as a protection of the patient's sense of hearing.

The environment for an incubator safe coil is different from those of normal coils: The temperature is higher (up to 39°C) and level of relative humidity may be elevated to 70%rh. This is not ideal for electronics, especially high voltage electronics like coils. Complete sealing of the electronics with a potting compound is a suitable method of protection (4).

Patient Positioning

Besides immobilization of the imaged section of the body, also the rest of the body should be immobilized to prevent moving artifacts which would result in a need for rescan. When "natural sedation" through feeding is sufficient, it is helpful to perform coil positioning when the patient is transferred into the MRI incubator at the NICU. This allows the patient some time to recover from the handling procedures during transport and the patient is not then disturbed again when arriving at the MRI site.

When scanning the head of a ventilated patient another geometric problem arises. The coil may collide with the y-piece or tubes of the ventilation system. The LMT neonatal head coil forms a bridge in the front ring leaving enough space for the ventilation system.

Careful cable routing is essential when scanning a patient. The normal struggle with "spaghetti syndrome" is topped by the absolute requirement that even

MRI-compatible cables may not be arranged in loops and may not touch the patient's body. Otherwise there is a risk of severe burns. The position of the tubing ports of the LMT nomag 1.5 supports straightforward cable and hose routing inside the incubator. Outside the incubator no cable may touch the magnet bore as this may also result in reduced imaging quality. The LMT nomag IC 1.5 provides guides for cables leading them along the incubator.

Specific Absorption Rate (SAR)

The international standard for MRI scanners (IEC 60601-2-33) requires a limitation of the transmitted power in relation to the weight of the body (or parts of the body) which are scanned. This rate is called SAR. The limits apply for environmental conditions of 24°C air temperature and a maximum humidity of 60%. Raising the humidity requires a decrease of the transmitted power.

For the adult body 1.5 W/kg are allowed for normal use, for the adult head 3 W/kg. As there is little experience with neonates, let alone pre terms, there is no requirement or recommendation on how to handle these. In addition there is a duty for MRI manufacturers to warn of problems when scanning patients with thermoregulatory problems. This is exactly the population intended to be scanned inside an incubator, and environmental conditions can deviate significantly from the standard calculation. Obviously this point needs special attention. During the first experiments with a prototype of the LMT nomag IC 1.5, temperature was monitored with a fiberoptic sensor attached to the patient's forehead. The temperature was continuously monitored and sequences were adjusted to limit the rise to 1°C. All imaging requirements could be fulfilled inside this limit (1).

REGULATORY AFFAIRS

Regulatory affairs describe all actions and documentation related to the approval of a medical device by governmental authorities.

For the EU, application of a CE mark is mandatory for placing a medical device on the market. The basic requirements of the EU directive 42/93/EU have to be fulfilled. One way to prove this is to comply with internationally harmonized standards. The LMT nomag IC 1.5 MRI diagnostics incubator is in conformance with the following standards:

1. IEC 60601-1: 1988 + A1:1991 A2:1995, Medical Electrical Equipment—General Requirements for Safety
2. IEC 60601-1-2:2001, Medical Electrical Equipment part 1–2, General Requirements for Safety—Collateral Standard: EMC Requirements and Tests
3. IEC 60601-1-4:2001, Medical Electrical Equipment part 1–4, General Requirements for Safety—Collateral Standard: Programmable Electrical Medical Systems
4. IEC 60601-2-20:1990 + A1:1996, Medical Electrical Equipment—Particular Requirements for Safety of Transport Incubators
5. ISO 10993-1 Biological Evaluation of Medical Devices Part 1 Evaluation and Testing

For the USA an approval by the FDA is mandatory, which requires the submission of a set of documents that prove the "safety and effectiveness" of a device. Under number K033565 the LMT nomag achieved approval by the FDA in November 2003.

In addition to the standard tests for incubators, the MRI-compatibility has to be validated. Due to the different magnetic and electromagnetic behavior of scanners, compatibility has to be tested and proven on a type by type basis. The criteria are described in more detail in the section on MRI-compatibility.

SYSTEM CONSIDERATIONS

Patients scheduled for MR imaging in an incubator are normally situated in the NICU. Only few hospitals will be lucky to have the NICU and the MRI-site "under one roof" or even better on the same floor (5). Thus transport is nearly always required. Due to the nature of the patients, changing from one incubator to another is stressful and should be minimized. As the change from a standard NICU incubator to the MRI-compatible incubator is unavoidable, it is desirable that more changes to and from additional transport incubators should be avoided. The transportability of normal incubators is limited. The casters do not provide a comfortable ride on uneven ground, additional equipment cannot be mounted, and an electrical and gas supply is not provided.

A suitable MRI incubator must serve as transport as well as for the MR imaging. The requirements for intrahospital transport are:

1. Gurney with sufficient comfort to provide soft transport for the most delicate patients
2. Mobile electrical and gas supply
3. Space for monitoring, ventilation, and suction.

All the above mentioned accessories should be MRI-compatible because this simplifies handling at the MRI site considerably when the gurney with all its attachments can be safely driven into the scanner room.

The devices mentioned are all available in MRI-compatible versions. The only intensive care equipment that is not available in a mobile and MRI-compatible version are syringe pumps.

One possible solution to overcome this problem is to keep the pumps outside the scanner room and prolong the lines to 4 or 6 m, or to use really old fashioned pumps with a spring loaded drive that are not dependent on any electronics. Both are solutions that require future improvement.

THE TECHNICAL CHALLENGE: 3T AND IMPROVED COILS

Every piece of technical equipment labelled "MRI-compatible" has its limitations regarding the field strength that does not influence the device, or vice versa. "This limit is transferred into a dispance limit specific to the MRI scanner type," (7).

Equipment that can be kept distant from the magnet, like a monitor, can profit from active shielding technology developed by the magnet manufacturers. For equipment like the incubator that operates only when inserted into the magnet there are other rules. Further development made the equipment MRI-compatible with the growing number of 3T scanners. Materials were reviewed regarding residual magnetism or "passive emissions," electronic filters were adapted to higher frequencies, and shielding is more efficient than ever.

An even greater step of improvement will be necessary for the scanners beyond 3T field strength which are already installed in research units, which may come to the hospitals in coming years. Further challenges are to improve coil technology (e.g. Designing array coils for optimize cardiac imaging) or to increase the overall usability of the system by improving transport or integrating, monitoring and other features into the incubation. This will reduce the "spaghetti syndrome" and will further improve the scanless integration of neonatal imaging into the daily routine of MRI units. The MRI-compatible incubator has been a technical challenge during the last few years and will remain so, as long as technical progress supports medical progress and helps to improve our lives.

REFERENCES

1. Whitby EH, Griffiths PD, Lonneker-Lammers T, et al. Ultrafast magnetic resonance imaging of the neonate in a magnetic resonance-compatible incubator with a built-in coil. Pediatrics 2004; 113:e150–e152.
2. Bluml S, Friedlich P, Erberich S, Wood JC, Seri I, Nelson MD, Jr. MR imaging of newborns by using an MRI-compatible incubator with integrated radiofrequency coils: initial experience. Radiology 2004; 231:594–601.
3. Sally BO, Marcia LL, Patricia WL. Maternal newborn nursing. 4th ed. Olds, London, Ladewig: Addison Wesley, Nursing, 1992.
4. Srinivasan R, Loenneker-Lammers T, Shah R. MRI compatible incubator for imaging pre- and term neonates poster. Proc ISMRM 2002; 10:799.
5. Maalouf EF, Counsell S. Imaging the preterm infant: practical issues. In: Rutherford M, ed. MRI of the Neonatal Brain. Philadelphia: W.B. Saunders, 2002:17–21.
6. ECRI, 'What's new in MR Safety: The Latest on the Safe Use of Equipment in the Magnetic Resonance Environment'. Health devices, 2005; 34:333–349.
7. Stokowski L, Laura RN, MS, et al. Ensuring safety for infants under going magnetic resonance imaging, Advances in Neonatal Care 2005; 5:14–27.

4.5

The Role of the Magnetic Resonance Imaging Post-Mortem of the Fetus and Neonate

Elspeth H. Whitby and Paul D. Griffiths
Academic Unit of Radiology, University of Sheffield, Sheffield, U.K.

THE ROLE OF THE MAGNETIC RESONANCE IMAGING POST-MORTEM OF THE FETUS AND NEONATE

Macroscopic and microscopic examination of organs and tissues after death can provide important information for the family of the deceased and the doctors that had been attending the patient in life. Understanding why a person died may play a role in the bereavement process for the family and confirming the nature and extent of the disease process is vital for understanding the pathology, continuing medical education, and assessing the accuracy of imaging methods. Historically the examination of the dead has been the leading method of learning anatomy and pathology and this continues in a more limited form today.

Radiological investigation of the fetus has been used for many years, usually involving plain-film radiography, occasionally supplemented by computed tomography (CT). The investigation of the fetus post-mortem has fundamentally different goals when compared to the adult case. Most often adult autopsy hopes to confirm/refute the presence of an acquired pathology and judge its extent. This may be purely for medical reasons or in some cases there may be a legal/criminal context. The fetal autopsy, in contrast, is usually performed to look for developmental abnormalities that produced spontaneous abortion or to produce an accurate classification of the abnormalities that led to a therapeutic abortion. The pattern of developmental abnormalities in conjunction with chromosomal and genetic studies is then used to advise the parent(s) about the risk of similar problems in future pregnancies. This is very much the case of second trimester losses although the later pregnancy and early neonate post-mortem cases have a much higher proportion of acquired pathology such as hypoxic ischemic damage. In fetal autopsy, therefore, there is major value in studying the macroscopic morphology of organs with microscopic investigations being less important, at least for developmental abnormalities.

There have been significant changes in the public issues around the fetal/neonatal autopsy procedure in the U.K. over the last few years. A number of high profile cases have been reported in the media where, it was claimed, tissue and organs had been retained by hospital and university departments without the consent of parents.

An extensive review of the claims revealed a widespread problem, with tissue frequently being retained for purposes other than individual case diagnosis (e.g., for research and teaching purposes) extending over many years. An early and predictable response to the headlines in the newspapers was a massive reduction in the number of cases in which fetal autopsy was agreed to by parents. This led to a reduction in the amount of information that was available to parents about possible chromosomal/genetic risk factors to future pregnancies. However, changes in the physical process of fetal autopsy have caused further problems in information gathering that is particularly relevant to brain abnormalities. The fetal brain is a difficult organ to process due to its high water content and virtual absence of myelin. In years gone by, the autopsy procedure involved removal the brain into formalin for 4–6 weeks to allow the tissue to fix and allow better sectioning and macroscopic and microscopic analysis. In the present environment a high proportion of those parents who do agree to autopsy insist on a rapid return of the whole body for burial, usually within 3–4 days. In most cases, therefore, the fetal brain is studied unfixed and in many cases analysis can not be performed or is incomplete (1). It should also be appreciated that many people have not been able to have full counseling about risk to future pregnancies because their personal or religious beliefs do not allow autopsy. In those cases information obtained during pregnancy is the only data on which to give parents advice.

A number of groups have investigated the possibility of performing MRI post-mortem with some technical success. One group investigated the use of post-mortem MRI in adults at the request of the local Jewish community (2) and has continued their work in conjunction with the local coroner's office. Other groups have performed post-mortem imaging of the fetus including the brain and spine in situ. One group from the Middlesex Hospital London, has previously reported 3-D imaging of the fetus *post mortem* with MRI (3) and the same group did perform an MRI versus autopsy study in 1996 (4). That paper described 20 aborted or stillborn cases where MRI was used to perform whole body imaging. The MRI was performed in situ, and presumably, on unfixed tissue. Technical details of the autopsy were not published but held by the Editor of The Lancet. They found agreement between MRI and autopsy in 8/20 cases and in 4/20 cases MRI provided more information when compared to autopsy. In the remaining 8/20 cases autopsy provided more information than MRI. The overall sensitivity for MRI detecting pathology in that study was 60% compared with 100% in the cases presented in our paper. This can probably be explained by the facts that we studied the central nervous system only and there has been a significant improvement in the MRI quality over the last few years. Woodward et al. (5) described the results of 26 post-mortem MRI examinations on intact non-fixed fetuses and compared the findings with autopsy results although the authors do not specify if fixed tissue was used. Their cases consisted mainly of body abnormalities as opposed to central nervous system, however they commented that MRI was particularly useful for assessing central nervous system structures. In that study 37/47 (79%) of major abnormalities were shown on MRI but only 1/11 minor abnormalities. We became interested in performing post-mortem fetal imaging because of problems raised in our in utero MRI program. In retrospect we did not appreciate the extent of the problems in pediatric pathology circles (6,7) and this was brought into sharp focus when we performed our in utero ultrasound versus MRI diagnostic accuracy studies. The vast majority of parents have agreed to have in utero MRI on the basis of the research studies we performed from 1999–2003.

One portion of that program was to ask women who were going to have termination of pregnancy on the basis of the ultrasound findings, if they would agree to a MRI examination of their fetus the day before termination. A high proportion of women agreed to this even though they knew there could be no benefit to their decision-making. The aim of that study was to corroborate the in utero MRI findings with the findings on autopsy following termination. However, it became apparent that the numbers in this study were going to be small (only 12 recruited and completed in 3 years) because the women were not agreeing to autopsy after the termination. This led us to question if post-mortem MRI could be used to provide the same macroscopic information of the fetal brain and spine when compared with fetal autopsy. We approached this by asking parents who had agreed to autopsy whether they would agree to post-mortem MRI just before the autopsy in all local cases, not just from the in utero MRI program. In all cases we imaged the fetal brain and in cases of suspicion of spinal pathology the spine was imaged as well. We then planned to compare the macroscopic findings on MR imaging with the autopsy results based on both macroscopic and microscopic studies.

The first part of the study aimed to compare 40 cases and the results of those have been reported elsewhere (1). All patients that were asked to enter the MRI study agreed and the 40 cases were enrolled inside 6 months. The aborted fetuses were brought to our institution of autopsy from a wide geographic extent with a wide range of demise to autopsy delays (mean 5 days but up to 14 days) but the MRI procedure was always performed less than 24 hours before the autopsy. The MRI procedures were performed on routine 1.5T clinical MRI systems using either the knee or wrist coil, depending on the size of the fetus. The fetus was transported from the pathology department and scanned within the sealed plastic containers, in which they are stored routinely in order to reduce the risk of contamination.

The first few examinations consisted of high-resolution fast spin echo T2 weighted, spin echo T1 weighted and gradient-echo T1 weighted volume imaging. The spin echo T1 weighted and volume imaging was stopped after the first few cases because they did not appear to provide any extra information in routine cases but were used on an ad hoc basis. The mainstay of our post mortem fetal imaging, therefore, involves T2 weighted imaging, which may appear to be sub-optimal in detecting developmental brain/spine pathology if experience is extrapolated from adult and pediatric neuroimaging. In those cases T1 weighted volume images are generally the most useful for a number of reasons, including the high anatomical resolution provided by the high matrix size and small partition thickness. However, the large difference in T1 relaxation times between the myelinated white matter and gray matter produces superb contrast resolution between the cortical ribbon and subjacent white matter. The situation is different in the second and third trimester fetus where there is very little myelin present. This, in conjunction with the relatively high water content of the entire fetal brain, means that there is negligible contrast between fetal gray and white matter on T1-weighted images. In distinction, exquisite anatomical detail can be obtained using FSE T2-weighted images where gray/white matter contrast is good.

There were many similarities between the problems encountered in starting to interpret fetal images post-mortem when compared to the in utero MRI program. The major problem was unfamiliarity with the normal structural changes in the brain and spine that occur, particularly during the second trimester. In the post-mortem cases, however, some assistance was already available as there are text-books of fetal cross-sectional anatomy using fixed and stained brain tissue through the second and third trimester. We used the text produced by Feess–Higgins and Larroche as our Ref. (8) and the high quality MR images obtained in our study closely matched the appearances of the fixed tissue preparations (Fig. 1).

Another advantage was that all our cases were going for formal autopsy after the MRI and if the brain and spine were called normal on autopsy we were able to build up a reference of normal images at different gestational ages. Samples of those normal examinations are shown in Figures 2–4 and those with abnormalities in Figures 5–11.

Analysis of the first 40 cases, comparing autopsy and post mortem MRI results of fetal brain and spine showed promising results. In eight cases autopsy of the brain did not give any usable information because of the poor state of the tissue. These cases could not be analyzed in the study because the MRI provided the reference standard, however, in all eight cases MRI provided high quality images that provided a macroscopic diagnosis—two of these cases are shown in Figures 5 and 6. In the other 32 cases there was complete agreement between autopsy and MRI in 31/32 and in the other case consensus could not be reached about the presence or absence of colpocephaly. We have now performed approximately 200 such examinations with comparable results and the pediatric pathologists that we work with are convinced of the value of the procedure. The two major areas of assistance for

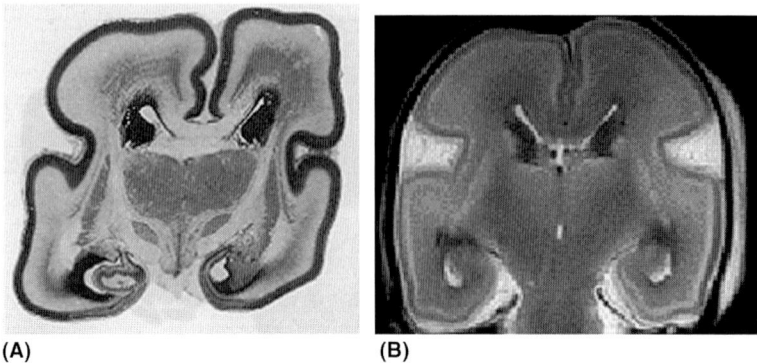

(A)   **(B)**

Figure 1. Comparison of a histological specimen (**A**) with an equivalent T2-weighted coronal MR image (**B**) both at 22 weeks gestational age showing the anatomical detail possible with MRI. At this maturity the hemispheric white matter is white due to the lack of myelin and the gray matter structures (including the cortical ribbon) are intermediate signal. The germinal matrix has a very low signal, as do the migrating neurons and glia within the white matter.

the brain are being able to target a specific area on autopsy that has been highlighted on MRI and also the ability of MRI to image the extra-axial spaces that are, by necessity, destroyed when a brain is removed. MRI of the spine is also highly advantageous because of the extensive procedure required to visualize the entire cord directly by autopsy.

As well as providing information that can be used in a clinical environment, post mortem MRI can give valuable insights into normal and abnormal brain development. We have already described in chapter 1.3 a method to study fetal cerebellar and bony posterior fossa growth and the support that provided for McLone's hydrostatic theory of Chiari 2 deformities (9). More recently we have reported the change in germinal matrix size over the second and third trimester. As described in chapter 1.2 the germinal matrix is the term used in clinical circles for the periventricular regions of the brain where neurons and glia are "born" and subsequently migrate to form the cortex and subcortical gray matter nuclei. The germinal matrix has characteristic imaging appearances, high attenuation coefficient on CT imaging, very low signal on T2-weighted images and high signal on T1-weighted images. These features are probably due to the high cellularity of the structure and the high protein content due to high nuclear/cytoplasmic ratios. As shown in Figure 1, the germinal matrix has much lower signal than the adjacent CSF in the ventricles and white matter on the T2-weighted imaging we use post mortem. It is possible to make accurate estimates of the size of the germinal matrix in relation to the overall size of the cerebral hemispheres. We have shown that the area of the germinal matrix adjacent to the frontal horn of the lateral ventricles changes considerably between 14–32 weeks (Fig. 12). The area of the germinal matrix increases rapidly between 14–19 weeks post last menstrual period and then appears to reach a peak for 2–3 weeks. After this time it reduces in size rapidly and by 32 weeks it is difficult to see any residual germinal matrix (unpublished data). It is possible to study the size of the germinal matrix in proportion to the size of the hemisphere by calculating A/T (where A is the square root of germinal matrix area and T is the hemispheric thickness) and plotting the ratio against gestational age (Fig. 13). This shows a linear negative correlation and one interpretation is that the growth of the cerebral hemisphere is solely related to cells being formed in the germinal matrix. This supports the known theory of the role of the germinal matrix but is difficult to study in fetuses in later pregnancy and neonates for two reasons: the germinal matrix is no longer functioning as a cell generator and hemispheric growth is influenced by other factors such as myelin formation.

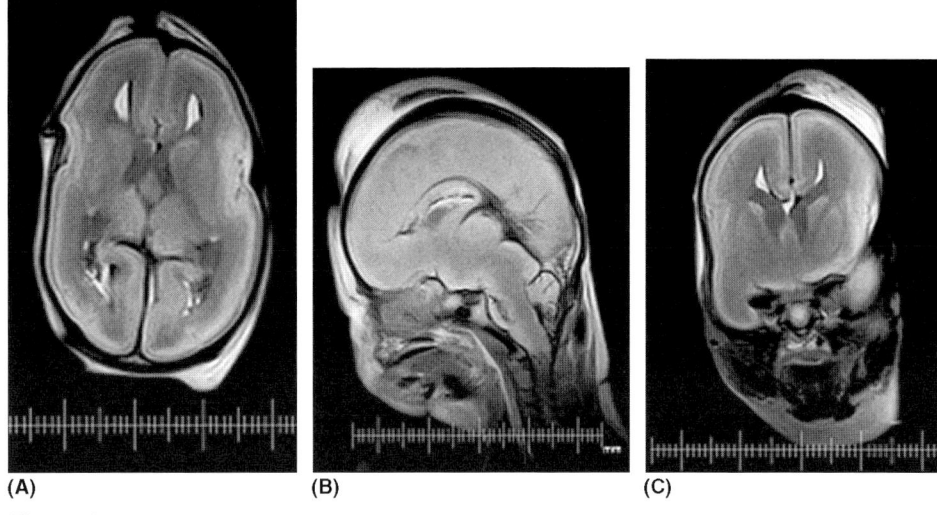

(A)   **(B)**   **(C)**

Figure 2.

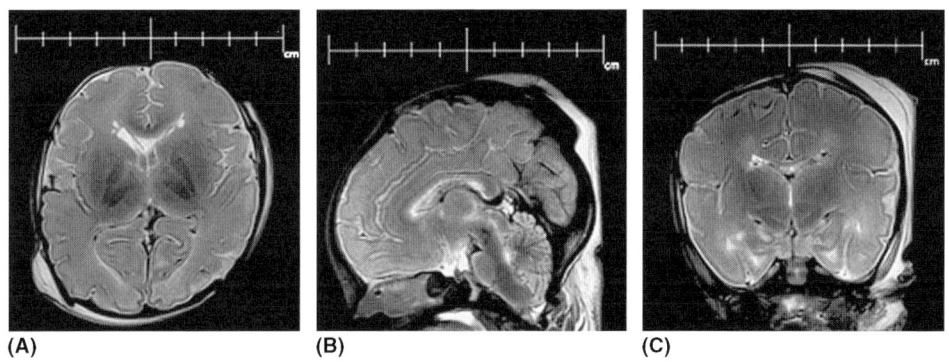

(A)   **(B)**   **(C)**

Figure 3.

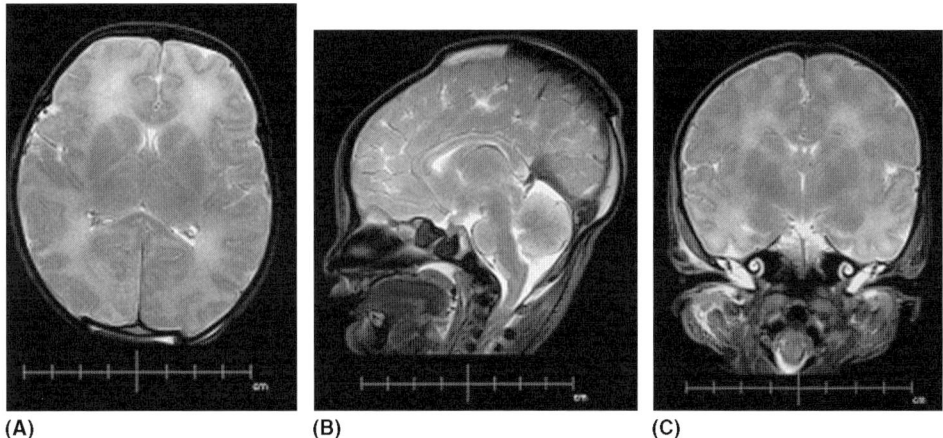

(A)   **(B)**   **(C)**

Figure 4.

Figures 2 to 4. Some of the changes in fetal brain morphology between 18 and 36 weeks gestational age (Figure 2, 18 weeks; Figure 3, 26 weeks; and Figure 4, 36 weeks). The most significant changes with increasing gestational age are: (1) increasing complexity of sulcation/cortical morphology, (2) increasing relative size of the cerebellum, (3) reducing volume of the germinal matrix, (4) increasing myelination.

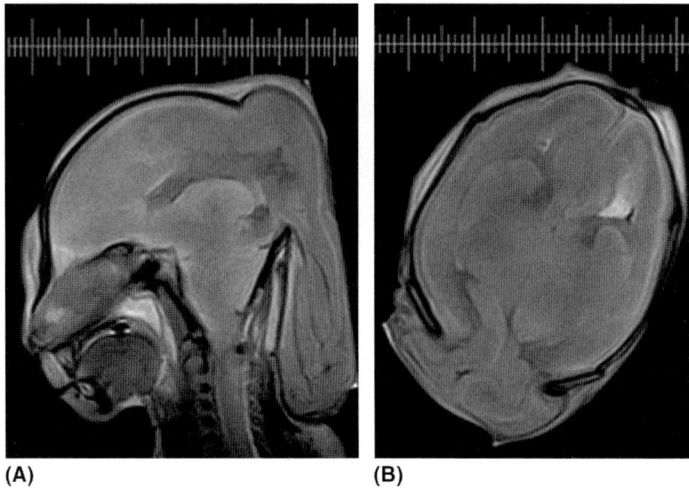

(A)   **(B)**

Figure 5. Parietal encephalocoele, (**A**) axial and (**B**) sagittal, showing a significant proportion of the brain herniating through a posterior defect.

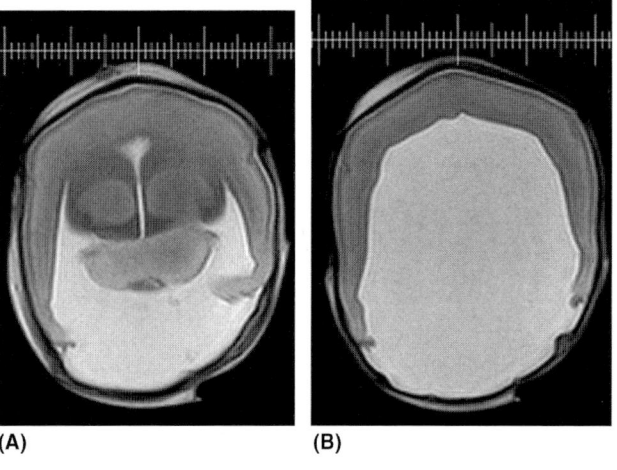

(A)   **(B)**

Figure 6. Alobar holoprosencephaly (**A**) and (**B**) axial, showing complete failure of separation of the cerebral hemispheres and ventricles. The thalami are fused.

It is also obvious from reviewing MRI of second trimester brains that there are structures in the developing white matter that have a lower signal than non-myelinated white matter fibers. Although we do not have histological confirmation at this point, we believe that the low signal in the white matter indicates migrating neurons and glia on the basis of matching the images with histological studies. This offers a method of studying normal and abnormal migration. We have seen brain malformations affecting one cerebral hemisphere only that show apparent reduction in cellular migration along with one or two cases that appear to have focal abnormalities of the germinal matrix and associated migration cone. Figure 14 shows one example with a small deformity of the developing cortex above it and it is likely (though not provable) that this was the precursor of a focal cortical dysplasia, such as polymicrogyria.

Disadvantages of Post-Mortem MRI

The evolving literature on fetal/stillborn post-mortem MRI suggests that macroscopic information can be obtained that provides the correct diagnosis in a high proportion of cases, at least for brain and spine. Previously we have already mentioned the particular

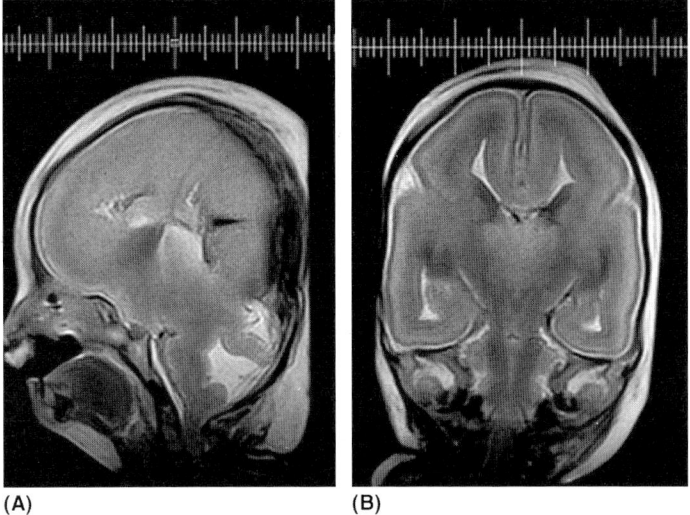

(A)   (B)

Figure 7. Dandy–Walker malformation (**A**) sagittal, (**B**) coronal, showing a large posterior fossa with vermian hypoplasia and a patulous connection between the fourth ventricle and a retrocerebellar cyst. Ventriculomegaly is not present.

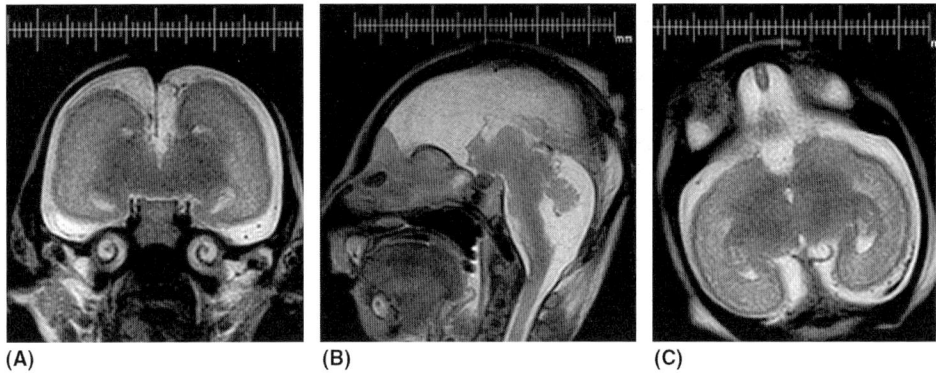

(A)   (B)   (C)

Figure 8. Microcephaly vera (**A**) axial, (**B**) coronal, (**C**) sagittal. Note the very small brain size (24 weeks) and no visible germinal matrix.

problems of handling fetal brain and spine tissue in an unfixed state, which leads to 20% of autopsies giving no usable information. We have not studied other regions of the body with post mortem MRI yet but we know that thoracic and abdominal viscera are not as difficult to process in an unfixed state, so the advantages of post-mortem MRI are likely to be less in purely diagnostic terms. There is no doubt that adequate studies will have to be done that include the thoracic, abdominal, and pelvic viscera in order to consider the effectiveness of post mortem MRI in a more holistic fashion.

There appears to be an indirect relationship between the length of post-mortem delay and the chance of producing usable information on autopsy, i.e., the longer the delay the more difficult it is to process the brain tissue. This is an issue because many hospital pathology departments have stopped performing autopsy of the fetus and stillborn child and refer them to regional centers. This often leads to autopsy being performed at 6–7 days or even later in some cases. Structural changes within the brain post mortem also affect the quality of post mortem MRI. As autolysis progresses the brain undergoes significant distortion from the weight acting on the dependant parts of

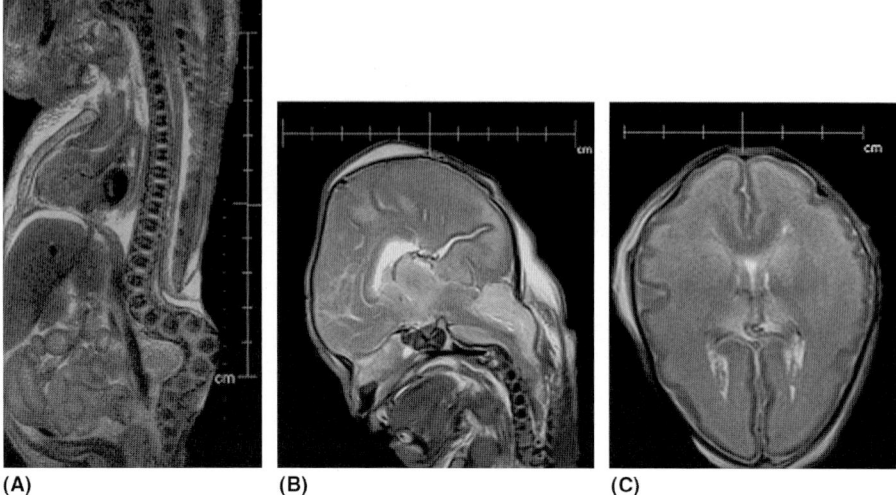

(A)   (B)   (C)

Figure 9. Lumbar myelomeningocoele and Chiari 2 malformation: (**A**) sagittal of lower spine, (**B**) axial brain, and (**C**) sagittal brain. The spinal cord shows connection with the skin surface via an abnormal placode, while the brain demonstrates an abnormal shape in the axial plane ("lemon-shaped") with gross caudal descent of the cerebellar tonsils.

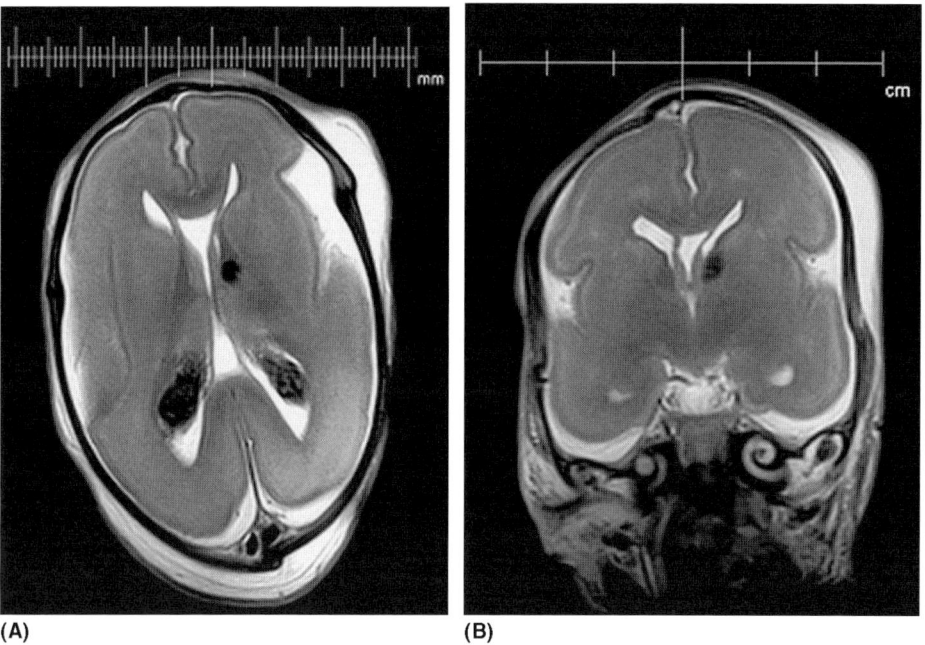

(A)   (B)

Figure 10. Germinal matrix hemorrhage (**A**) axial and (**B**) coronal, showing a small hemorrhage (low signal) in the left germinal matrix in the caudato-thalamic notch with intraventricular extension.

the brain. In those cases it may be difficult or impossible to make accurate anatomical diagnoses. There have been no formal studies as to the time that post-mortem MRI should be done after demise, but we have made two observations on the basis of our cases to date. First, MRI appears to be able to provide usable information in cases with moderate post-mortem delays (4–7 days) when the subsequent autopsy fails to give

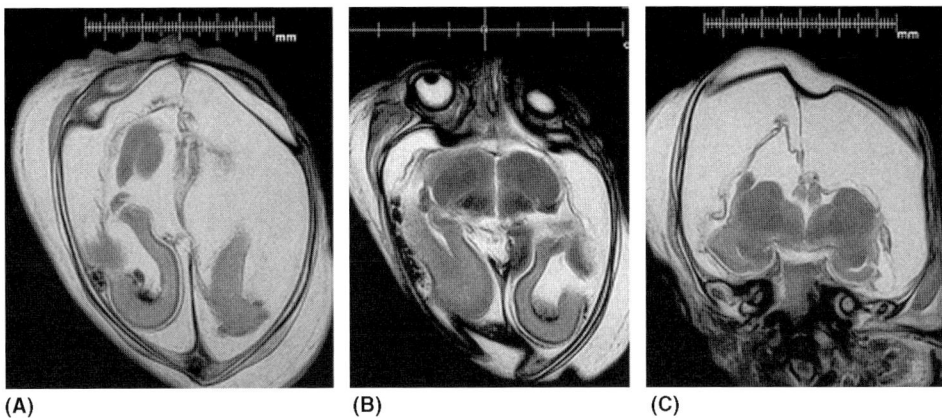

(A) (B) (C)

Figure 11. Hydranencephaly (**A**) and (**B**) axial and (**C**) coronal, showing extensive destruction of the cerebral hemispheres but with relative sparing of the occipital lobes and subcortical structures.

structural data. Second, MRI is rarely degraded by post-mortem delays of three days or less, although this does depend on other factors such as storage process and the method of therapeutic abortion used.

One obvious disadvantage of post mortem imaging as an alternative, rather than an adjunct, to formal autopsy is the lack of histological information provided by microscopic examination of samples. What is not clear is the contribution of that information to the final diagnosis at different ages. The vast majority of adults die of acquired pathology from a wide range of causes. We know from MRI of patients that MRI has high sensitivity (detects an abnormality) but often low specificity (can't tell what it is) and this leads to patients being biopsied, with or without total resection, to provide the diagnosis. There is no reason to suspect that MRI of adult corpses will be any different, but it is still difficult to define in what proportion of cases the histological information changed the diagnosis made on macroscopic examination, although it is likely to be high. Imaging of the second trimester fetus is different as the majority of abnormalities when they are present are developmental in nature and most frequently have obvious macroscopic manifestations. It seems likely that the overall contribution of histological examination in those cases will be considerably lower. The third

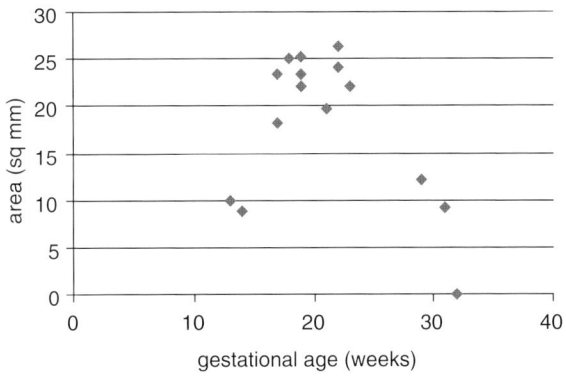

Figure 12. Area of germinal matrix plotted against gestational age of the fetus measured on post mortem MRI. The germinal matrix appears to have a maximum size at around 20 weeks followed by a rapid reduction.

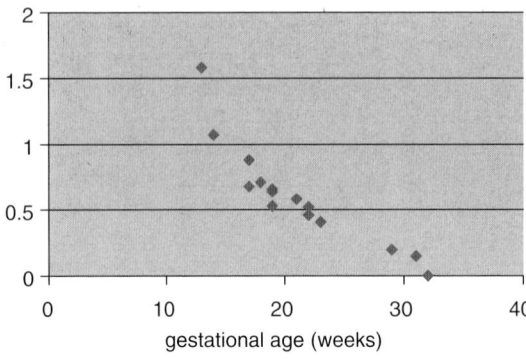

Figure 13. A plot showing the relationship between germinal matrix area and hemispheric size (A/T) against gestational age in weeks. There is a reasonable negative linear relationship between reduction of germinal matrix size and hemispheric growth in the pre-myelinated brain.

trimester fetus and stillborn child present a slightly more complicated picture. Although malformations are still well represented there is a significant representation of acquired disease, mainly hypoxic ischemic, where histological confirmation may be valuable. Again the precise contribution of microscopic analysis is unknown.

In many cases issues about the relative disadvantage of not having histology are redundant for the investigation of fetus post-mortem at the time when the vast majority of parents are not giving consent for autopsy. This seems unlikely to change and it is our opinion that information gathered from any other means that helps with informing parents of risk to future pregnancies can only be considered an advantage. One refinement is possible that may be acceptable to parents and pathologists and that involves image-directed biopsy. Examples of how this might work are: post-mortem MRI is performed routinely and if a mass lesion is seen in the brain (e.g., a hematoma) biopsies are taken, under image guidance with MRI-compatible needles if the lesion is small or freehand if large. Alternatively, MRI may show a generalized abnormality of cortical formation and a full thickness biopsy of a portion of hemisphere taken to allow histological confirmation of the precise type of malformation. This approach would fall into the category of minimally invasive autopsy.

There are many other practical problems to be considered if MRI is shown to be valuable as an alternative or adjunct to formal autopsy. In many countries, particularly the U.K., access to MRI for living patients is limited with long waiting times and it could be argued that post-mortem MRI should not be performed at the expense of clinical examinations. During the period of our studies we had access to research-dedicated scanners and so this was not an issue for us. It appears likely that a large volume,

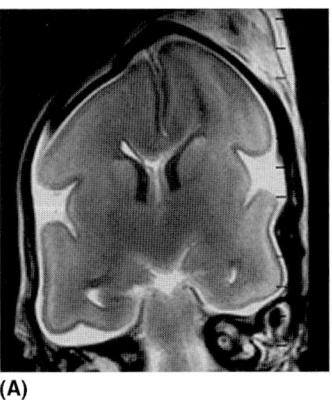

(A)

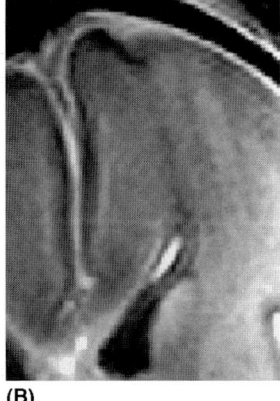

(B)

Figure 14. Post-mortem coronal T2-weighted image (**A**) with magnified view of the cortex (**B**) in a 23-week fetus that underwent spontaneous abortion. Note the dark streak of tissue extending from the tip of the left germinal matrix to the cortex that shows a well-defined dimple. This may represent the early stages in the development of a focal cortical dysplasia.

multicenter study into the value of fetal/stillborn MRI will be performed in the U.K. and the results of that study will influence the way forward. There are three possible outcomes: MRI is of no value (in which case the discussion ends), MRI is a suitable alternative to autopsy, or MRI is viewed as an adjunct to autopsy. The last two options would require extra access to MRI and the expected volume would be greater than the number of autopsies performed at present, as we predict that large numbers of parents who would not agree to autopsy would request post-mortem MRI. The next issue would be where and how to perform the procedures. There is no doubt extra scanners would be needed in the centers doing this work. At present fetal autopsies are referred to regional centers and we would see a few regional or supra-regional centers doing the post mortem MRI. Should post-mortem be performed on the same MRI scanners that are used for clinical workload? We do not see any health and safety issues here but it is inevitable that fewer patients will be scanned. One alternative would be to site dedicated units in the mortuary environment and for fetal/neonatal work these could be smaller, cheaper systems than the large whole body clinical systems. The major commercial MRI manufacturers do appear to be somewhat resistant to developing this type of system at present.

The other practical problem, of equal importance, is who would report the post-mortem MRI examinations? Worldwide there is a shortage of radiologists, which is particularly marked in the U.K. where current estimates state that a threefold increase in numbers is required to attain the per capita mean on mainland Europe. Pediatric radiologists, who are perhaps best equipped for this work, are an exceptionally rare commodity. The range of gestational ages studied, including early second trimester, however, is out of the experience of all clinical radiologists and significant training would be required. One alternative would be to train pediatric pathologists to interpret the imaging. This would have many advantages, including detailed knowledge of fetal anatomy and the ability to analyze any specimens taken from image-directed biopsies.

There are many unresolved issues surrounding post-mortem MRI but there is a high chance that this will become an important clinical issue over the next ten years.

REFERENCES

1. Griffiths PD, Variend D, Evans M, et al. Post mortem magnetic resonance imaging of the fetal and stillborn central nervous system. AJNR 2003; 24:22–27.
2. Bissett R. Magnetic resonance imaging may be an alternative to necroscopy. BMJ 1998; 317:1450.
3. Brookes JAS, Deng J, Wilkinson IDW, Lees WR. Three-dimensional imaging of the postmortem fetus by MRI: early experience. Fetal Diagn Ther 1999; 14:166–171.
4. Brookes JAS, Hall-Craggs MA, Lees WR, Sama VR. Non-invasive perinatal necroscopy by magnetic resonance imaging. Lancet 1996; 348:1139–1141.
5. Woodward PJ, Sohaey R, Jackson DP, Klatt EC, Alexander AL, Kennedy A. Post mortem MR imaging: comparison with findings at autopsy. Am J Roentgenol 1997; 168:41–46.
6. The Chief Medical Officer. Report of a census of organs and tissues retained by pathology services in England. London, The Stationery Office, Department of Health 2000.
7. The Chief Medical Officer. The removal, retention and use of human organs and tissues from post mortem examination. London, The Stationery Office, Department of Health 2001.
8. Feess-Higgins A, Larroche JC. Development of the Human Foetal Brain: An Anatomical Atlas. In: Feess-Higgins A, Larroche JC, eds. Paris: INSERM CNRS, 1987:13–189.
9. Griffiths PD, Wilkinson ID, Variend S, Jones A, Paley MNJ, Whitby E. Differential growth rates of the cerebellum and posterior fossa assessed by postmortem MR imaging of the fetus: implications for the pathogenesis of the chiari 2 deformity. Acta Radiologica 2004; 45:1–6.

Index